# Praise for Dee McCaffrey

"The biggest threat to America is the rising epidemic of obesity and type 2 diabetes. Dee McCaffrey's practical plan is part of the solution. Having lost 100 pounds herself and kept it off for over 20 years, Dee's guidance is a proven success. But it's more than a diet book. Dee has done an excellent job of providing a blueprint for a healthy way of eating that will add energy, vitality, and years to your life."

— Michael T. Murray, ND, coauthor of
   *The Encyclopedia of Natural Medicine*

"Dee is a wealth of information on healthful living. In *The Science of Skinny*, Dee identifies healing foods like organic apple cider vinegar and other power foods that can contribute to your health and longevity."

— Patricia Bragg, ND, PhD, pioneer health crusader,
   health educator, author, and nutritionist to Hollywood stars

# The Science of
# SKINNY

# The Science of
# SKINNY

## START UNDERSTANDING YOUR BODY'S CHEMISTRY—AND STOP DIETING FOREVER

### Dee McCaffrey, CDC

Da Capo
LIFE
LONG

A Member of the Perseus Books Group

Designed by Trish Wilkinson
Set in 11 point Minion Pro by the Perseus Books Group

Cataloging-in-Publication data for this book is available from the Library of Congress.

First Da Capo Press edition 2012
ISBN 978-0-7382-1557-0 (paperback)
ISBN 978-0-7382-1557-8 (e-book)

Published by Da Capo Press
A Member of the Perseus Books Group
www.dacapopress.com

Da Capo Press books are available at special discounts for bulk purchases in the U.S. by corporations, institutions, and other organizations. For more information, please contact the Special Markets Department at the Perseus Books Group, 2300 Chestnut Street, Suite 200, Philadelphia, PA, 19103, or call (800) 810-4145, ext. 5000, or e-mail special.markets@perseusbooks.com.

10  9  8  7  6  5

*Michael and Kristine*
*Words cannot express my overflowing gratitude for your*
*immeasurable love and support. This one is for both of you.*

# Contents

## PART 2: THE SKINNY

# Introduction

*What moves [individuals] of genius, or rather what inspires their work, is not new ideas, but their obsession with the idea that what has already been said is still not enough.*

—Eugène Delacroix

When I tell people that I repeatedly failed at dieting for the majority of my life, but eventually claimed victory over my lifelong battle with obesity, the first question I am asked is, "What did you do?" Most expect me to name a popular diet program or weight-loss surgical procedure, but the answer is deeply personal and intrinsically richer than expected. While studying chemistry in college, I was literally brought to my knees by a savage awareness that processed foods were killing me. At age thirty, carrying 210 pounds on my 4′10″ petite body frame, I was invited to make a change.

By disposing of my diet mentality, and reaching beyond the conventional approaches to nutrition, I developed *a way of eating for life* that gave me a freedom with food I had never experienced before. One bite at a time, I studiously removed processed foods from my life and replaced them with the real foods our body is designed to eat. Within thirteen months of making that fateful change, I lost 100 pounds and have kept them off for twenty years and counting.

Along the way, I discovered a passion. While climbing the industry ladder in my chemistry profession, I spent nearly all of my off time sharing my weight-loss experience with others: explaining the relationship between food and health, and teaching them how to shop and prepare healthful meals for themselves and their families. Eventually, with the loving support and prompting of my husband and partner in health, Michael, I channeled that moonlight activity into a second career as a nutritionist, and together we became advocates for a healthier food environment for all Americans.

Over the past two decades, my passion has not waned; however, navigating people into healthier lives has grown increasingly more challenging. While I have continued to keep processed foods out of my life, the food industry has been adding more to everyone else's, and obesity has become our nation's most serious health problem. From my unique perspective as a scientist, nutritionist, and former obese person, I have sadly witnessed the rise in obesity from many directions—sitting alongside my friends in weight-loss support group meetings, where an alarming number of them continue to gain weight even after years of attendance; in nutrition counseling with clients who range from chronically overweight to morbidly obese; teaching overweight children why eating sugary breakfast cereal is not the best way to start the day; and from the scientific literature concerning obesity and health. In all cases, I have observed something gravely disturbing: not only has the girth of our nation expanded to levels never before seen in human history, but the weight gain itself is *unnatural*.

According to *F as in Fat: How Obesity Threatens America's Future 2011*, a report from the Trust for America's Health (TFAH) and the Robert Wood Johnson Foundation, more than two out of three states, thirty-eight total, have obesity rates over 25 percent, and twelve states now have obesity rates above 30 percent. A mere four years ago, only one state was above 30 percent. The rates of both diabetes and high blood pressure also have risen dramatically over the last two decades.[1] In the report, Jeff Levi, PhD, executive director of TFAH, said, "Today, the state with the lowest obesity rate would have had the highest rate in 1995. There was a clear tipping point in our national weight gain over the last twenty years."[2] A tipping point indeed.

Prior to the 1950s, a person would certainly gain weight from eating too many calories. But the weight gain of today is characterized by forces no early-twentieth-century glutton ever had to contend with. Highly refined carbohydrates, processed cooking oils, and an unbelievable myriad of food additives have been linked to unforeseen and powerful chemical reactions in the body and the brain, inducing obesity at rapid and alarming rates. This type of obesity is not just a matter of too many calories and not enough exercise. It is aggressive, stubborn, and more deadly than ever. Its complications are many, and most of its causes are the result of food chemistry gone mad.

I have long suspected something was amiss. Back in 1989, prior to my weight loss, I was working m⋯ ⋯ay through college as a chemist at an environmental testing labora⋯ ⋯to practice my chemical pronunciation skills, I became famil⋯ ⋯s of all the chemicals being used in the lab to test for ⋯ ⋯n in water and soil samples. One evening at hor⋯ ⋯v favorite (and very frequent) indulgences: ⋯ ⋯—the only baking skill required was to aa⋯ ⋯I had done it at least a hundred times.

But this time was a⋯ ⋯eknownst to me, my eyes were drawn to the small p⋯ ⋯he box where the ingredients were listed. Mind you, in 198⋯ ⋯igredient lists was not a common practice, and especially not mine. ⋯ read through the list, skimming past the sugar and flour, my eyes fell upon three words I never expected to see in my angel food cake—sodium lauryl sulfate. *Sodium lauryl sulfate? Isn't that what we use in our tests at the lab?*

My suspicions were confirmed when I returned to work the next day. The detergent-like chemical being used to test smelly water samples was indeed the exact same chemical I had been eating in every bite of my angel food cake. This did not sit well with me, and I began to wonder what effect sodium lauryl sulfate was having on my body. Could it, and perhaps other chemical food ingredients, be a contributing factor to my obesity? Back then, answers to those kinds of questions were not easy to find, and all I had to go on was my chemist's instinct. Following that instinct changed the course of my life, and eventually formed the basis for *The Science of Skinny*.

In the years that followed, I learned a great deal about food—how perfect it is in its natural state, and how deranged it becomes when we take it apart, add chemicals to it, and consume it in unnatural ways. As I have adapted to living in a lean, healthy body, I've come to understand the true meaning of the word *skinny*. The dictionary's definition (very lean or thin), and our culture's shallow application of the word—skinny lattes and skinny jeans—does not apply here. Being lean or thin does not always mean that a person is healthy. We all know lean and thin people who are very unhealthy. However, it is undeniably true that when people are optimally healthy and free of disease, they will always be blessed with a thin body. Therefore, because weight loss should be thought of as a path to overall wellness, I've elevated the status of the word and given it a whole new meaning—optimal health. As you read this book, keep that definition in mind every time you see the word *skinny*.

By now you've realized that *The Science of Skinny* is not a diet book—in fact, it was first published under the title *Plan-D: The Amazing Anti-Diet*—nor is it a "last resort" for those like myself who have struggled with their weight for a long time. Rather, it is a natural, organic health plan to get your body back to the place where it functions best. This new and improved version of my original book retains much of the same information, but in light of the ever-changing world of health and nutrition, I have added new science, new recipes, and more detail to the content. I have rewritten whole sections of the book to reflect new insight I have gleaned from my experiences working with clients and reader feedback I have received over the past two years. What hasn't changed is that this book will set you on a path of lifelong learning about nutrition and the healing effects of whole foods, so that you can join with the thousands of others who have used this plan to get skinny. You will learn how to eat for long-term health, and you will do it in a way that is tasty and enjoyable—without reliance on calorie counting or other dieting tactics. In fact, you may need to rewire your brain and let go of the diet mentality as I did, to clear some space for new concepts and scientific truths about food, fat, and healing.

If you do not need to lose weight but are interested in improving your health through nutrition, you are in for a treat. You'll learn how to feed yourself and your family with high-quality foods, while building an arsenal of nutritional knowledge that will sustain you for the rest of your life.

You will choose among a wide variety of foods to support your body's main detoxifying and fat-burning organ (your liver), and eat proper portions to achieve balanced body chemistry. Balanced body chemistry is essential for maintaining weight, for assimilating nutrients, eliminating waste, and warding off disease. The meaningful fitness routine outlined in the plan is moderate and designed to assist in balancing your body chemistry. You will better understand food and appreciate it as an instrument of personal healing. Nourishing yourself according to *The Science of Skinny* principles becomes a wise, mature, and loving act of awareness, cultivated through a gentle "one day at a time" approach.

The nutshell of *The Science of Skinny* is this: *eat foods in their closest to natural form as possible*—avoiding refined foods, artificial sweeteners, and chemical food additives—and you will reap the benefits of a happy mind and a skinny body. This lifestyle is part of a flowering movement in our culture that Michael and I have named "processed-free" living. Others have described it as *clean eating* or *holistic nutrition*. Processed-free living is an individual's enlightened and sincere desire to avoid, as much as possible, refined carbohydrates, processed oils, and the more than three thousand synthetic chemicals that are added to the foods most Americans eat each day. And while we do this earnestly, this lifestyle is not to be approached with black-and-white thinking or a lofty goal for perfection. The willingness to strive for *progress*, not perfection, will bring about results simply by eating processed-free foods to the best of your ability.

Making the decision to eat processed-free foods can sometimes seem confusing and daunting. If you've ever wondered whether Newman-O's are really better for you than Oreos, you're not alone. Recognizing the need for clarity when it comes to natural foods, and to provide nutrition education to both young and old, we established Processed-Free America—a nonprofit organization committed to providing education, support services, and a national awareness of the effect processed foods have on our health. *The Science of Skinny* is the culmination of the work we have been doing over the past decade, which includes the success stories of people who have transformed their health by following its tenets.

Within these pages, I will tell you exactly what you need to know about food, fat, and permanent weight loss. In the first part of the book, I share my own personal health and weight-loss journey—the struggle and eventual triumph—and will delve into the specifics of how I overcame my love affair with fast foods, doughnuts, and chocolate. I will also tell you what I have learned over the years since then, about how the chemicals in those foods were probably more responsible for my weight problems than I ever realized.

Next, I will introduce you to the Laws of Skinny Science—the tenets upon which optimal health and lasting permanent weight loss are built. I will explain to you why sugar, flour, and canola oil should be banned from your kitchen, and how the right combination of foods can work wonders for your metabolism. You will learn a great deal of science (in layman's terms), as I draw upon my chemistry background to illustrate and emphasize the importance of eating foods in their closest-to-natural form. Many nutritional myths will be debunked. You'll understand why coconut oil is not the dietary demon it was made out to be, and why it's taking back its crown as the king of healthy oils. I'll explain why the National Academy of Sciences has declared that there is no safe amount of trans fat, and that if there is one thing you do to improve your health, it is to eliminate this devastating artificial oil from your life. Next, the specifics of the Processed-Free Plan for Balanced Eating and Living are outlined in detail, including all of the scientifically proven Skinny Superfoods and supplements. I have also made sure to include information for children and vegetarians.

For those who need structure when it comes to eating, I have provided portion guidelines and menus, and a list of approved processed-free food products. I have also provided seventy of my special recipes, as well as tips on how to modify your favorite recipes into Skinny cuisine. You'll learn that staying skinny is doable in restaurants if you're choosy and ask the right questions, and that dining while traveling or staying in others' homes is easier than you think. I also provide you with information about support groups in your area, should you decide to join with like-minded individuals who desire to eat processed free.

Finally, after reading this book you may find yourself inspired to make a difference in the lives of others by sharing what you've learned. You may also want to do what you can to stop the proliferation of harmful additives in the food supply. In this last section I provide information about how to join with me in the crusade for a healthier food environment.

Throughout the writing and researching for this book, I made many handwritten notes to keep my thoughts in order. Writing out "Science of Skinny" over and over again became laborious, so one day I jotted down "S.O.S." As soon as it went on the paper, it dawned on me that this book may just be the answer to a distress call. As you read its pages, you will find that to "save (y)our ship," you need do nothing more than approach eating as intelligently as the foods themselves have been designed by nature. If you have intuitively turned to nutrition as a means to better health, if you want to understand how and why foods affect us, and if you want to learn more about the role of food in the human story—then this book may become very important to you. Let it be the lifeline that leads you out of the murky processed-food waters into a vibrant new life.

# PART 1
# THE SCIENCE

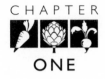
# From Junk Food Junkie to Natural Food Expert

*Twenty Years of Sustained Weight Loss*

> *The most beautiful experience we can have is the mysterious.*
> —ALBERT EINSTEIN

I want to share my story with you—some of it may mirror your own, some of it may seem familiar for other reasons. What I want you to know is that, no matter what is in your past or family history, you are not destined to be unhealthy or overweight. If anyone was a candidate for that, I'm certainly the poster child. My family history suggests I was a likely candidate for obesity and early death; diabetes is rampant on my mother's side, heart disease on my father's side. My maternal grandmother weighed 300 pounds when she passed away; my other grandmother suffered a sudden, fatal stroke at the age of fifty-two. Current genetic theory would suggest the odds of escaping degenerative disease and maintaining a healthy body weight throughout my lifetime were stacked against me from my very first breath.

The oldest of three, I was born in San Francisco, California, in the summer of 1961 to working-class parents of Irish and Mexican American descent. We

3

ate like every other American family during the 1960s—meat, potatoes, white bread, white rice, and canned vegetables. Although Popeye was among my favorite cartoon personalities, I was not able to stomach canned spinach with the vigor that he did. In fact, most vegetables made their way into my napkin, to be stashed in the garbage when my mother wasn't looking.

Toward the end of my kindergarten year, my parents bought their first, newly built home in San Jose, California—an area now famously known as Silicon Valley. As a child growing up in suburbia, I was very active and remained a normal, healthy weight. I had a great appreciation for physical activity and being outdoors; I loved riding my bike and climbing trees (in fact, I was known for climbing anything that presented a challenge!). The wooded creek bed running behind our neighborhood provided me with many hours of solitary walks, when I would lose myself in daydreams and songs.

## From Healthy, Active Child to Compulsive Eater

I openly admit that I am a recovered compulsive eater—a condition characterized by a compulsion to eat when not hungry or frequent episodes of uncontrolled quantity eating. My first recollection of compulsive eating is when I was five years old—I stole a Tootsie Pop from the corner store. Like most mothers, mine had an eagle eye for anything out of the ordinary, so before I was able to tally how many licks it takes to get to the center of a Tootsie Pop, she marched me down the street to apologize to the storekeeper for stealing his inventory. The memory of that confession marks a turning point in my story—at the age of five, I was already sneaking and stealing food, and hiding to eat it.

Compulsive eating usually starts in early childhood when eating patterns are formed, or as the result of a significant emotional or physical trauma. In either circumstance, most people who become compulsive eaters have never learned the proper way to deal with stressful situations and instead use food as a coping mechanism. And so it was with me. My parents had a stormy marriage, and as a result, at around the age of nine I lost my desire for outdoor activity. Rather than playing outside with my friends after school, I preferred to be alone and kept most of my feelings to myself.

I began eating more food than I needed as a way of avoiding feelings and conflict—to comfort my fears and to suppress my anger at a situation over which I had no control. I remember sneaking slices of bread and hiding in my room to eat them. My sister and I hid chunks of salami in our kitchen cupboard and snuck bites when Mom wasn't looking. I stole change from my mother's purse and secretly bought candy when we went to the grocery store. At family celebrations and holidays, I gorged on all the goodies without inhibition.

My parents' inevitable divorce became final when I was eleven—the age, which photos reveal, I was officially "overweight." My mother did her best to provide a stable home and balanced meals, but at every opportunity I overate. Eating made me forget about the emptiness I felt when my father left, and unconsciously food became my principal source of happiness.

As my weight crept up, I became self-conscious of my body. As early as fifth grade, I refused to wear dresses to school because I didn't want the other kids to make fun of my fat legs. In junior high, one of my friends described my legs as "logs with kneecaps," a phrase that took up permanent residence in my memory.

In high school I joined the tennis team to increase my physical activity, but despite my good skills and enjoyment of the sport, I continued to gain weight. Other activities such as singing in the choir and performing in musicals brought intermittent joy into my otherwise troubled existence, but I never felt that I truly fit in anywhere. Those were especially painful years, as I became increasingly aware of what I was missing out on because I was fat. Secretly, I longed to be popular—but the shame of being overweight repressed me, so I related more to food and books than to my peers. I compensated by excelling in my classes, convincing myself that I didn't need friends. Food was my best and most reliable friend. I could always count on food to make me feel better, but I was never happy about being fat.

Without my dad's income, our family economics sharply declined. Fortunately, my mother knew how to stretch a dollar, especially when it came to food. Often working two or three jobs to make ends meet, Mom fed us by shopping at the discount grocery store, and on a few bleak occasions we ate from donated food boxes. I learned to cook "the basics" such as rice, hamburger, and spaghetti with sauce mix from a packet. Boxed pizza mixes (the kind that came with a can of pizza sauce and the just-add-water dough mix), boxed mac and cheese, canned vegetables, and an assortment of other processed foods were also part of my early culinary repertoire.

To her credit, Mom drew the line at most snack foods and overtly un-healthy stuff. She did not regularly buy the sodas, sugary cereals, chips, cook-ies, or other treats that were staples in the homes of our neighborhood friends. Those were saved for special occasions or when we had extra money. Our staple snack was popcorn, which Mom herself popped in a large pot on the stovetop. We used the fresh peaches from the trees in our backyard to make pies and jams, and baked our own cookies and cakes from scratch, using good old white sugar and white flour. As was the norm back then, eat-ing at fast-food establishments was a rare but welcome treat.

## Natural Foods Not for Me

During the mid-1970s, my mom developed an interest in natural foods, making a valiant effort to overhaul our processed-foods diet.

We started shopping at the health food store, where the tie-dye-clad clerk's name was Sunshine and most of the food was fresh or in bulk bins. Aside from a natural candy bar called Gypsy Boots, made of dates, carob, and shaved coconut, my siblings and I didn't take well to healthy sweets made with raw honey. Nor could we sanction any meal that included brown rice, whole wheat pizza crust (or anything whole wheat, for that matter), granola, tofu, and—heaven forbid—raw vegetables (ugh!). Our taste buds were dedicated to hot dogs, spaghetti, and white bread. The experiment failed miserably!

Mom gave in, and we went back to eating the way we were accustomed. We did make one permanent change—we switched to "brown bread" (white bread with a smattering of whole wheat flour in it, so that it wasn't com-pletely white). We could tolerate that, but at any opportunity outside the home, I chose white bread. I now know that I was addicted to it, and that addiction continued to rage into my adult years.

Blame it on the hippies; blame it on the times—whatever the catalyst, my mom changed after the divorce. Part of the experimentation with nat-ural foods came from information she gleaned through her study of natural health and spirituality. Mom began reading to us at bedtime from the Bible and taught us to pray, not for worldly things, but for peace and comfort in our lives. She started using herbal remedies and foods as medicine for aches, pains, and colds. As the eldest of my siblings, I took a great interest in the information. As a teenager, I did not have much use for such things. As an adult, however, the prayers and remedies my mother passed on to me became invaluable tools that were instrumental in helping me overcome my life's greatest challenge.

When I was sixteen, a move to the other side of town required me to change high schools in the middle of my junior year. Shortly afterward, because of a series of unfortunate events, we were homeless. We lived in shelters for six months before my mom was able to get herself back on her feet and move us into our own place.

My compulsive eating behaviors rapidly progressed during that year. A part-time job at a Dairy Queen provided me with a steady supply of sweet treats and greasy foods, as well as my own pocket money, which I used to buy more junk food. After changing high schools, I lost my enthusiasm for academics and started skipping classes. A fledgling cigarette smoker since junior high, I morphed from the sporadic splurges into a full-blown smoker during my senior year.

Despite my foray into quasi–juvenile delinquency, I graduated from high school with National Honor Society standing. Although my parents had always encouraged me, and it was my sincere intention to attend college after high school, I had no money or guidance to get me there. While my grades were high enough to garner me acceptance to two prominent universities, I clearly was not destined to follow that path. Instead, I started working full-time and moved out on my own. It was then that my compulsive eating and weight soared. By the time I turned eighteen, I was officially obese.

During my early adolescence, I had mastered the art of soothing any uncomfortable feelings with food—in fact, I'd buried them to the point that I no longer recognized that I felt *anything*. This destructive pattern continued because I never learned to trust that uncomfortable feelings eventually pass, or that I could be capable of soothing myself without food. Even though my mother had taught me to pray and worked to instill good dietary habits in me, my emotional pain was too great and I was distracted by our domestic upheaval.

Learning to bury feelings with food at a young age had a targeted amnesic effect on me. By the time I reached adulthood, I had no idea why I loved to eat so much. I had done it all my life and didn't know any other way. Even more baffling was that I could control and eat single portions of some foods (e.g., green beans), whereas I had strong cravings for other foods and felt compelled to eat another serving . . . and then another . . . and another. Sugary foods—doughnuts, pastries, cookies, and of course chocolate—were those I was compelled to eat the most. Peanut M&M's were my favorite. I could inhale a whole one-pound bag in one evening.

## What? A Gallstone?

When I was eighteen, I began to experience sharp abdominal pain. After several tests, the doctor told me that I had a large gallstone and that I would have to undergo surgery to have my gall bladder removed. *What?* I was only eighteen! How could *I* have a gallstone? I thought only fat old ladies got gallstones.

Turns out fat young ladies get them, too. My instructions for diet, upon release from the hospital after surgery, were, "Do not eat fatty foods." That's it. Nothing further. So I went home and white-knuckled my way through two weeks of no French fries or potato chips. That was the extent of my abstinence from fatty foods.

By age nineteen, my weight had climbed to 180 pounds; that was when I went on my first diet. I lost 40 pounds over the course of a few months and then quickly gained it back, plus more, in half that amount of time. Over the next decade, I tried everything from the latest fads and miracle programs to crazy diets I made up myself. My story is typical—I never lost enough to reach a healthy goal weight, and I always gained back more than I lost. By my late twenties I had dieted my way into seemingly permanent obesity, and my weight hovered steadily above 200 pounds—that's nearly twice the normal weight for someone my height.

It was always my dream to attend college. At age twenty-one—without a clear vision of what I wanted to be when I grew up—I enrolled in general education courses at the local community college. During my introductory chemistry class, I fell in love with the science. The world of chemistry fascinated me. I earned an A+, and for the first time in a long time, I had confidence in myself. I declared my major in chemistry and eventually transferred to a university to complete my bachelor's degree.

It was thrilling to be in college, but I also had a lot of responsibilities at my full-time job. My primary method for managing the stress and pulling all-night study sessions was to eat anything and everything I wanted. And all I wanted was to eat junk food. Super Big Gulps, pizza, ramen noodles, sandwiches, and chocolate sustained me during my first years of school. Nary a vegetable or a piece of fruit passed my lips.

## Chemist in Training

During my second year at the university, I was offered a paid summer research internship in the chemistry department. The work honed my research and analytical skills while broadening my scientific interests. I began to see future possibilities for my career.

Life went on. College continued. A blossoming romance led to an engagement and then marriage. We were both still in school and working. After the research internship ended, I secured a part-time chemistry position at an environmental testing laboratory. My job duties entailed performing chemical tests on water, soil, and air samples taken from areas near notable sources of environmental pollution or from environmental monitoring sites. These included—but were not limited to—ground water; well water; wastewater treatment facilities; construction sites; land development areas; agricultural runoff from farming; military bases; factories; industrial waste; and the soil, streams, lakes, and ponds surrounding chemical storage tanks.

The tests I used were established and regulated by the U.S. Environmental Protection Agency (EPA) to detect the presence of specific organic pollutants such as industrial solvents, pesticides, herbicides, fertilizers, metals, volatile organic compounds, fossil fuel emissions (e.g., gasoline and diesel), and many others. I learned the federal regulations governing the use and disposal of these chemicals, and the maximum government-allowed residual and exposure levels for humans. This job inspired me to focus my college major on environmental chemistry.

## Bingeing My Brains Out

As much as I wanted to lose weight, by this point, I had given up dieting and succumbed to my insatiable appetite. I snacked all day and gorged on large meals and sweets at night. A typical binge consisted of eating beyond the point of being full, so stuffed that I could barely move. Passing out on the couch from the toxic overload was a frequent occurrence, and when I woke up I vowed that I would never again eat so much—only to find myself making the same vow days or even hours later.

One afternoon in February 1992, overstuffed from a supersize lunch, I ransacked the pantry searching for something more to quell my cavernous cravings. Tucked away in a far corner behind the auxiliary canned goods, I spotted my "fix"—a bag of stale candy left over from the previous Halloween. I remembered my reasoning for purchasing that particular bag of candy for the trick-or-treaters—it was a type of candy I despised, so that was supposed to keep me from eating it. Yet, there I was, four months later, diving into that bag of candy with the same rapacious madness of an alcoholic sucking the last drops from a whiskey bottle recovered from the trash.

In the midst of devouring this disgusting, despicable candy, a ray of clarity pierced my foggy brain: *Something is seriously wrong with me.* I was bright, intelligent, and on the brink of a promising future. To the outside world my life seemed normal, but in reality I was spiraling out of control. My brains and strong character were no defense against the cunning and baffling power of compulsive eating. Silently suffering from a God-shaped hole in my soul, I was incapable of loving myself enough to effect a change. And because I was unable to truly share myself with others, inside I was tortured by isolation and loneliness.

## Cognitive Dissonance

After working at the lab for several months, I became acutely aware of three things: (1) *thousands* of chemicals are dumped into our water, air, soil, and food every day; (2) some of the chemicals I was using in my lab to test for pollution were the same chemicals found on the ingredient lists of the processed foods I was eating; and (3) each person has a responsibility to revere and care for our environment (our planet and our body).

I began to experience a phenomenon social psychologists call cognitive dissonance. Cognitive dissonance is an inner disturbance felt when a person holds two contradictory ideas simultaneously. The ideas, or cognitions, in question may include attitudes and beliefs, and also *the awareness of one's behavior*. The theory of cognitive dissonance proposes that people have a motivational drive to expel dissonance. They do this by either changing their attitudes, beliefs, and behaviors; or by justifying, rationalizing, blaming or denying.[1] Justification and rationalization, as they relate to compulsive eating, are forms of denial—a refusal to believe or give in to the truth of one's situation.

My cognitive dissonance was brought on by a growing enthusiasm for cleaning up the environment and a deep disgust of the chemical waste in our world. Yet I could not even clean up my own world, my own environment—my body. I had not yet become disgusted with the "pollution" I was dumping into my body every time I drank a Dr Pepper, ate a Big Mac, and smoked a cigarette. But the drone of dissonance was getting louder.

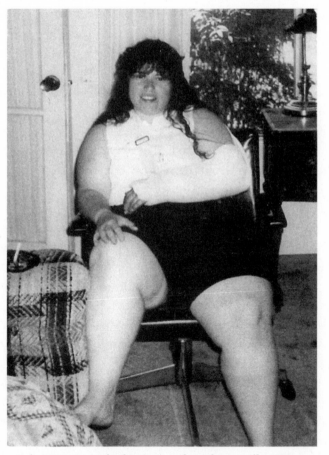

July 1990: I weighed 210 pounds and was still gaining.

## It's Not About the Backpack

A month after the stale candy episode, I was on a field trip with one of my college classes that involved hiking up a steep hill. The dissonance hadn't yet reached decibel levels, so I foolishly thought it would be easy to hike up a hill. Never mind the fact that by this time I was a pack-a-day cigarette smoker and my weight had climbed to somewhere over 210 pounds. Needless to say, it was more than a struggle to pull my body up the arduous slope. Within minutes, my classmates—who were all in much better shape than I was—had scaled past me and were jubilantly enjoying the glorious view from the top of the hill.

At the halfway point, I stopped climbing because I could hardly breathe. My legs were hurting and my heart was pounding. What happened next was what I consider to be *the* most humiliating experience of my life. As I stood there trying to regain composure, the attractive hike leader had to come back down the hill to see if he could assist me in some way. With genuine concern, he offered his hand and asked, "Can I take your backpack?" *As if the backpack were the problem.*

To keep my pride intact, I thanked him but continued on without his assistance. However, my spectacle had drawn attention, so as I inched my way up the hill, huffing and puffing, all eyes were on me. Everyone was waiting for the slow fat girl to reach the top.

Just as I finally joined the rest of the class, my foot slipped out from under me and I fell—flat on my rear. Mortified beyond compare, I turned and looked away from the crowd. At the top of the hill, looking out over the beautiful San Francisco Bay, I felt like the lowest thing on earth. In that moment, a wave of realization washed over me. Dissonance broke and stripped denial from me. My life stood starkly in front of me, demanding my attention. The physical condition of my body was symbolic of how I had let everything in my life get out of control. *I had let this happen. No one else was to blame. What was I going to do?*

Then, I heard a voice. I don't know whether it came from inside or outside of me. Its message was loud and clear: *Change your life or die.*

Those words frightened me in a way I cannot describe. There were many times in my life when I feared I would die at an early age of my obesity. I had frequent chest pains, and even though the doctors assured me I had no signs of heart disease, my family history always made me suspect. Stiff hip joints and nocturnal back pain were evidence that my body was degenerating, and when I allowed myself to notice, I knew that I was already spiritually and emotionally dead.

Over the next few days, the experience haunted me like a springtime version of the Ghost of Christmas Future. With each visit, I heard its beckoning mandate: *Change your life or die*. I attempted to squelch the fear by turning to the only method I had ever known to cope with fear—I ate. And I continued to eat until the day came when the desire to remain the same was more painful than any ill-conceived suffering I might have to endure as a result of putting down the fork.

That day was Friday, April 3, 1992. On that day the motivational drive to reduce dissonance shifted something inside me. I had what can only be described as a profound inner change—what the psychologist Carl Jung called a "vital spiritual experience." The old attitudes, ideas, and emotions of my compulsive eater self, which until then had been the guiding forces of my existence, were willingly cast aside. In exchange, I gradually allowed myself to explore new ways of thinking and acting. Instead of wasting my days struggling with food and weight, I started learning and living. I began to believe in myself and became committed to changing my life.

## Natural Foods, Take Two

The first step in changing any behavior is awareness, so I began to examine my eating history. Previous attempts to lose weight had failed because they were rooted in a flawed diet mentality. Instead of *changing the types of foods* themselves, I only tried to eat *less of the same foods* that had historically made me fat! Temporary efforts to eat less bread and ice cream, fewer cookies and French fries, were always just that—temporary. The problem with that approach was that because I was addicted to those types of foods, I was never satisfied with less of them, and I eventually reverted to eating larger and larger quantities.

To lose weight and not have it return, I needed to change my whole approach to eating and adopt the change as a permanent way of life. While embarking on this endeavor, I was fortunate to become affiliated with a weight-loss support group in which small factions of its members were refraining from eating all forms of sugar and flour. At first this seemed daunting, but I saw success in those who had been living sugar and flour free for many years. People like me who had struggled their entire lives with obesity, now lived in a normal-size body—some of them 150 to 200 pounds lighter—without desire or pangs of deprivation for the starchy sugar-laden foods we had all grown up eating.

Seasoned members claimed that sugar and flour were addictive substances that, when eaten on a regular basis, caused cravings that led to over-eating. Furthermore, many of them claimed that their migraine headaches, arthritis, and diabetes had vanished after giving up flour and sugar. Walking through the fear that threatened to sabotage my commitment to change, I decided to give it a try. The first new action I took in my weight-loss process was eliminating all forms of refined sugar and flour from my life. Thirty days later, I had dropped 20 pounds.

Simultaneously, I began to educate myself about food. I spent countless hours in the library reading nutrition books, and countless more hours in the kitchen creating healthier versions of my favorite foods. Because of my work in the lab, I had become intimately familiar with the chemical names and toxic properties of the majority of common environmental pollutants, particularly those used in and on America's food supply. I made the connection that pesticides, preservatives, flavorings, colorings, and refined carbohydrates affect body chemistry in such a way that balanced health was difficult to sustain. It was this understanding that led to a deeper level of surrender—I began to read every food ingredient list with scrutiny in an effort to avoid as many food additives as possible.

From all of the reading and with the help of my organic chemistry background, I developed my own healthy eating plan and followed it as if my life depended on it. I stopped eating all of the foods that had historically been problems for me. These included anything made with refined sugar and refined white flour (no more white bread or M&M's), fatty meats, fried foods, and fast foods. In their place, I added new foods I'd never tried before (and even those natural foods I never liked before) into my meals. A white rice lover to the core, I was convinced I'd never be able to embrace brown rice. But it quickly became a favorite staple, along with broccoli, apples, yogurt, oat bran, and—you guessed it—whole wheat! As the new foods began to cleanse my body of years of poor eating, my taste buds began to change. To my utter surprise, I actually began to *crave* vegetables!

I adopted a healthy mind-set of abstaining from processed foods for the current day only, and sometimes minute by minute. As a neophyte, the prospect of giving up unhealthy foods for a lifetime was overwhelming, but I was confident that I could stick to my healthy plan for just one day.

Nutritional responsibility and accountability were my new guiding principles. I kept a record of everything I ate, and chronicled my feelings in a journal. A food scale, measuring cups, and measuring spoons became essential kitchen tools for helping me determine proper portion sizes. Ironically, these healthy boundaries freed me to truly enjoy eating in a way I never had before.

Having a set plan for eating is not much different than having a pre-planned driving route to get from point A to point B. The route keeps you from getting lost or distracted from your destination. Planning meals ahead of time kept me focused on my goal so as not to get distracted by my emotional fluctuations of the day. In essence, it taught me how to separate food from feelings and put food in its proper perspective. The eating plan became my anchor—the one constant in my ever-changing life.

## Soul Food

Overcoming compulsive eating must happen on a soul level. My excess weight was but a symptom of a deeper problem. My difficulty was that I ate food as a way to fill many voids in my life, thus leading to an unhealthy relationship with food. No plan for healing that relationship was successful when it was based on diet alone. The God-shaped hole in me needed nourishing, too, so I began to feed it with "soul" food. It began with a simple prayerful request, one that I have said every day since:

> Please infuse me with the courage, willingness, and strength to make wise and healthy food choices today.

To me, this prayer is a daily surrender of my compulsive behavior concerning food. By letting go, I increase my capacity for more meaningful ways of nourishing myself. This mental and spiritual practice is quite different from dieting, because its goal is to heal the soul as well as the psyche. It is a daily, ongoing process that, combined with healthful eating, expels the desire to eat compulsively.

Taking walks alone was another form of soul food—a lost love recovered from my childhood. I started with slow, short walks, and quickly worked my way up to brisk, aerobic, sixty-minute walks. Walking helped build and strengthen my body, as well as build and strengthen my relationship with myself. It gave me the nourishment and energy to change and reshape my life. As the days, weeks, and months passed, I watched my shadow on the ground get smaller and smaller, while my spirit inside grew larger and larger.

Another spiritual discipline instrumental in my weight loss was the practice of journaling. It enabled me to identify what certain foods represented in my emotional life. I used writing as a tool to dig up the feelings I had buried over the years, so they could no longer have power over me. I also learned that the discomfort I felt when going on a diet—that sense of deprivation—was not about food and never had been. Writing exposed the pieces of my life that were painfully absent or had been taken from me, and revealed exactly how I had used food to fill those voids. For instance, eight months into my new lifestyle and 80 pounds lighter, I binged on a huge amount of popcorn. Earnestly wanting to understand why, I journaled everything I could remember about eating popcorn—specifically my earliest memories.

I discovered that popcorn represented love and closeness with my family before the divorce; therefore, my mental craving for popcorn was an emotional craving for love and closeness. From then on, whenever I craved a particular food, I did this writing exercise to help break the emotional attachment. Slowly over time, I worked hard to identify my weaknesses and erase the conditioning that had trapped me for so long.

## Discovering My True Life's Purpose

In just over a year, I trimmed more than 100 pounds from my 4'10" frame—*nearly half my body weight*—and dropped nine pant sizes, going from a size 22 jeans to a size 4! Simultaneous to reaching my goal weight, I graduated from college with a bachelor's of science degree in environmental chemistry.

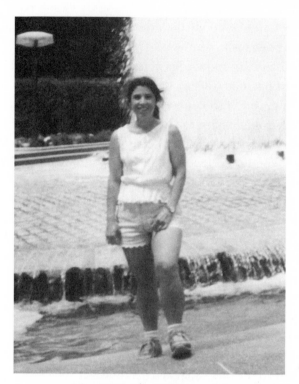

May 1993: I lost 100 pounds!
I weighed 110 pounds!

Days before the popcorn binge, I quit smoking and haven't desired a cigarette since. The unwavering belief in myself, the commitment to a daily eating and exercise plan, the release of those awful emotional attachments, and a deep sense of wholeness gave me confidence, self-esteem, and freedom from shame and humiliation. I had reclaimed my true self that was buried so deeply for so many years. There have been many ups and downs in my life since then, but I have rarely succumbed to finding comfort, celebration, or relief in excess food.

What started as a hollow desire to be skinny has become so much more than I would have ever prayed for on that fateful day overlooking the San Francisco Bay. My weight loss infused me with a true sense of purpose and a passion for helping others achieve optimal health. I have dedicated myself to serving others in this capacity, and I live a gratified life from sharing my experience, strength, knowledge, and hope with others. Each day that I eat well, I am well—and I embody the principles of true health and healing—which attracts others who want what I've found.

Eager to expand my knowledge of food, in 2000 I enrolled in the nutrition program at Bauman College. Once I entered the world of food science, healthful cooking, and diet counseling, I knew I had found my niche. My chemistry background became extremely valuable in helping me to understand not only the inherent chemical nature of food itself, but also the many aspects of how foods and food additives interact with the body to create health or disease.

My studies taught me a very important truth: *eating foods in their closest to natural form is our best medicine.* Although degenerative disease may be too far advanced in some people for complete reversal, because of what I have learned and witnessed, I am convinced that all people can *greatly improve* their state of health. By following scientific and historically proven health principles and eliminating processed foods, an individual can embrace a way of eating that will lead to regeneration of the entire body, mind, soul, and spirit.[2]

Many would say that my weight loss is the result of eliminating processed foods from my diet. That is true; however, I believe that it is more the result of listening to the inner voice that called me to change my life, and of my willingness to avail myself to the power and wisdom of that voice. Some good friends have taught me to "seek the serenity to accept the things I cannot change, the courage to change the things I can, and the wisdom to know the difference." Such serenity and wisdom can bring a measure of happiness. But without the courage to change the things one can, a greater measure is missed.[3] Processed-free living involves that greater measure.

Finally, while my own journey has been personal and unique, at the very core I am just like you. I have been there—unhealthy and in the depths of hopelessness. If I can change, so can you.

My intention now is to use my experience to educate and enlighten you, so that you can find a healthier and more life-affirming relationship with your body and the food you eat. Welcome to processed-free living. Welcome home.

## Are You a Compulsive Eater?

Poor food choices and unhealthy eating behaviors are common practices in our fast-paced, convenience-oriented lifestyles, but most people who are overweight can make the positive changes outlined in this book once they put their mind to it. However, some individuals with chronic food compulsions and/or strong food addictions need more specialized help.

My work with others has clearly demonstrated that many compulsive eaters can lose weight by adhering to a sound eating plan for a period of time, but if they don't simultaneously learn how to deal with their addiction to food they will most likely return to compulsive eating (often times by overeating or binging on *healthy* foods) and gain the weight back. Until the root causes of the disorder are addressed, the compulsive eating will never be arrested.

In my nutrition counseling practice, in addition to promoting processed-free eating, I recommend that those who are compulsive eaters do themselves a favor by experiencing an established support group with many members who have already achieved freedom from compulsive eating and maintenance of a healthy body weight. Overeaters Anonymous (OA) is recommended; it is patterned after the same well-respected 12-step program used in food-addiction treatment centers around the world. The Anonymous programs are designed to help individuals transition from unhealthy behaviors of all kinds into healthy and balanced lives.

There are OA meetings in every part of the world, and in nearly every city in the United States. Many online and telephone meetings are also available. There are no dues or fees for attendance; contributions to local groups is voluntary. To find a meeting in your area, log on to www.oa.org or call 505-891-2664.

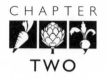
# Smart Scientists and Our Not-So-Distant Ancestors

*The way we eat has changed more in the last fifty years than in the previous ten thousand.*

—MICHAEL POLLAN, AUTHOR OF
*IN DEFENSE OF FOOD: AN EATER'S MANIFESTO*

In 2001, I was introduced to the work of distinguished neurosurgeon Russell Blaylock, MD. His compelling book *Excitotoxins: The Taste That Kills* presented startling evidence that substances added to foods and beverages overexcite neurons to the point of brain cell damage, and eventually, brain cell death. He cited over five hundred studies to make the case against two such excitotoxins—monosodium glutamate (MSG) and aspartame (found in Equal)—as the causative factors in Alzheimer's, Parkinson's, multiple sclerosis, and other neurodegenerative diseases.

However, a more relevant and unexpected revelation in Dr. Blaylock's book answered my lingering question about whether food additives contribute to obesity. He cited key evidence from a 1969 paper published in *Science* by Dr. John Olney, a medical doctor and neuropathologist, which showed that MSG injected into newborn rats affected a part of the brain that caused them to become grossly obese. The effect was not from excess food intake, but from a biochemical disturbance created by the MSG. Repeated and more recent studies have shown that this MSG-induced obesity occurs in most animal species, including monkeys, proving this phenomenon is not exclusive to rats. In fact, the effect is so well established and reproducible, scientists now routinely use MSG to purposefully induce obesity in animals to study the effects of obesity and its complications.

In subsequent writings, Dr. Blaylock has explained that this type of obesity is very difficult to diet and exercise off because the metabolism and fat-storing mechanisms in the animal's body are gravely affected. Additionally, animals fed MSG develop ravenous appetites and prefer carbohydrates and sugars to other foods—clear markers of food addiction. He believes that MSG is one of the main causes for our nation's obesity crisis.

By the time I read Dr. Blaylock's book, I had been working as a chemist for twelve years. For nine of those years I had maintained my weight loss, educated myself in nutrition, and mentored many people into healthier lives. I was more knowledgeable on the subject of health than were many health professionals, but frankly, the news about MSG blew me away. As I would later find out, this information was only a small speck inside a prodigious Pandora's box. There was more to be revealed.

In the past fifty to one hundred years, our food supply has changed—dramatically. We have gone from growing, harvesting, and preparing our own food with our own hands, to mass-producing concoctions that are made in food laboratories. Artificial sweeteners, artificial colorings, flavor enhancers, stabilizers, hormones, antibiotics, genetically modified foods, preservatives, and pesticides have infiltrated our pantries and eateries, stripping us of our birthright of good health. While obesity and its related illnesses have garnered the attention of the world's health experts, the number of normal-weight people suffering from digestive disorders, arthritis, osteoporosis, cancer, and heart disease—all illnesses relating to poor diet—is just as staggering.

It is astounding that in the name of science, we have blindly and tragically denounced many of our traditional real foods as unhealthy, and replaced them with synthetic look-alikes. Out of fear of rising cholesterol levels and heart disease, we have swapped real eggs for Egg Beaters, and real butter for margarine. The healthiest oil of all—coconut oil—was unjustly kicked to the curb, while the highly processed, genetically engineered canola oil has reigned supreme in the mind of misled consumers. Many nutritional myths have been accepted as dogma and have led us down a sordid path of trans-fat and sugar-induced self-destruction. This is what smart scientists and food activists at Yale University call a toxic food environment.[1] Traditional wisdom and sheer intuition would tell us that not only is it unnatural to re-place real food with chemical concoctions, it simply cannot be sustained.

To help me better understand the effect of food on human health, I needed to look back in human history, to a time when people weren't con-cerned about their weight or the ingredients in their food. Most of today's common health problems were rare as little as one hundred years ago. An-thropologists and researchers agree by and large that our modern diseases *did not exist* in traditional cultures where people's diets consisted of high-fiber foods such as fresh vegetables and fruits, legumes, whole grains, healthy fats, and lean protein sources.[2] Therefore, to learn and develop a way of eat-ing for life, I researched the role of food in the human story, and used the traditional diets of our not-so-distant ancestors as my guide.

To illustrate, I'd like to introduce you to the work of two very smart sci-entists who have profoundly influenced my own work. These American icons, Weston Price, DDS, and Francis M. Pottenger Jr., MD, devoted their lives to investigating and disseminating information on the relationship between optimal health, nutrition, food choices, and the evolutionary trend toward a processed, refined, mass-produced food supply. Their work covers over one hundred years of study, observations, and research, which spans the globe and is as relevant today as it was when their studies were first con-ducted. It is my intention to enlighten you as I was by the nutritional truths gleaned from their extensive studies and teachings.

## Dr. Price and the World's Skinniest People

After receiving his degree in dentistry from Harvard in 1893, Weston Price became a prominent, well-respected dentist, professor, and researcher in his field. He taught thousands at dental schools and wrote textbooks on dentistry that became standards at universities throughout the country. Al-though dentistry was his career, Dr. Price is most likely the greatest nutri-tionist who ever lived.

During his years in private practice, Dr. Price began to notice that the children of his patients were developing dental problems that their parents had not experienced at that same age. In addition to having more decay, the children's teeth were crowded and crooked because they didn't fit properly into the dental arch.

These problems were nonexistent just ten or fifteen years earlier, which caused him to wonder why it was happening now. He also noticed that the condition of the teeth reflected a person's overall health. A mouth full of cavities always accompanied a body either full of disease, or with a generalized weakness and susceptibility to disease. In Price's time, tuberculosis was the major infectious illness, and he noticed that the children with the rotten teeth were the ones who were increasingly affected by TB.

Considering possible reasons, Dr. Price suspected that some deficiency in the modern Western diet of the day was the cause of the problem. Solid scientific evidence indicates that all three symptoms Dr. Price noticed in his young patients signal physical degeneration and an increased vulnerability to diseases such as heart attacks and cancer.

Dr. Price knew that the observations of anthropologists had long documented the excellent teeth found in primitive cultures. Being rather well-off financially, he and his wife, Monica Price, RN, decided to travel the world to study primitive societies. They were specifically looking for healthy peoples who had not yet been touched by civilization—who still ate entirely according to native ways. In the early 1930s such groups were still around. They often lived in close proximity to fellow villagers and people of the same ancestry who were just beginning to adopt modern diets. Throughout the world in the 1930s, groups in the early stages of modernization were using foods imported from Western countries—sugar, white flour, canned foods, and refined vegetable oils. This combination of old and new enabled Dr. Price to see and record a picture of a disappearing world.[3]

## A Worldwide Journey

Dr. Price and his wife traveled to isolated villages in the Swiss Alps, to cold and blustery islands off the coast of Scotland, to the Andes Mountains in Peru, to several locations in Africa, to the Polynesian islands, to Australia and New Zealand, to the forests of northern Canada, to the Everglades and cypress swamps of Florida, and even to the Arctic Circle. In all, they visited with fourteen groups of native peoples.

In every village they went to, Dr. Price conducted dental and physical exams, and documented all of his findings. He recorded the components of each group's daily diet, and even preserved samples of the various foods his research subjects ate, so as to later conduct chemical analysis of those foods. To further document his observations, Dr. Price and his wife took eighteen thousand photographs.

Weston Price's discoveries were remarkable. He found entire cultures with beautiful straight teeth—including the children. An American medical doctor living among the Inuit and northern Indians told Dr. Price that in thirty-five years of treating the natives, he had never seen a single case of cancer among those who only ate their traditional foods. He observed that any native he treated with tuberculosis had been eating modern foods, and that when he sent them back to their native villages and native foods, they usually recovered. In every culture where the people were immune to dental and degenerative disease, chemical analysis of their foods showed them to be rich in nutrients poorly supplied in the modern diet.

Dr. Price recorded his findings from his travels to all fourteen countries in his book *Nutritional and Physical Degeneration*, published in 1939. Many in his profession viewed his work as profound and significant. So, too, did many anthropologists; for years, the book was required reading for anthropology classes at Harvard.

What is clear from Dr. Price's studies is that there is a definite connection between consumption of traditional and natural foods and the maintenance of good health. This connection is emphasized by studies of groups who followed their traditional diet and lived near relatives who had adopted a more westernized diet. This gave Dr. Price the opportunity to compare the health of two related groups whose only difference was their diet. Dr. Price was even allowed to examine skeletal remains of ancient people in various groups he studied. In Peru alone, "he examined 1,276 successive skulls without finding one with the narrowed dental arches of modern people."[4]

Before discussing Dr. Price's specific findings, I want to clarify what the groups were eating, when I refer to traditional foods versus those of a more modern diet. The following table demonstrates the drastic differences between them.

## Table 2.1  Traditional Diets vs. Modernized Diets in 1930

| Foods in Traditional Diets | Foods in Modernized Diets |
| --- | --- |
| All traditional diets studied were rich in *animal foods** containing *saturated fat* and *cholesterol* such as butter, eggs, fatty fish, wild game, and organ meats. The fats in these foods are rich in the fat-soluble vitamins A, D, E, and K | Consumption of naturally raised meats and seafood declined, while the increase of canned meats and seafood increased.<br><br>Artificial vitamins were taken to make up for deficiencies. |
| Raw dairy products: milk, yogurt, butter, cheese | Pasteurized, homogenized milk and dairy products made from this milk |
| Tropical fruits, raw honey, pure maple syrup | Refined sugar or corn syrup |
| Legumes, sprouted grains, raw nuts and seeds soaked in water, naturally leavened breads | White flour products, roasted nuts |
| Cold-pressed oils | Refined or hydrogenated vegetable oils |
| Naturally preserved, fermented vegetables, fruits, beverages, meats, and condiments | Canned foods<br>Additives and colorings |

*Unlike the meats eaten today, the animals eaten in traditional diets were pasture raised (grass-fed) without hormones or antibiotics.

SOURCE:  The Weston A. Price Foundation, Principles of Healthy Diets, www.westonaprice.org/basics/principles-of-healthy-diets#traditional.

Diets would vary from country to country. For example, in the Lötschental Valley in the Swiss Alps, the villagers lived primarily on the butter and cheese made from raw unpasteurized milk, *roggenbrot* (rye bread) from rye grown in the valley, berries, and occasional beef.

Populations that lived near seas and oceans, such as Gaelic peoples of the Outer Hebrides, Inuit, and the Maori of New Zealand, all consumed large amounts of seafood. Additionally, while the Maori had a variety of plant foods and fruits, Inuit only gathered nuts, berries, and some grasses in the short summer months and depended almost 100 percent on animal products. The Gaelic were limited to growing oats and used them as a major part of their diet.

Diets of the tribes in Africa that were studied greatly varied. In the Sudan, the diet consisted of fermented whole grains with fish, red meat (particularly liver), vegetables, and fruit. A number of other tribes throughout Africa were primarily agricultural and their diet comprised corn, beans, sweet potatoes, bananas, and millet, along with some fish and milk, whereas the Muhima tribe raised cattle and lived on meat, milk, and wild plant foods.

Some commonalities among all diets that Dr. Price noted were the daily use of fermented foods, which ranged among cheeses, yogurt, grain drinks, fish, and seaweeds. Additionally, native diets were rich in fats, particularly animal fats; whether from insects, eggs, fish, game animals, or domesticated herds, primitive peoples knew that they would get sick if they did not consume enough fat. The consumption of saturated fats is necessary for the body to assimilate and utilize proteins. Finally, the foods were natural, unpasteurized, pesticide free, and unprocessed, with no added sugar, white flour, preservatives, additives, or colorings.[5]

## Dr. Price's Amazing Findings

In every group he visited, Dr. Price did what he was best at—he counted cavities and examined the natives' teeth. Imagine his surprise to find, on average, less than 1 percent of tooth decay in all the peoples he visited! He also found that these people's teeth were perfectly straight and white, with high dental arches; and that they had well-formed facial features. And there was something more astonishing: none of the peoples Price examined practiced any sort of dental hygiene; not one of his subjects had ever flossed or used a toothbrush! However, kinsmen of groups studied who had left their isolated village and had spent time in modern cities eating modernized foods, experienced large amounts of dental diseases.

The Lötschental Valley, nearly a mile above sea level in an isolated part of the Swiss Alps, had been for more than a dozen centuries the home of some two thousand people when the Prices first visited in 1931. At this time in Switzerland, tuberculosis took the lives of more people than did any other disease. Yet, astonishingly, no deaths had occurred from tuberculosis in the history of the Lötschental Valley, despite frequent exposure to the disease. Dr. Price noted this was evidence of a good diet and natural forces at work.[6]

In general, Dr. Price found, in contrast to what he saw in America, no incidence of the very diseases that plague modern people who consume a processed-food diet: cancer, heart disease, diabetes, hemorrhoids, multiple sclerosis, Parkinson's, Alzheimer's, osteoporosis, and so on. But groups who no longer only ate their traditional diet were highly susceptible to tuberculosis and other degenerative diseases.

Dr. Price saved and preserved a variety of foods obtained from each country that he sent back to the United States for analysis of the vitamin and mineral content. The results showed that the traditional foods contained *ten times* the amount of fat-soluble vitamins (A, D, E, and K), and *four times* the calcium, minerals, and water-soluble vitamins found in the Western diets of the 1930s.

Dr. Price also noticed another quality about the healthy people: they were happy, hardy, and strong, despite the sometimes difficult living conditions they had to endure. Whereas depression was not a major problem in Dr. Price's day, it certainly is today: ask any psychiatrist. While certain villagers sometimes fought with neighboring villagers, within their own groups, they were cheerful and optimistic and bounced back quickly from emotional setbacks. These people had no need for antidepressants.

There are so many more stories and details about specific groups and foods Dr. Price studied than I can include in this chapter. But, what I can summarize for you from the highlights of his findings is that one's health—both physical and dental—is directly related to food choices. Poor nutrition leads to chronic and degenerative diseases, and contributes to the development of obesity.

The good news that I have personally experienced, and seen with my clients, is that when people change their poor food choices and adopt a processed-free lifestyle, they get *skinny*.

## Dr. Pottenger's Skinny Cats

About the same time that Weston Price was traveling the globe, a medical doctor in California was conducting a very extensive nutritional experiment with domestic cats. While attending medical school, Dr. Francis M. Pottenger Jr. developed a "hatred" for the way civilized man treated himself and his children. He wondered why people so capable of advancing their technology, failed so miserably in promoting their biological health. He felt a driving need to know and understand how people could maintain good health and eliminate chronic illness. This missionary zeal led him to focus his medical career toward the field of nutrition. After graduating from medical school in 1930, he went to work with his father, also a physician, at the Pottenger Sanatorium, a facility internationally recognized for its outstanding treatment of tuberculosis. Good nutrition was one of the key components of the treatment.

Dr. Pottenger's most famous and enduring project was a ten-year study (1932–42) to determine the effects of processed foods on the health of domestic cats. It is this study that contributed to proving that poor diets change DNA and create disease traits that affect future generations. The study was prompted by the high death rate among his laboratory cats undergoing operations to remove their adrenal glands. At the time, adrenal extract from cats was used to calibrate the strength of medication given to tuberculosis patients.

In preparing his cats for surgery, Dr. Pottenger fed them what he believed was the optimum diet for cats. It consisted of raw milk; cod liver oil; and cooked scraps of liver, tripe, sweetbreads, brains, heart, and muscle. However, despite feeding them what he considered a healthy diet, many of these cats did not seem healthy; they exhibited nutritional deficiencies and a high percentage of them did not survive the surgery.

Concerned with the cats' poor postoperative survival, Dr. Pottenger noticed the cats showed a decrease in their reproductive capacity; also, many of the kittens born in the laboratory had skeletal deformities and organ malfunctions.

By a quirk of fate, as the number of cats donated by his neighbors kept increasing, he couldn't handle the demand for cooked meat scraps. So he ordered raw meat scraps from a local meat-packing plant. Always a scientist, Dr. Pottenger fed these raw meat scraps to a segregated group of cats so that he could observe any change. Within a few months, this group appeared healthier, its kittens more vigorous, and these cats had a higher survival rate after their operation.

The contrast between the two sets of cats was so startling that it prompted Dr. Pottenger to conduct an experiment to verify these facts scientifically. Because pathological problems in cats eating cooked meats were similar to those in his TB patients, he believed a controlled-feeding experiment with animals would isolate variables of importance in human nutrition as well. This experiment is now famously known as the Pottenger Cat Study.

As explained in his book *Pottenger's Cats,* he very carefully designed the study to research these questions:

- Why did the cats eating raw meat survive surgery at higher rates than did cats eating cooked meat?
- Why did cats eating raw meat appear healthier and more vigorous?
- Why did a diet consisting of cooked foods not provide adequate nutrients?
- What was the relationship of these findings on human nutrition?

His study encompassed four generations involving nine hundred cats. Each cat's record was carefully documented with its own chart that tracked its history, weight, development, diet, and outcomes. The experiments met the most rigorous scientific standards of their day.

## The Cat Study: Some Startling Revelations

All the cats were supplied the same basic minimal diet, but the major portion of their diet varied. Two separate feeding experiments were conducted to determine the effect of raw versus cooked foods. The first feeding experiment involved two groups of cats. One group received a diet of two parts raw meat, one part raw milk, and cod liver oil. The second group received two parts cooked meat, one part raw milk, and cod liver oil. The second feeding experiment involved four groups of cats. One group received a diet of two parts raw milk, one part raw meat, and cod liver oil. The other three groups were respectively given two parts pasteurized milk, evaporated milk, or sweetened condensed milk; one part raw meat; and cod liver oil. (The cod liver oil was routinely included as a rich supplemental source of vitamin A.) Four generations of cats were carefully studied over the course of ten years. Dr. Pottenger was hoping to demonstrate the health effects of eating raw foods (the natural diet for cats) versus eating cooked and processed foods over successive generations.

Table 2.2 clearly summarizes the health effects on the cats studied. All four generations of the cats fed raw meat and raw milk remained healthy throughout their normal life span. The groups of cats receiving either cooked meat or processed milk developed diseases and illnesses earlier in their life

## Table 2.2  Summary of Dr. Pottenger's Ten-Year Cat Study

| GROUP | A & B | C | D | E | F |
|---|---|---|---|---|---|
| | | | Food Received | | |
| | Raw milk<br>Raw meat<br>Cod liver oil | Raw milk<br>Cooked meat<br>Cod liver oil | Pasteurized milk<br>Raw meat<br>Cod liver oil | Evaporated milk<br>Raw meat<br>Cod liver oil | Sweetened condensed milk<br>Raw meat<br>Cod liver oil |
| First Generation | Remained healthy throughout their normal lifespan. | The first generation of all four processed food groups developed diseases and illnesses near the end of their lives. | | | |
| Second Generation | Remained healthy throughout their normal lifespan. | The second generation of all four processed food groups developed diseases and illnesses in the middle of their lives. | | | |
| Third Generation | Remained healthy throughout their normal lifespan. | The third generation of all four processed food groups developed diseases and illnesses in the beginning of their lives; many died before six months of age. | | | |
| Fourth Generation | Remained healthy throughout their normal lifespan. | There was no fourth generation in any of the processed food groups; either the third generation parents were sterile, or the fourth generation cats were miscarried before birth. | | | |

The experiment included nine-hundred cats over four generations. Six different feeding groups were studied. All groups were supplied the same basic minimal diet, but the major portion of the diets were varied. Groups A and B were fed whole foods (raw milk and raw meat in varying proportions). Group C received cooked meat and raw milk. Groups D, E, and F were given increasingly processed types of milk: pasteurized, evaporated, and sweetened condensed milk plus raw meat. The group receiving sweetened condensed milk showed the most marked deficiencies.

span with each succeeding generation, to the point where they were no longer able to reproduce their species. The cats eating only raw food were disease free and healthy, generation after generation after generation. They reproduced easily and were well coordinated—when dropped from up to six feet or thrown, they always landed on all four feet. Miscarriages were rare and the cause of death was generally old age. Autopsies invariably revealed normal internal organs.

The cats eating the cooked and processed foods had myriad health problems that grew with successive generations. Often by the third generation, their bones became so soft as to be actually rubbery. The diseases of old age—vision problems, infections of internal organs and bones, arthritis, heart problems, underactivity of the thyroid gland, and inflammation of the joints and nervous system—were common. Coordination was poor; when tossed a short distance, the cats had trouble landing on all four feet. Pneumonia and lung abscesses were the most usual causes of death in adults; pneumonia and diarrhea were the usual causes in kittens. The cats fed sweetened condensed milk developed much heavier fat deposits and showed the most marked nutritional deficiencies of all the groups.

At autopsy, analysis of the bones of processed foods–fed cats determined calcium and phosphorous content to second- and third-generation kittens to be one-third to one-half that of the raw meat–fed kittens. Females often showed small ovaries with a congested uterus; males frequently showed testes that had failed to develop the ability to produce sperm.

The miscarriage rate among first-generation processed food–fed cats was about 25 percent; among the second generation, about 70 percent. No fourth generation of kittens was born to the groups fed processed food in the years of the study. In the third generation, the cats suffered from most of the degenerative diseases encountered in human medicine; the kittens always died before reaching six months of age.

Dr. Pottenger also studied and documented the effect of the mother cat's diet on her nursing kittens. He found that when normal, healthy kittens were born, their state of health was either maintained or reduced based on the diet fed to the mother cat. In other words, if the diet of the nursing cat was changed from the raw components to the less healthy diet, she could not pass on adequate nutrients to the nursing kittens. This directly impacted the health of the kittens. The milk the kittens received from mothers on the unhealthy diets was deficient in nutrients and that reinforced the deficiencies with which the kittens were born. However, if the deficient kittens were given feedings in which proper nutrients were provided during the nursing period, improvements to their general condition occurred.

## What Pottenger's Study Means for Humans

The results of the cat study clearly show that nutrition impacts health and that genetic weaknesses do develop over time. Those weaknesses develop when generation after generation continues to depend on a diet that is devoid of correct nutrients. That impact can be lessened only when a diet with proper nutrients is adopted! Also, a healthy diet may halt or prevent illnesses and degenerative diseases. (That point is clearly shown in both Dr. Pottenger's cat studies and the research conducted by Dr. Weston Price.)

As for applying his results to human nutrition, Dr. Pottenger said, "While no attempt will be made to correlate the changes in the animals studied with malformations found in humans, the similarity is so obvious that parallel pictures will suggest themselves."

The Pottenger Cat Study gives insight into why children today are getting degenerative diseases that used to only show up in humans at an age of fifty years or older. What's alarming about this study is that the levels of health get progressively worse with each generation, just as we are seeing with humans. It takes approximately twenty years to beget a generation of humans, so to conduct the same study through four generations would take over eighty years. Of course no such study is being done on humans, but it's easy to observe that there has been a tremendous increase in heart disease, cancer, arthritis, and autoimmune diseases over the last eighty years.

Does this make you wonder why so many children are now developing cancer, diabetes, and other rare medical conditions that were once only found in adults? Could our processed foods be the reason why Generation X is experiencing high rates of infertility? Think about it—a fertility clinic was all but unheard of a mere fifty years ago.

However, Dr. Pottenger's study is not a gloom-and-doom story. Quite the contrary. He proved that diseases are *not* inherited; rather only the *tendency or potential* of a disease is passed on from parents to offspring. The disease tendency is transferred by way of the genetic code (DNA), and will only manifest as a disease if there are factors that exploit that weakness (poor diet, for example).

Throughout the study, Dr. Pottenger pulled some of the sick cats out of their processed-food groups and put them into the raw-food groups. The results showed that within a short amount of time, the sick cats got well. And more than that, the disease tendencies no longer manifested in the DNA of subsequent generations when those generations continued on the raw diet.

My understanding of the results of the Pottenger Cat Study is that we have the ability to improve our health simply by improving our diet. We can reverse disease traits that have been passed on to us if we take the necessary steps to correct nutritional deficiencies.

## The Parallels Between the Work of Dr. Pottenger and Dr. Price

The health problems of the cats Dr. Pottenger studied provided parallels with the human societies that Dr. Price studied. The cats that ate processed foods developed the same diseases as did humans eating refined foods. These cats also developed the same dental malformations that children of people eating modernized foods did, including narrowing of dental arches with attendant crowding of teeth, underbites and overbites, and protruding and crooked teeth.

Humans don't have the same nutritional requirements as cats, but we have strong empirical evidence that both species need a significant amount of particular high-quality foods to reproduce and function efficiently.[7]

The work of Weston Price and Francis Pottenger was combined in 1952 and is maintained and expanded on today through the public education mission of the Weston A. Price Memorial Foundation. I encourage you to visit the foundation's website (see Chapter 17), which is a storehouse of cutting-edge articles and research on whole foods nutrition.

In the coming chapters, I will spotlight more smart scientists and other crusaders whose work is helping to reform and restore our nation's food supply to one that more closely resembles the high-quality foods of the skinniest people in the world.

## Jen's Story

After years of wrong-headed thinking regarding food, I feel like I've finally "gotten it." It's been about four months since my doctor strongly suggested I try Dee's plan. It was an eye-opener, and scary, but I took the leap. Twenty-five pounds are gone! My head is clearer with this new way of life. I'm not as sluggish as I used to be. I'm excited to see my doc again to see what else my body is doing well these days.

We're bombarded with all sorts of different messages as to what's "healthy" and what's "best" and what's going to change our lives and be our magic pill. It's work; it's a choice that has to be made every single day. It isn't easy . . . nor should it be. But here I am . . . twenty-five pounds lighter with a desire to stop polluting my body. A desire to truly live as opposed to just coasting along in a fog. Finally . . . there really IS a light at the end of this tunnel.

—*Jen Hammack, age 33, professional photographer*

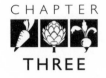
# The Laws of Skinny Science and Nature's Perfect Foods

*Eating has a spiritual function, for it fills us with nature's life force. As we digest and assimilate its contents, the essence of our food becomes a part of us.*

—EDWARD BAUMAN, MED, PHD,
FOUNDER AND PRESIDENT OF BAUMAN COLLEGE

Scientists have many different tools available to them when trying to explain how nature and the universe at large work. One of those tools is observation, from which scientific laws, or natural laws as they are sometimes called, are discovered. A scientific law is a concise statement about the results of repeated observation of phenomena that always apply under the same conditions. One example of a scientific law is Newton's law of gravity. Every time you throw a ball into the air, it will come back down. Likewise, there are biological laws that govern our body and our health. Those laws, just like the law of gravity, have been in place since time immemorial, and the last time I checked, they haven't changed. When we eat food in its closest to natural form, we get skinny; when we don't, we get sick. These are not new concepts; however, health is still a mystery to most people.

Through years of repeated observation, both personal and intellectual, I have come up with what I call the Laws of Skinny Science. They are mainly explanations of the biological laws mentioned above. Your understanding of each of these laws is critical to your ability to get and stay skinny. Each of these laws will be discussed more fully in later parts of the book, where you will gain a deeper appreciation for the delicate balance between what we eat and how it ultimately affects our health. While each of these laws is critical in helping you develop a *way of eating for life*, the most important by far are the first two laws, which I will focus on in the remainder of this chapter. They are the foundation upon which the other laws are built, and you will begin to see just how important it is to leave the design of food up to nature, rather than to humans.

The Laws of Skinny Science are:

1. Healthful eating is about respecting how our body is designed. (See pages 38–40.)
2. Whole, natural foods are "perfect packages" uniquely designed to nourish our body. (See pages 40–41.)
3. Refined sugar and refined flour are so far removed from their natural state that our body doesn't recognize them as foods; they are toxins that rob us of our health. (See Chapter 4.)
4. You must eat fat to lose fat. (See Chapter 5.)
5. Food additives don't honor how our body is designed; they are catalysts for poor health and should be avoided. (See Chapter 6.)
6. A body can only be skinny when its alkalinity is balanced. (See Chapter 9.)
7. The "calories in, calories out" argument is tragically flawed. (See Chapter 10.)
8. The amount of vegetables you eat is directly proportional to the amount of weight you will lose and the amount of health you will gain. (See Chapter 12.)

## Doing Your Body a Lifelong Favor

The reason we are suffering in great numbers from diet-related diseases is that we're not taught to honor two of our most precious gifts—our body and the whole, natural foods that are designed to sustain it. Which brings us to the first Law of Skinny Science: Healthful eating is about respecting how our body is designed.

Your body is an amazing machine that works hard every day to keep you alive. Given time and the right ingredients, it has an inherent ability to heal itself. The operative words here are "the right ingredients." The human body was specifically designed to function best on foods that have either not been changed from their original form, or been only minimally changed. Those foods include vegetables and fruits; legumes; nuts and seeds; and lean, free-range wild or pasture-raised animal proteins, including eggs, raw dairy, and wild fish. Dr. Price's study of societies' eating their traditional diet revealed that the skinniest people in the world did not die from the diet- and lifestyle-related illnesses that are killing most people today, mainly because their food wasn't taken apart or tainted with chemicals foreign to their DNA. Our not-so-distant ancestors ate "perfect packages"—foods in their closest-to-natural form.

So just what is it about whole, natural foods that make them so optimal for our body? To understand this, we must first examine the inherent perfection of food. Studying food and nutrition has given me a great appreciation for its design and its designer. When we examine how food exists in nature, it is undeniable that our food was provided for us by an intelligent nature and does not occur by random chance.

Perhaps one of the reasons we've allowed processed foods to become so dominant in our culture is that we don't really understand the power and value of foods in their whole form. Although the study of nutrition is one of the oldest sciences, it is still one of the biggest mysteries. It was only a hundred years ago that vitamins and minerals were discovered to exist in foods. Up until that time, scientists and doctors of the day could only make educated guesses that there had to be *something* in foods that provided us with health and well-being.[1]

Today, about forty-seven basic nutrients have been identified as being necessary for our normal growth and the maintenance of human life. These comprise the micronutrients (vitamins and minerals) and the macronutrients (essential fatty acids, the amino acids that make up proteins, carbohydrates, and water). Collectively, these nutrients are like our twenty-six letters in the alphabet. From those letters, we can literally make thousands of different words. Likewise, from these basic forty-seven nutrients, our body can synthesize (or make on its own) proteins, vitamins, fats, hormones, enzymes, and neurotransmitters.

An estimated ten thousand different compounds are created in the body just from these forty-seven nutrients—all of which are essential to the maintenance of our health. All forty-seven nutrients must be present in our diet because they work together, synergistically. Therefore, the lack of any one of these nutrients might result in the underproduction of hundreds of those vital compounds. Imagine how many words would be affected if the letter *e* were suddenly missing, or deficient, from the alphabet. When we are lacking the essential nutrients in our diet, disease and degeneration begin to form. The effect of deficiencies and underproduction of vital compounds can take days, years, or even decades to show up as disease symptoms.

But even when we get the minimum of these essential nutrients, we are not optimally healthy, especially when we are taking them into our body in synthetic and processed forms.

## Embracing Nature's Perfect "Packaged Foods"

There is something more in whole foods that we need to honor, something science still has not been able to explain. This is the second Law of Skinny Science: Every food that grows on the planet is uniquely and precisely packaged and designed for our body.[2]

No two foods are exactly the same. Each food contains differing amounts and types of nutrients that, when certain foods are eaten together, provide our body with complete and balanced nutrition. Additionally, the foods themselves contain specific combinations of vitamins, minerals, phytochemicals, fibers, and enzymes that work together synergistically to help our body digest those very foods. For example, as you will learn in the next chapter, the minerals required by our body to digest sugar are calcium, phosphorous, chromium, magnesium, cobalt, copper, zinc, and manganese. Sugarcane in its natural form is rich in these minerals, as well as many vitamins, which all work with natural sugarcane's fiber and enzymes to help our body digest the naturally occurring sugars. Similarly, other plant foods such as fruits, carrots, and beets also supply our body with the specific nutrients needed to properly digest their sugars.

Another example of the perfect design of food is found in seed-bearing plants. Rex Russell, MD, a board-certified diagnostic radiologist known for his work promoting whole-foods diets, explains, "A scientific examination of seeds indicates that they could not have developed by random chance." Seeds (which include grains, beans, and nuts) grow everywhere in the world, in any climate, and reproduce quickly. They have a long storage life: kernels found in Egyptian tombs can still be sprouted after four thousand years. Nutritionally, if they are not processed or refined, these intelligently designed seeds meet nearly all of our nutritional needs, as they are filled with vitamins, minerals, fibers, and even protein.[3]

## Fruits and Vegetables—The Givers of Life

Consider also the perfection of fruits and vegetables. The vast array of colors in fruits and vegetables owes to their high content of a special family of nutrients called phytochemicals, alternately called phytonutrients. These important compounds give plant foods their colors, flavors, and disease-fighting abilities. The more intense the color of a fruit or vegetable, the greater the concentration of phytochemicals. Like the scientists of a century ago who had only begun to discover vitamins and minerals, nutrition researchers today have only skimmed the surface in identifying these powerful compounds. Thousands of phytochemicals have been identified, yet many more remain a mystery. It is estimated that there are *thousands* of different phytochemicals in a typical fruit or vegetable. Tomatoes alone are believed to contain an estimated ten thousand different phytochemicals! While these nutrients are not considered essential by the medical community in the same way that vitamins and minerals are, that could only be due to the fact that we don't know enough about them. One Harvard scientist has proposed that the health benefits of at least one phytonutrient, epicatechin, is so important that it should be classified as a new vitamin. Norman Hollenberg, a professor of medicine at Harvard Medical School, has spent years studying the benefits of cocoa drinking on the Kuna people in Panama. He found that the risk of stroke, heart failure, cancer, and diabetes is reduced to less than 10 percent in the Kuna, where the people drink up to forty cups of natural cocoa a week. Natural cocoa contains high levels of epicatechin.[4]

Vitamins are defined as essential to the normal functioning, metabolism, regulation, and growth of cells; deficiency of a vitamin is usually linked to disease. Currently, epicatechin doesn't fit that definition, but again, not enough is known about the role phytonutrients play in maintaining optimal health. It may be that stroke and some diseases are the result of epicatechin deficiency, or perhaps of a phytonutrient deficiency in general.

The word *vegetable* comes from the Latin word *vegetare*, meaning "to enliven or animate." The name describes the very essence of the purpose of vegetables, which is to provide our body with life. Fruits also fulfill this purpose; however, it is vegetables that contain some of the most powerful life-giving qualities, which scientific studies have proven can prevent, as well as treat, many diseases, especially chronic degenerative illnesses such as heart disease, cancer, diabetes, and arthritis. Our ancestors ate an abundance of vegetables; hence, until recently, cancer and other diseases were a rare or nonexistent occurrence in human history. Many of the people who have followed the Processed-Free Eating Plan have experienced the tremendous healing effects of vegetables by including an abundance of them in their daily meals.

In many cases, fruits and vegetables provide the same, if not better, remedies for common ailments than do medications. For instance, doctors often prescribe taking an aspirin every day to prevent heart problems. But studies have shown that taking an aspirin every day actually increases the risk of other serious problems, such as hemorrhagic strokes. This is because the main ingredient in aspirin, salicylic acid, is chemically manufactured and does not work the same way in the body as does naturally occurring salicylic acid.[5] If doctors would prescribe fruits and vegetables instead, the harmful side effects of synthetic aspirin could be avoided. Later you'll find out that dark chocolate has been shown to be more effective than taking an aspirin to thin the blood.

Not only do fruits and vegetables contain salicylic acid, but they also help the body make more of its own natural salicylic acid. Studies have shown that people who do not take aspirin but eat an abundance of vegetables and fruits, have the same levels of salicylic acid in their blood as do patients taking low doses of aspirin but not eating an abundance of vegetables and fruits. Fruits and vegetables provide just the right amount of salicylic acid to prevent both kinds of strokes—those caused by unnecessary clotting (which leads to heart attacks) and hemorrhagic strokes. Eating just three vegetable servings a day decreases the incidence of strokes and heart attacks by a significant amount.[6]

## Life Force Energy

When you break a bone, a doctor will set it and put it in a cast, but the doctor doesn't heal the bone. Nature does. There is an intrinsic force in our world that mends bones and works behind the scenes to restore order. This invisible force is the basis for long-term health and healing. In ancient Chinese medicine, this force, or energy, was named *chi* or *qi*. The Japanese term for it is *ki*. In India they call it *prana* and in Hawaii it is known as *manna*. African Bushmen call it *boiling energy*. In the West we refer to this timeless force as Life Force Energy. All cultures and traditions recognize that Life Force Energy needs to be able to flow freely and abundantly into our body for us to experience the full range of physical, emotional, and spiritual well-being. So where does this energy come from? It comes from our food!

Phytochemicals in plant foods absorb sunlight in the visible region of the electromagnetic spectrum, causing them to be vibrantly colored. Green veggies owe their color to a special phytochemical called chlorophyll. Chlorophyll is the green pigment of all green plants, including leafy vegetables such as lettuces, spinach, and kale; broccoli and most other cruciferous vegetables; wheatgrass; and the algae superfoods spirulina and chlorella. The colors in plants are a form of stored energy, which is housed in the plant's cells. When we eat colorful fruits and vegetables, we experience a noticeable difference in our energy levels. This is because the energy in the food is transferred to us. Therefore, the more fresh and alive the food is, the more energy we receive.

While technology has made great strides in extracting vitamins, minerals, and enzymes from foods and putting them into powders, capsules, and meal replacement bars, there is still something missing from those altered foods. We cannot extract the life-giving energies from plants and put them into a pill. There is simply nothing on the planet more perfect and as good for us as the Life Force Energy in natural foods.

## How Phytonutrients Prevent Cancer

The formation of cancer is a multistep process, and phytonutrients do their good work to fight cancer by blocking one or more of those steps. For instance, cancer can begin when a cancer-causing molecule—from the foods or beverages you consume, the air you breathe, or the products you rub on your skin and hair—comes into your body and invades a cell. But if a phytonutrient is already swimming around in your bloodstream, it can also reach the cell and activate enzymes that sweep the carcinogen out of the cell before it has a chance to do any damage. Sulforaphane, a phytonutrient found in broccoli, is known to block both breast cancer and prostate cancer cells.[7]

Other phytonutrients prevent cancer in other ways. Citrus fruits and berries contain flavonoids, which prevent cancer-causing hormones from latching onto cells in the first place. Isoflavones, found in legumes, kill tumors by cutting off the blood flow needed to nourish them. Indoles, found in cabbage, Brussels sprouts, broccoli, and cauliflower, enhance detoxification and make it easier for the body to flush out toxins. Saponins, found in kidney beans, garbanzo beans, and lentils, prevent cancer cells from multiplying. P-coumaric acid and chlorogenic acid, found in tomatoes, block chemicals from combining to create carcinogens. The list goes on and on.[8]

Because each type of phytonutrient works in a different way, we need to eat a wide variety of plant foods. Consider the synergistic effect of all the different actions of the different phytonutrients on cancer—from whisking carcinogens out of cells, preventing hormones from latching onto cells, cutting off blood flow to tumors, and interfering with the creation of carcinogens. Meals that contain a variety of plant foods ensure an abundant supply of phytonutrients. On the other hand, if all we eat are a few of the same vegetables over and over, we're missing out on some of the best cancer-fighting agents. That's why you can't just eat lots of broccoli, but no tomatoes or legumes, and expect to prevent cancer.

By following the guidelines outlined in the Processed-Free Eating Plan, it will be easy to get a healthy dose of phytonutrients at every meal. Every plant food that has been tested has been found to contain these amazing substances. Moreover, some phytonutrients do not appear to be destroyed by cooking or other food manipulation, unlike many vitamins, and are in fact enhanced by certain changes. Isoflavones found in soybeans, for instance, are only available for absorption by our body when the soybeans are fermented to make products such as tempeh and miso (fermented soy foods are the only soy foods I recommend). Similarly, the phytonutrient lycopene, found in tomatoes, is a more potent cancer fighter when the tomatoes have been cooked. And phenethyl isothiocyanate, found in cabbage, remains intact even when the cabbage is made into coleslaw or sauerkraut. However, many antioxidants are lost during cooking, so it's important to eat as many raw fruits and vegetables as possible. It is also important to eat the edible peels and skins of fruits and vegetables such as apples, carrots, potatoes, cucumbers, and kiwis, as this is where many of the phytonutrients are contained.[9]

## Cooperation with Nature—Our Best Ally

I recently came across a copy of a cookbook that was first published in 1968, called *Ten Talents: Natural Foods Cookbook and Health Manual,* the title of which sums up this chapter nicely. What intrigued me the most about this book was not the recipes, but the extensive instructions on nutrition and how to eat to be skinny. In the foreword, written by Frank J. Hurd, MD, also one the authors, it is stated:

> All of us are hungry for those necessary requirements that our "All knowing Creator" designed our bodies to have, to maintain a healthy, vigorous and responsive body. We can no longer depend upon nature alone to supply the human body with its vital life forces. We must cooperate with nature by having a thorough understanding of our physiology and bodily needs. Then, and only then, can we reap from nature that which will keep us in health.[10]

Our designer cared for us and our nutritional needs by specifically designing and providing food in a perfect form. That is the second Law of Skinny Science. It was only when we forgot how perfect it is, and thought we could make it better, that we began to experience problems with our health. The next chapter is a clear example of this statement.

## Colleen's Story

In 2007 I was suffering from severe arthritis in my hips and back, to the point where it was too painful to walk most days. I also had horrible nasal allergies. My doctor recommended Dee's Processed-Free Eating Plan as a nutritional therapy (she had been to see Dee for her own arthritis and had great results from following the plan). Although I was also carrying 65 extra pounds, I thought that was just age related, so I wasn't thinking that I needed to lose weight—I just wanted relief for my arthritis.

Within three days of following the plan, I noticed I had less joint pain as I walked to my mailbox. I continued to eliminate processed foods, refined sugars, and wheat products, and increased my intake of vegetables, fruits, and healthy oils. I also made sure to eat salmon several times a week. To my surprise, not only did my arthritis pain disappear, my extra weight literally melted off, and my allergy symptoms decreased significantly. Within four months, I lost 65 pounds.

My body has been pain free for four years now, and my weight has remained steady at a wonderful 125 pounds. But what's even more wonderful is that my skin glows, my hair is shiny, and I no longer suffer from allergies. I've even been able to do yoga exercises regularly.

The things I have learned from this plan have been invaluable. I now understand the effect food has on my body's pH, and I know which foods will help keep me healthy and pain free, so even when I go out to eat at a restaurant I can make the right choices. As a result of eating processed free, my body desires the healthy foods more than it desires the unhealthy ones.

—Colleen Politi, age 57, therapeutic musician

CHAPTER

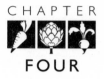

FOUR

# A Scientist's View
# of Sugar and Flour

*[Sugar] ought to be against the law—and white bread also.*
—WILLIAM DONALD KELLEY, DDS, AT A 1971 MEETING
OF THE MID-MANHATTAN CHAPTER OF THE INTERNATIONAL
ASSOCIATION OF CANCER VICTIMS AND FRIENDS

The initial reason for eliminating white sugar and white flour from my life was the strong personal evidence that I was addicted to the stuff. Many books have been written on the subject of sugar and food addiction, and it is now a widely accepted fact that some people experience peculiar brain chemistry, similar to that of an alcoholic, which causes them to react differently than other people do when they ingest refined carbohydrates. As you know, I am one of those people. Even though I readily accepted this fact for myself, I continued to research and explore beyond the food addiction model, because even non-food-addicted people who eat refined carbohydrates are suffering in large numbers from diet-related illnesses. Being a scientist, and wanting to reach both populations, I needed a more compelling reason for convincing people to eliminate sugar and flour from their lives. Twenty years ago, finding scientific information about the effect of sugar and flour on the body was like looking for a needle in a haystack. The information was there, it just wasn't widely publicized, and still isn't even to this day. More recently, the scientific and medical communities have discovered a lot more about what sugar and white flour do to the body, and the scientific truth is not so sweet. A spoonful of sugar may help the medicine go down, but you wouldn't need any medicine at all if you cut the sugar and flour out of your life for good. The effect of sugar on your body goes far beyond empty calories and tooth decay—it is, according to several medical experts, a scary toxin. White flour has its own set of devastating effects on the body, but it hasn't received as much attention from the scientific community as sugar has. I'm going to touch on both, starting with the seductively sweet poison.

Nearly two hundred years ago, the average American consumed less than ten pounds of refined sugar per year. Today, we gobble and slurp down about 156 pounds of sugar per person in that time. That's thirty-one five-pound bags for each us! A 2010 study published in the *Journal of the American Medical Association* concluded that sugar intake significantly contributes to ill health and specifically increases triglyceride levels that lead to heart disease. After examining the added sugar intake and blood fat levels in more than 6,100 adults, the researchers found that people consumed an average of 21.4 teaspoons of added sugars a day, and those with the higher intakes were more likely to have lower levels of HDL (good) cholesterol and higher levels of triglycerides. A separate national health survey in 2010 found that teenagers aged fourteen to eighteen consume a whopping 34 teaspoons of added sugar a day.[1] The "added sugars" in question included table sugar, brown sugar, high-fructose corn syrup, honey, molasses, brown rice syrup, agave syrup, evaporated cane juice, and other caloric sweeteners in prepared and processed foods—for instance, in soft drinks, iced tea, candy, pastries, cookies, and canned fruits. The sugars in whole fruit, 100% fruit juice, and other whole foods were not included in the numbers.

Eating 21.4 teaspoons of added sugar a day equates to pouring 7 teaspoons of sugar onto each of your three meals a day. The adult study prompted the American Heart Association to change their "use sugar in moderation" stance of the past, and to make specific recommendations about the amount of added sugar that can be consumed in a heart-healthy diet. The numbers they came up with were 6 teaspoons per day for women and 9 teaspoons per day for men (they didn't set any recommended limits for children or teen-agers). These recommended amounts are still way too high, because sugar creates more havoc in our body than just adding empty calories and promoting tooth decay, even when consumed in small amounts. According to nutritionist Nancy Appleton, PhD, author of six books on the dangers of eating refined sugar, including the best seller *Lick the Sugar Habit*, "Every teaspoon of refined sugar you eat works to throw the body out of balance and compromise its health."[2] The study findings are only the latest in a vast body of sugar-disease connections that have been well documented in medical journals throughout the world.

Seductive and sweet, refined sugar is more a drug than it is a food—it is a poison. Aside from quickly adding pounds of fat to our belly, butt, and thighs, sugar interferes with many body functions and slowly and deleteriously robs us of important nutrients. The result is a myriad of complications and degenerative diseases such as allergies, arthritis, gallstones, colitis, depression, gout, diabetes, hypoglycemia, heart disease, osteoporosis, obesity, and cancer (particularly breast cancer and colon cancer), to name just a few!

## Raw Sugarcane: Nature's Wonder Food

To understand what happens to sugarcane when it is refined (and why it does such dastardly deeds), you must first come to know the beauty of sugarcane in its raw natural form. It is a prime example of a perfect-package whole food. Sugarcane is a plant—a tall grass with a stout, jointed, and fibrous stalk that looks similar to bamboo. Therefore, like all other plant foods, sugarcane is brimming with vitamins, minerals, fibers, enzymes, and phytonutrients. If you walked into a field of sugarcane and cut off a piece to chew on, not only would you would experience a yummy, sweet, yet dark-flavored treat, but you would also get nourished. Yes, *nourished*. Sugarcane is rich in the minerals calcium, chromium, cobalt, copper, magnesium, manganese, phosphorous, potassium and zinc. It also contains iron and vitamins A, C, $B_1$, $B_2$, $B_3$, $B_5$, and $B_6$. In addition to vitamins and minerals, sugarcane contains a high concentration of phytonutrients, antioxidants, and numerous other health-supportive compounds. The refinement of sugarcane removes all of these wonderful nutrients, leaving a nutritionally empty substance. I will discuss the refinement process in more detail a little later.

In most countries where sugarcane is cultivated (Brazil and India are the top two producers, though it is grown in over one hundred countries), it is consumed in the raw form. The locals suck or chew on an exposed end of the raw sugarcane to extract the juice. The juice can also be extracted in larger quantities for drinking, by feeding the stalks through a slow-moving roller pressing machine. Sugarcane juice is consumed worldwide, and is a traditional food with a profound presence in the local cultures where it is grown. The locals drink it with a pinch of sea salt and lemon juice, for a natural high-energy drink whose value goes far beyond its sweet taste.

If you've ever had the pleasure of drinking freshly extracted fruit or vegetable juices, you know the health value of doing so. Freshly extracted juices contain live enzymes and nutrients that are easily absorbed by the body for quick nourishment. As sugarcane is a grass, its juice is a high-potency equivalent to wheatgrass juice, only with less chlorophyll and more sugar content. Even so, sugarcane juice contains only about 15 percent total sugar content—the rest of the juice consists of water brimming with all of those vitamins and minerals mentioned before, plus an abundance of phytonutrients (including chlorophyll), antioxidants, proteins, soluble fiber, and a host of other organic compounds.

Several scientific studies have revealed that sugarcane is extremely high in a unique mix of compounds called polyphenols.[3] Polyphenols are a large class of phytonutrient compounds with powerful antioxidant properties and numerous health benefits. When consumed as a "whole package," the polyphenols in sugarcane juice work in harmony with the vitamins, minerals, and other cofactors to slow down the absorption of its sugars into the bloodstream, resulting in a very low-glycemic food. The glycemic index (the effect a carbohydrate has on blood glucose levels) of sugarcane juice is on the order of 30 to 40, depending on the geographic location and the nutrient content of the soil it is grown in. On the glycemic index scale, low-glycemic foods rank between 0 and 55 and are released into the bloodstream slowly and gradually. They are typically safe for diabetics. To give you a comparison, the glycemic index of peanuts or broccoli is 15, and unsweetened apple juice is 40. Refined sugar has a glycemic index of 64 (nearly twice that of raw sugarcane juice).

## What Is the Glycemic Index?

The glycemic index (GI) is a measure of the effects of carbohydrates on blood sugar (glucose) levels. Carbohydrates that break down quickly during digestion, releasing glucose rapidly into the bloodstream, have a high GI; carbohydrates that break down more slowly, releasing glucose more gradually into the bloodstream, have a low GI. One of the absolute keys to achieving effective weight loss is to maintain blood sugar levels within a healthy range. By doing so, you also prevent heart disease, improve cholesterol levels, prevent insulin resistance and type 2 diabetes, and prevent certain cancers.

### Table 4.1 Glycemic Classifications

| Classification | GI range | Examples |
| --- | --- | --- |
| Low GI | 55 or less | Most fruits and vegetables, legumes (beans, peas, lentils), whole grains, nuts, seeds, dairy products, raw sugarcane, coconut sugar, sugar alcohols, and fructose |
| Medium GI | 56-69 | White sugar, whole wheat products, basmati rice, corn, sweet potatoes, baked potatoes with skin, and sucrose |
| High GI | 70 and above | White bread, most white rice, rice cakes, pastas, breakfast cereals, potatoes without skin, gluten-free breads, and glucose |

SOURCE: International Table of Glycemic Index, www.mendosa.com.

Processed-free eating does not necessarily rely on the glycemic index, as it does have its drawbacks and limitations. The glycemic response is different from one person to another, and even in the same person from day to day, depending on blood glucose levels, insulin resistance, and other factors. Some processed foods can have a low glycemic index with detrimental effects on health, for instance, chocolate cake (GI 38), ice cream (GI 37), or pure fructose (GI 19); whereas whole foods such as baked potatoes with skin (GI 69) and watermelon (GI 80) have a high GI but possess other beneficial health properties. It is more important to note that most processed and refined carbohydrates have high GIs, which adds to the other numerous reasons why they should be avoided.

The low glycemic effect of sugarcane juice is actually the least of its health benefits. Its high concentration of antioxidants makes it something of a superhero among foods. Several studies have shown that the antioxidants in sugarcane juice help fight against viral and bacterial infections, boost the immune system, protect against diseases of the liver, and are effective at fighting against cancer, especially prostate and breast cancer.[4] An Australian study also showed that it stabilizes blood sugar levels and promotes weight loss in obese rats.[5] It's hard to believe that a food so good and perfect in its natural form could go so wrong. Refining sugarcane juice unleashes a deranged version of sucrose, transforming the sweet and salubrious Dr. Jekyll into the seductively wicked Mr. Hyde.

## How Sugar Is Processed

There are thirty-seven different known varieties of sugarcane, and they all have considerable differences in the color of the stalks. Regardless of color, the refinement process is not pretty. Sugarcane processing happens in two stages. The first stage begins with that beautiful sugarcane. At the factory near where the sugarcane is grown, the juice is pressed out, using large roller mills similar to an old-fashioned wringer washing machine. As the sugarcane juice gushes out, it is collected in large vats. The fibrous stalks are saved and used as fuel to boil water. Unlike the sugarcane stalks used to press the yummy juice for consumption, the sugarcane stalks used for refinement are not cleaned prior to pressing. At this point the juice is crude, with dirt from the fields, small fibers from the stalks, and of course all the colorful plant pigments. Sugar refiners call this juice "dirty," therefore it needs to be "cleaned."

To clean the juice, it is treated with a compound called calcium hydroxide, commonly known as slaked lime—a white, chalky powder (not the same kind of lime that is the green citrus fruit!). As it is technically nontoxic, slaked lime is used in water and sewage treatment, and has many commercial and food uses as well. When added to liquids, it forms a fluffy solid (like a tuft of wool) that aids in the removal of smaller particles from water, resulting in a clearer product. Adding slaked lime to sugarcane juice settles out most of the dirt, which is then removed before the juice is heated by steam to evaporate off most of the water. Without the majority of its water content, the sugarcane juice becomes a dark, thick syrup, still rich in most of the nutrients contained in the raw sugarcane juice, including the polyphenols.

To remove the rest of the water, the syrup is placed into a very large pan and boiled. The boiling destroys the enzymes and some of the nutrients. As more water is boiled off, tiny sucrose crystals, called seedlings, are added to the syrup to initiate crystallization. These microscopic seedlings act as a surface for the sucrose contained in the syrup to attach and form into bigger crystals. If you've ever made rock candy, you know this process, except instead of a string or stick, the surface for crystals to form are the sucrose seedlings. Once the crystallization is complete, the crystals are removed from the syrup, but they still have some syrup clinging to them, so they are spun dry in a centrifuge (similar to how most of the water is removed from your laundry during the spin cycle.) Hmm . . . lots of laundry analogies here, perhaps that's because sugarcane processing is similar to removing dirt from clothing. Except in the case of sugarcane, the "dirt" is all the healthy nutrients!

The crystals are then given a final dry with hot air, producing crude raw sugar (not to be confused with the product Sugar in the Raw, or other sup- posedly raw types of sugar; those will be discussed later in this chapter). The syrup (now called molasses) contains most of the remaining nutrients, and some of the sucrose that was not crystallized out. Likewise, the raw sugar crystals still have some of the nutrients in their outer coating, while the crys- tal interior is 99 percent pure sucrose.

The crude raw sugar is soft and brown, with a dark, distinctive taste that most people are not accustomed to. The locals sometimes consume it, but the vast majority of it is shipped to refineries in North America, Europe, and Japan, where it is further processed into white sugar. The molasses is usually turned into food for cattle (to fatten them up faster; more on that later also), or sent to a distillery where alcohol is made. Molasses is also sold for human consumption.

The second stage of processing is called refinement, wherein the crude raw sugar is "cleaned up," "purified," and made ready for the end user. It is first mixed with heavy syrup (not the original molasses that it was sepa- rated from), and heated to a temperature that is warm enough to dissolve the crystal's outer coating but keep the rest of the crystal intact. The outer coating, you may remember, contains the last bit of nutrients from the original sugarcane juice—but of course sugar refiners need to remove it because it is seen as "less pure" than the crystal interior. The crystals are then separated from the syrup by centrifuge.

You would think at this point we'd be done, right? Haven't all of the nutrients been removed? Nope, there's more. To ensure that any "impurities" that may be inside the crystals are removed, they are subjected to even more dissolving, producing a syrup. The syrup is clarified by adding slaked lime again, along with phosphoric acid, which reacts to produce a compound called calcium phosphate. Calcium phosphate has the ability to entrap and absorb any "impurities," and then it floats to the top of the syrup where it can be skimmed off. In order to have this chemical reaction remain stable, other harsh chemicals are added in to the syrup. The clarified syrup is decolorized by filtering it through charcoal filters (most refineries use charcoal from the bones of dead animals). The syrup is boiled again, and then repeatedly crystallized and centrifuged to produce refined white sugar.

Sounds horrible, right? It is! There is not a speck of anything remotely resembling the original sugarcane in this substance. And I don't say that lightly—it is a *substance*, not a food. Remember, raw sugarcane juice contains only 15 percent sucrose, balanced by an abundance of nutrients. Refined white sugar is 99.8 percent pure sucrose balanced by nothing. This is where the term "empty calories" comes from—calories with no nutrition.

If you're thinking that refined sugar made from white sugar beets, called beet sugar, is any better for you, think again. It's basically made the same way, with a few less steps. It, too, does not resemble anything of the original plant from which it is derived.

## The Truth About Sugar

Now that you know the stark differences between raw natural sugarcane and refined sugar, you will be able to understand why refined sugar is bad news for your body. The problems sugar causes are far reaching, yet few researchers have been willing to publicly incriminate sugar for the poison that it is. But as a nation full of sick and obese people, we can't afford to be ambiguous about it any longer. Following are the scientific truths about sugar, which will help you understand the third Law of Skinny Science: Refined sugar and refined flour are so far removed from their natural state that the body doesn't recognize them as foods—they are toxins that rob us of our health.

## Your Body Does Not Need Refined Sugar

To function properly, our body needs only the equivalent of 2 teaspoons (8 grams) of blood sugar (glucose) circulating through our bloodstream at any one time. This small amount of glucose is easily obtained by digesting proteins, essential fats, and complex carbohydrates such as vegetables and whole grains. Compare the 2 teaspoons of sugar your body needs at any one time to the 21.4 teaspoons (85.6 grams) the average adult consumes daily. Most people are completely unaware of the amount of sugar in their diet, which makes it easy to understand how they can rack up so many teaspoons. In one form or another, sugar is found in almost all packaged foods. Despite its falling sales numbers, high-fructose corn syrup is still one of the most common forms of refined sugar, followed by cane sugar, beet sugar, and honey. Two new "natural" sugars—evaporated cane juice and agave nectar—are showing up on the ingredient lists of many "health foods," but they're not really natural or healthy. These, and other sugars, are lurking in many foods that you might not even consider sweet. For example, you might be surprised to learn that:

- Many meat packers feed sugar to animals prior to slaughter. This improves the flavor and color of cured meat.
- Sugar (in the form of corn syrup and dehydrated molasses) is often added to hamburgers sold in restaurants to reduce shrinkage.
- The breading on many prepared foods contains sugar.
- Before some salmon is canned, it is often glazed with a sugar solution.
- Some fast-food establishments and restaurants serve poultry that has been injected with a flavorful processed honey solution.
- Sugar is used in lunch meats, bacon, and canned meats.
- A special pharmaceutical grade of sucrose is manufactured for use in prescription drugs, vitamins, cold remedies, and nutritional supplements.
- Sugar is found in such unlikely items as soups, bouillon cubes, and dry-roasted nuts.

- Some iodized salt contains sugar (in the form of dextrose).
- Some brands of vanilla extract contain sugar or corn syrup.
- Seasoning mixes, such as taco seasoning, sauce mixes, and salad dressing mixes, often contain some form of sugar.
- Condiments such as ketchup, mustard, and mayonnaise contain sugar.
- Nearly all fat-free salad dressings contain more sugar than do the regular versions.[6]

Sugar is also found in many other foods such as crackers, tortillas, bagels, bread, canned beans, canned vegetables, frozen entrées, pickles, peanut butter, macaroni and cheese, spaghetti sauces, and breakfast cereals (including those that don't taste overtly sugary). Sugar sweetens jams, jellies, pork and beans, relish, flavored yogurts and milks, canned fruit, and salad dressings, not to mention chocolate and an endless list of desserts.

Human evolution has not yet caught up with the sugar industry. For many thousands of years, humans survived without eating refined sugar at all. Even the naturally occurring sugar in fruits was only eaten when the fruit was in season, maybe one or two months out of the year. The past two hundred years of refined sugar consumption is but a moment compared to thousands of years, and the body is just not equipped to metabolize such large amounts of sugar on a daily basis. Our body does its best to adjust, but becomes overworked and exhausted, and eventually begins to degenerate, manifesting in a host of diseases.[7]

## Sugar Is an Addictive Substance

Have you ever eaten a piece of broccoli and found that you just couldn't stop? Do you have urges for eggplant and find it hard to satisfy your craving unless you eat it? Do you wait hours in line for the perfect apple, or drive across town because you heard a new shop now carries the most scrumptious oranges? Most people would probably say no to all of the above. On the other hand, isn't it true that people do find that after eating one cookie or one M&M, they just can't stop?

What is it that makes a person *crave* a food? The same thing that makes someone crave a cigarette, a drug, or alcohol—a chemical dependency. And sugar is nothing but a chemical, the legal heroin of the food family. Nearly all addictive substances start as something natural, and are then refined into unnatural chemical forms of the starting substance. After all, heroin is nothing but a chemical: the juice of the poppy is refined into opium and then refined into morphine and finally to heroin. As you just learned, the juice of the cane or beet is refined into molasses and then refined into brown crystals and finally to strange white crystals. This highly concentrated form of sugar *does not exist anywhere in nature*, not even in the original sugarcane or sugar beets themselves!

The idea of sugar addiction has sparked controversy among scientists for many years, but they began to change their views after a Princeton University study titled "Sugar and Fat Bingeing Have Notable Differences in Addictive-Like Behavior" was published in the March 2009 *Journal of Nutrition*. The study posed the question, "Why do people not binge on broccoli?" and set out to find the answer. The researchers were able to solidly demonstrate that sugar affects the brain differently than other foods do, and specifically found that sugar stimulates the same beta-endorphin receptor sites in the brain that are stimulated by cocaine, nicotine, opiates (such as heroin and morphine), and alcohol. These receptor sites are in the emotional center of the brain responsible for the release of "feel-good" neurotransmitters called opioids and dopamine. It was also confirmed that bingeing on sugar results in physical withdrawal symptoms and cravings, similar to what occurs with other drugs and alcohol.[8]

Drug addictions are typically characterized by three steps: increased intake of the drug to maximize pleasure, withdrawal symptoms when access to the drug is cut off, and an urge to relapse back into drug use. Rats on sugar have similar experiences. In the study, researchers withheld food for twelve hours and then gave rats food plus sugar water. This created a cycle of bingeing whereby the animals increased their daily sugar intake until it doubled. When researchers either stopped the diet or administered an opioid blocker, the rats showed signs common to drug withdrawal, such as teeth-chattering and the shakes. Early findings also indicated signs of relapse. Rats weaned off sugar repeatedly pressed a lever that previously dispensed the sweet solution.[9]

I never had teeth-chattering shakes when I went through sugar withdrawal, but I do know it can sometimes be temporarily uncomfortable. Sugar addiction is just as difficult to overcome as any other addiction. If you think you may be addicted to sugar, processed-free eating is the best way to overcome it.

## Sugar Depletes Calcium and Upsets Body Chemistry

Although most people don't understand their body's nutritional or digestive requirements, *our body knows* what it needs. That's why raw sugarcane is brimming with enzymes and nutrients. By contrast, refined sugar is devoid of these nutrients and the built-in enzyme systems that exist in raw sugarcane (and other naturally sweet foods, such as fruit). So when you eat a cookie made with refined sugar, your body freaks out. It *knows* that to properly digest the sugar, it needs these missing nutrients and the corresponding enzymes. Therefore, your body is forced to adapt by pulling stored nutrients (especially calcium) from your bones, tissues, and teeth, just to digest the sugar in the cookie you just ate. This is called leaching.

Most of us are fed sugar from the time we are children. Imagine having calcium and other minerals leached out of your bones and teeth on a daily basis over a period of years, without adequately replacing them through a healthy diet. You may end up with crooked teeth (like Dr. Price's young patients), or a calcium deficiency in your midyears or perhaps even younger. Your doctor may prescribe a calcium supplement, but it won't do any good because as long as refined sugars are continually eaten, essential nutrients, including calcium, are unavailable to your body. The depletion of calcium leads to a whole host of health problems, including obesity.

In addition to keeping our bones and teeth strong and healthy, minerals are used to help us maintain proper body chemistry (alkalinity). Many people think that they can eat anything they want as long as they exercise and take their vitamin and mineral supplements daily. But eating sugar creates acid in your body fluids and changes your body chemistry in such a devastating way that many of those essential nutrients will be unavailable to your body. Body chemistry and alkalinity will be discussed in more detail in Chapter 9.

## Sugar Suppresses Your Immune Response

Your immune system is your body's only defense against foreign invaders such as viruses and bacteria. It is your white blood cells that have the ability to attack and destroy these invaders. Nearly all forms of sugar interfere with the ability of white blood cells to perform their job. In one study, when healthy volunteers consumed a large amount (100 grams) of refined sugar, their white blood cells' ability to destroy bacteria was impaired for at least five hours.[10]

Ironically, sugar is in almost every over-the-counter cough syrup, cough drop, and flu remedy designed to help us fight coughs and colds. Sugar is also in commercially sold chicken soup, another remedy we take when our immune system is already compromised!

## Sugar Consumption Leads to Heart Disease, Obesity, Diabetes, and Cancer

On a spring evening in 2010, while I was flipping through the TV channels, the title of a show on the University of California channel piqued my interest—*Sugar: The Bitter Truth*. Within one minute of tuning in, I was glued to the TV. In a presentation by the Mini Medical School for the Public, Dr. Robert Lustig, a professor of pediatrics in the division of endocrinology at the University of California–San Francisco School of Medicine, and leading expert on childhood obesity, gave one of the most thorough and scientific examinations of sugar I had ever seen (and I have been following the science on sugar for a long time.) He detailed the damage caused by both sugar and high-fructose corn syrup (which he called "the most demonized additive known to man") and asserted, in no uncertain terms, that there is no difference between the two—they are both "poisonous toxins" that disrupt the function of insulin in the body, leading to obesity.[11]

Sugar (sucrose) is a compound consisting of one glucose molecule bonded to one fructose molecule. For comparison, think of salt (sodium chloride), which consists of one sodium atom and one chlorine atom. When you eat salt, it gets broken down in your stomach into its individual components, sodium and chloride. So when you eat too much salt, your blood levels of sodium go up, which can lead to high blood pressure. When you eat sugar, it gets broken down in your stomach into its individual components, glucose and fructose. If it's a refined form of sugar, such as white sugar or high-fructose corn syrup, the breakdown happens immediately and a flood of glucose and fructose are released directly into the bloodstream. If the sugar is still in its natural state, bound up in a whole food such as raw sugarcane juice or a piece of fruit, the breakdown happens more slowly and the glucose and fructose do not flood the bloodstream.

In response to glucose coming in to the bloodstream, the pancreas secretes a hormone called insulin. Insulin's job is to make sure that your blood glucose levels don't go above the 2 teaspoons at any one time that I mentioned earlier. Insulin takes most of the excess glucose out of the bloodstream and transports it to the cells of all the organs in your body to be used for energy immediately. Your cells have specific receptor sites for allowing insulin to bring glucose into the cell to be converted into energy right away. This is why sugar gives you fast, quick energy. Only a small amount of glucose does not go to the cells; instead it is transported to the liver, where it is converted into a compound called glycogen, which the body can burn for energy at a later time.

The other part of sugar, the fructose, goes directly to the liver and gets stored as fat. None of it goes to the cells for energy. When small amounts of sugar are consumed, it's not a big deal.

However, when we eat a lot of sugar, and eat it all day long, that creates an overload. Our body is not designed to deal with large amounts of glucose. When excessive glucose enters the bloodstream, the pancreas can't gauge how much glucose is coming in, so it overproduces insulin to make sure that there's enough. As a result, too much glucose is taken out of the bloodstream and your blood sugar levels go too low (below the 2 teaspoons). The result is a quick burst of energy followed by a fast drop in energy (blood sugar crash). At the same time, because the excess glucose can't be used for energy immediately, it goes to the liver to be stored as fat. And of course all of the fructose goes to the liver for fat storage. This is why people are getting so fat.

The daily average of 21.4 teaspoons of sugar in the typical American diet is far and above what the body was designed to handle. The pancreas responds to all of this blood sugar by pumping out more and more insulin. What ends up happening, and what Dr. Lustig was so passionate about explaining, was that this glut of sugar overloads the pancreas and the insulin produced becomes less effective at removing excess glucose from the bloodstream. Also, even though insulin is still being produced, the cell receptor sites that normally allow insulin to bring glucose into the cell to be converted into energy, fail to respond. This condition is known as insulin resistance, and can lead to diabetes. Insulin resistance causes higher triglyceride levels and blood pressure, lower levels of the good cholesterol, and can worsen with continued intake of sugar. This is called metabolic syndrome and is a major predictor for the development of heart disease.

In his April 13, 2011, *New York Times* article "Is Sugar Toxic?" Gary Taubes writes, "One of the diseases that increases with obesity, diabetes and metabolic syndrome is cancer. The connection between obesity, diabetes and cancer was first reported in 2004 in large population studies by researchers from the World Health Organization's International Agency for Research on Cancer. It is not controversial. What it means is that you are more likely to get cancer if you're obese or diabetic than if you're not, and you're more likely to get cancer if you have metabolic syndrome than if you don't. . . . Cancer researchers now consider that the problem with insulin resistance is that it leads us to secrete more insulin, and insulin (as well as a related hormone known as insulin-like growth factor) actually promotes tumor growth."[12]

If you're interested in watching Dr. Lustig's ninety-minute presentation (and I highly recommend that you make the time to do so), it can be viewed in its entirety at UCTV.com or on YouTube. The video has become somewhat of an Internet sensation, gathering more than 1.5 million views since it was first posted on July 30, 2009. I'd say that's a clear indication that people are beginning to understand that eating sugar has more far-reaching effects than its being empty calories.

## Sugar Is a Cancer Fuel

The World Health Organization's admission that sugar causes cancer is concern enough for alarm. But sugar's role in cancer is even more insidious. In 1920, Otto Warburg, a German biochemist and Nobel Prize–winning doctor, discovered that normal cells get their energy for reproduction from oxygen, while cancer cells reproduce by fermenting glucose (sugar). In other words, cancer cells require sugar to perpetuate their growth. When you eat sugar, you are actually feeding cancer cells. Additionally, if you don't eat enough Life Force Energy foods loaded with cancer-fighting phytochemicals, it is almost certain that the stage is being set for cancer to develop in your body.

To stop cancer cells from growing, they need to be starved. Additionally, cancer cannot grow in the presence of an alkaline body chemistry. As I have discussed, sugar is one of the major contributors to upset body chemistry, creating an acidic rather than an alkaline environment in the body.

## Joe's Story

At 248 pounds on a 5′9″ frame, I was diagnosed as a type-2 diabetic in 1999, and subsequently worked with my doctor to get my blood levels back in check by losing some weight and starting an exercise program. However, I did not change my way of eating . . . I just cut back on the quantities. In 2005 I lost 40 pounds but struggled to maintain it. As happens with most of us who lose weight without changing our eating habits, the loss was not sustainable, so by 2009 I had gained half of my weight back and my blood sugar was completely out of control again. I'd stopped testing my blood. . . . I was in denial and badly needed a wake-up call.

At the gentle suggestion of my wife, I attended the May 2009 Diabetes Expo. While waiting in line for a frozen yogurt, we stood near a booth representing one of the pharmaceutical companies. The man working there asked if he could check my blood. I said, "Sure." He ran the test and said, "My man, you should be dead! Your blood sugar is 240!" Needless to say, I decided to skip the frozen yogurt!

Just across the aisle, a dynamic, energetic, petite woman was demonstrating how to select and prepare healthy foods for diabetics. It was Dee McCaffrey. My wife and I sat in the front row and were educated, entertained, and enthralled with the idea that *by changing what we ate,* we could lose weight, better control my blood sugar, and *maintain the weight loss!*

Dee discussed what to eat and what to avoid, and explained *why*. We finally understood what was causing my body to react to my diet with elevated blood sugar levels. When we got home, we threw out *all* of our processed food, including white sugar, white flour, and chemically enhanced convenience foods, and stopped going to fast-food restaurants. Using Dee's great recipes, we changed how we cook our favorites and added her favorites to our daily diet. We started reading labels, avoiding things

*continues*

## Joe's Story *continued*

like refined carbohydrates, foods with high-fructose corn syrup, and chemicals with names we could not pronounce. We learned to choose packaged foods carefully, based on healthy ingredients with high fiber and low sugar ratings. We started incorporating as many different fresh vegetables as possible into our diet and chose organic whenever we could. We found that we actually liked raw or lightly cooked vegetables! And we used all of the lemons our beautiful backyard tree could produce!

Following Dee's plan, the weight started falling off, my blood sugar stabilized, and I am happy to report that I dropped from 210 to 180 pounds, have kept it off one year, have tons of energy, and find that it is easy to eat this way when you make up your mind to avoid processed foods. I now test my blood daily. Following Dee's plan and coordinating with my doctor, my A1C readings dropped from the high 9s to a 6!

Every once in a while when I have a craving for something sweet, my wife makes a batch of Dee's chocolaty "Allowable Sin" to satisfy my sweet tooth. We keep them in the freezer and they are amazing!

Diabetes is a killer disease. This plan truly saved my life!

—*Joe, age 58, professional musician*

## Getting the Sugar Out of Your Life

I hope by now you realize that you must remove refined sugar from your life if you want to be skinny and healthy. If you eat in restaurants, you should know that you are probably getting some form of sugar in your food, either in the seasonings, sauces, salad dressings, or the meat. The only way to make sure you are not eating sugar is to read the ingredient list of any food that comes prepared or in a package. Because of the prevalence of sugar in the food supply, you probably won't be able to avoid it entirely without becoming a complete neurotic. However, you should make every effort to eliminate it as much as possible.

Ingredients are listed in order of their predominance by weight in a food product. In other words, when reading an ingredient list you should know that the ingredient that weighs the most is listed first, and the ingredient that weighs the least is listed last. Some people subscribe to the idea that if a form of sugar is listed after the third ingredient, the sugar in that food product is not in a significant amount. *This is a flawed method for avoiding sugar.*

One of the most deceptive methods that food companies use to deal with a load of sugar in a food product is to use a variety of different sugars in lesser amounts, or to distribute sugars among many other ingredients, so that no one sugar appears in the top three. For example, a manufacturer may use a combination of sucrose, high-fructose corn syrup, corn syrup solids, brown sugar, dextrose, and other sugar ingredients to make sure none of them is present in a large enough quantity to attain a top position on the ingredient list. If the sugars were combined on the product's ingredient list, sugar might very well be the first (most predominant) ingredient on the list!

Check ingredient labels for these forms of sugar:

| | |
|---|---|
| Agave | High-fructose corn syrup |
| Barley malt | Invert sugar |
| Beet sugar | Maltodextrin |
| Brown sugar | Maltose |
| Cane sugar | Maple syrup |
| Cornstarch | Modified food starch |
| Corn syrup | Molasses |
| Corn syrup solids | Organic cane sugar |
| Crystalline fructose | Raw sugar |
| Dextrose | Refiner's syrup |
| Evaporated cane juice | Rice syrup |
| Evaporated cane sugar | Rice syrup solids |
| Fructose | Sorghum syrup |
| Fruit juice concentrates | Sucrose |
| Glucose | Sugar |
| Honey | Turbinado sugar |

One way to tell if a product has a lot of sugar in it is to look at the nutrition fact panel for the number of grams of sugar per serving. If a product has a high number of grams of sugar per serving, it's a sure bet that sugar has been added.

A nutrition fact panel will not distinguish between naturally occurring sugar and added sugar. For instance, one cup of plain yogurt has 15 grams of sugar listed, but those sugars are from the naturally occurring lactose in the milk. On the other hand, one cup of vanilla-flavored yogurt has 28 grams of sugar, nearly twice the amount! That means that nearly half the sugars have been added to the yogurt. The only way you will know whether sugars have been added is to read the ingredient list to see if any sugars are listed.

As a general rule, I recommend staying below 8 grams of sugar per serving on packaged items such as cereals, granola, crackers, breads, crackers, and so on. One teaspoon of sugar is the equivalent of 4 grams of sugar.

## Skinny Sweeteners

I've explained how refined sugars behave in your body. But what about natural sugars?

Many people have a false understanding about sugars in general. The popular notion is that sugar is sugar—whether it comes from white sugar, whole sugarcane, honey, or a piece of fruit—and that it all behaves in the body the same way. *This is not true.* The naturally occurring sugars in whole sugarcane, fruits, milk products, and even maple syrup and raw honey have an advantage over refined sugars in that they are balanced by a wide range of nutrients that aid in the utilization of the natural sugars contained within them.

As humans, we have a natural desire for the taste of sweet foods. There is nothing wrong with acknowledging that desire and satisfying it *on occasion*. However, when we do indulge our sweet tooth, we need to do it with sweet foods that will nourish us, rather than deplete us. Therefore, we want to keep in mind the nutrient value and the health benefits of the sweet foods we choose. The Processed-Free Eating Plan incorporates the *occasional* use of the following natural sweeteners:

### Stevia

The sweetness of stevia comes from the leaves of a perennial herb that the Paraguayan natives call "sweet leaf." *It is not a sugar*—it is an herb that just happens to be sweet. Just one teaspoon of the liquid extract has the same sweetness as one whole cup of sugar. Stevia has been used for over 1,500 recorded years as a traditional remedy for diabetes and gum disease among the indigenous people of Paraguay and other South American countries.

The scientific research shows that the leaves of the stevia plant contain many nutrients, including chromium, calcium, magnesium, potassium, iron, beta-carotene, vitamin C, niacin, and protein. They contain several other compounds called glycosides, which are responsible for the intensely sweet taste but do not provide calories. The main glycoside in stevia is called stevioside. Research shows that the body does not digest or metabolize glycosides; therefore they are not converted to glucose. This important property makes stevia an ideal sweetener for diabetics. In fact, scientific research shows stevia has the ability to actually heal the cells in the pancreas, thereby improving glucose tolerance in people with diabetes. According to the generations of people who have used stevia as part of their daily diet, stevia has also been proven to regulate blood sugar.[13]

In addition to its natural sweetening qualities, stevia has many health benefits. There have been over five hundred scientific studies performed on stevia since it was discovered by Western Science in 1899. The results of the studies reveal that stevia has the following positive effects on human health when added to the daily diet:

- Stevia is effective in regulating and normalizing blood sugar levels in people who suffer from diabetes and hypoglycemia.
- Stevia aids the weight-loss process because it contains no calories, and may therefore be used in recipes that satisfy the sweet tooth and balance the diet, eliminating feelings of deprivation or lack of variety. A small amount of stevia will help reduce cravings for sweets and fatty foods.
- Stevia inhibits the growth of oral bacteria. This may explain why regular users of mouthwashes and toothpastes containing stevia are less susceptible to colds and flu. Studies also show improvement with bleeding gum problems.
- Stevia can be applied externally to the skin to rapidly heal wounds and cuts, and to clear up eczema, dermatitis, and acne.
- Stevia contains inulin, a natural fiber that stimulates the growth of helpful intestinal bifidobacteria. This may explain why stevia improves digestion and soothes an upset stomach.

- Unlike any other sweetener, stevia has been reported to have antiviral properties and may also lower blood pressure.[14]

Stevia is my sweetener of choice and *the only* sweetener I recommend for *daily* use (you'll find that some of my recipes call for other natural sweeteners, but these are occasional treats). Use stevia to sweeten teas, yogurt, oatmeal, smoothies, and anything else you like!

## Raw Honey

Throughout history, honey has been regarded as "nature's gold"—a medicinal food capable of healing the body and soothing the spirit. Honey has a long history as a component of folk remedies for many ailments, including colds, coughs, and digestive difficulties. In East Indian Ayurvedic medicine, honey is used as a blood purifier, a decongestant, and a kidney tonic.

For those who believe that honey is just another type of sugar, its nutritional profile may be surprising. Although honey is comprised of nearly 80 percent natural sugars, it also contains small amounts of protein, the B vitamins thiamine, riboflavin, and niacin, vitamin C, calcium, potassium, iron, and other minerals, and enzymes.

Honey also has antibacterial properties. Bacteria cannot survive in raw honey, whereas refined sugar and refined honey create an ideal breeding ground for harmful bacteria. Raw honey is also a rich source of antioxidants, which stop disease-causing free radicals in their tracks. Research presented in January 2008 at the First International Symposium on Honey and Human Health revealed that phytonutrients found in raw honey have been shown to possess cancer-preventing and antitumor properties. Three particular antioxidants discovered in raw honey prevent colon cancer in animals.[15]

Most of the honey found in supermarkets is not healthy. It is basically the refined white sugar version of honey, which makes it just as bad for us. When honey is heated (pasteurized) and processed, its cancer-fighting antioxidants are destroyed, along with many of its natural enzymes and nutrients. Therefore, the best way to enjoy the benefits of honey is in its natural form: raw, unfiltered, and unpasteurized. You can find raw honey in natural food markets, specialty shops, and farmers' markets. Some raw honey is solid and some is liquid; it depends on the variety.

## Pure Maple Syrup

This is not pancake syrup, which is an artificially flavored processed food. Pure maple syrup is derived from various maple trees by tapping the tree bark and allowing the sap to flow out freely. The sap is clear and almost tasteless and very low in sugar content when it is first tapped. It is then boiled to evaporate the water, which concentrates the sugar and creates the flavor and color profile of the syrup. The darker the color, the longer the syrup has boiled, shifting it further from its original state.

Pure maple syrup contains fewer calories and a higher concentration of minerals than honey, although it contains no protein or vitamins. Maple syrup is an excellent source of zinc and manganese. The latter is essential for helping antioxidants disarm free radicals in the cells. In addition to acting as an antioxidant, the zinc contained in maple syrup can decrease the progression of atherosclerosis. Zinc and manganese are both important for strengthening the immune system, as many types of immune cells in the body depend upon them.

Maple syrup has a wonderful rich flavor and is the secret ingredient in my famous wheat-free chocolate chip cookie recipe. Enjoy maple syrup on oatmeal, mixed into yogurt, or mixed with some flaxseed oil to top your French toast or pancakes.

## There's No Comparison to Pure Maple Syrup

Pure maple syrup can strengthen the immune system and aid antioxidant functions in the body. Its ingredient list, which contains only one, cannot be matched by artificial substitutes. Check out this ingredient list on a bottle of a leading brand of artificial pancake syrup, taken from the company's website:

**Ingredients:** corn syrup, high-fructose corn syrup, water, cellulose gum, caramel color, salt, sodium benzoate and sorbic acid (preservatives), artificial and natural flavors, sodium hexametaphosphate.

This is supposedly food?!

## Unsulfured Blackstrap Molasses

Blackstrap molasses is the dark, thick, viscous liquid that comes from processing raw sugarcane into its more refined form. While not a whole food, this sweetener is actually good for you. Unlike white sugar and corn syrup, which are stripped of all nutrients, blackstrap molasses contains significant amounts of the health-promoting nutrients found in the original whole sugarcane, including polyphenols. One tablespoon of blackstrap molasses provides up to 20 percent of the daily value of calcium, magnesium, potassium, and iron. It also contains copper, manganese, selenium, chromium, B vitamins, and protein. I recommend buying organic, unsulfured blackstrap molasses. It is made from mature sugarcane and does not require treatment with sulphur dioxide, a preservative, used during the extraction process of other types of molasses.

## Brown Rice Syrup

Brown rice syrup is an amber-colored syrup with a mild butterscotch-like flavor. It is prepared by fermenting brown rice with special enzymes to disintegrate the natural starch content of the grain. Once the process is complete, the fermented liquid is strained off and the rice is allowed to slowly cook until it reaches a smooth, liquid consistency. The health benefits of brown rice syrup come from its main ingredient, the brown rice, which contains protein, bran, and fiber. The bran also contains the minerals magnesium, manganese, and zinc. The syrup therefore is rich in protein and fiber, which help slow down the absorption of the natural sugars contained in the syrup. Brown rice syrup has a light flavor and is only half as sweet as sugar.

## Organic Whole Cane Sugar

Unrefined, organic, whole cane sugar can almost be considered a whole food. Rapadura is the Portuguese name, referring to a form of raw, unadulterated, dried sugarcane juice that is formed into a large brick. Sucanat is a U.S. trade name for *Sugar Cane Natural*. According to a representative from the ASSURKKAR Sugar Company in Costa Rica, the two sugars are exactly the same, they are just sold by two different companies.

Whole cane sugar is produced by first pressing the juice from the sugarcane and then bringing the juice to a low boil to form a syrup. At this point, the process goes differently than for white sugar. Instead of adding seedling to the syrup, the syrup is poured into an open device and is stirred with paddles while over low heat. The sugar crystals begin to form naturally (as opposed to being aided by seedling) as the water evaporates. The sugar is then ground in a sieve, leaving a dark brown, grainy sugar. It has not been cooked at high heats (like all other sugars) nor spun to change it into crystals, and the molasses has not been separated out. This sugar is produced organically and does not contain chemicals or anticaking agents.

Because this sugar is dehydrated at low heat and is not separated from the molasses, many of the nutrients naturally present in the sugarcane juice have been retained, including the polyphenols. That is *the* most important property of this type of sugar that cannot be claimed by any other type of "raw" sugar on the market. A 100-gram serving of organic whole cane sugar contains 1,000 milligrams of calcium, 13 milligrams of potassium, and 90 milligrams each of magnesium and phosphorous. It also contains 100 milligrams of vitamin E, and trace amounts of the B vitamins, iron, manganese, copper, and zinc. Refined white sugar contains none of these; therefore organic whole cane raw sugar is a much healthier alternative.

The granules are a dark brown color, round, porous, and easily compressed, and can replace refined white sugar cup for cup in recipes. Some of my recipes call for organic whole cane sugar. It can be purchased in natural food markets or online.

Beware of a pair of sneakily similar terms. Read literally, "evaporated cane juice" or "evaporated cane sugar" would simply mean that the sugarcane juice has been evaporated, leaving the sugar crystals with their nutrients still intact. Technically, that would be the same as rapadura or Sucanat. However, that is not the case for the type of "evaporated cane juice" that is being used in food products. According to the CEO of ASSURKKAR, the term is wrongly used in the food industry—"prostituted" he put it. "Nowadays the food companies are trying to sell more 'natural' products, so they use the most impressive or high-impact wording to call the customers' attention" he said.

When it comes down to it, the "evaporated cane juice" that is being used in food products is unequivocally the same as refined white sugar. The subtle difference in composition between the two is simply the "evaporated cane juice" has a smidge more vitamin A, C, and calcium (in a 100-gram sample). However, neither of these amounts are anywhere near what exists in the natural sugarcane or the more unrefined rapadura and Sucanat.

The "evaporated cane juice" that is used in food products is a cream-colored, nearly white, fine crystal. Visually it is clear that it has been refined. Yet it is readily available for purchase in natural food markets.

## Coconut Nectar and Coconut Crystals

While stevia is my go-to sweetener for daily use, coconut nectar and coconut crystals are my new favorite sweeteners to use in recipes. Coconut nectar is a sweet sap that comes from the flowers of the coconut tree, not from the coconut itself. It is a completely raw, unrefined sweetener. The only processing is the low-heat evaporation to remove water and thicken the nectar. It does not taste like coconut—rather, its taste is mild, similar to caramel or butterscotch. But the best thing about coconut nectar is its low-glycemic effect. Its fructose content is only 1.5 percent when collected from the blossoms. As the sap is dried and thickened, removing much of the water, the fructose content of the final product is still only about 10 percent. Its glycemic index is 35, making it relatively safe for diabetics. It contains enzymes, vitamins, minerals, proteins, and other nutrients (including vitamin C).

When the coconut nectar is air-dried down to its crystalline form, the end result is coconut crystals, also known as coconut sugar or palm sugar. Coconut crystals have a naturally brown or sandy color, closely resembling organic whole cane sugar, and are also loaded with vitamins and minerals.

## Luo Han Guo

The Chinese have used the *luo han guo* fruit as a natural sweetener and healing remedy for many centuries. They call *luo han guo* the "longevity fruit" because the steep mountain fields in Guangxi Province, where it is grown, have an unusual number of residents that live to be one hundred years old or more. *Luo han guo* has almost no effect on blood sugar levels, with only 2 calories per serving. The fruit is used only after it is dried, and can be ground into a powder that contains natural substances called mogrosides (from the same family of glycosides found in stevia). These natural compounds make *luo han guo* three hundred times sweeter than sugar, and like stevia's glycosides, they are also responsible for some of the health benefits associated with the fruit. Many promising studies are being conducted, which are confirming the nutritional and healing properties of *luo han guo*. The mogrosides in *luo han guo*:

- Are under investigation as potential tumor inhibitors[16]
- Have antioxidant properties[17]
- May help manage diabetes because of their inhibitory effects on blood sugar levels[18]
- May defend against heart disease[19]

Like stevia, *luo han guo* can be purchased in powdered form in packets or in larger containers or as a liquid extract. Use it in recipes and to sweeten foods.

## Xylitol and Erythritol

Xylitol and erythritol belong to a class of compounds known as sugar alcohols, or polyols, which are an interesting form of carbohydrates. Their molecular structures are kind of like a hybrid between a sugar molecule and an alcohol molecule (hence their name), although they are neither. In addition to xylitol and erythritol, some of the more common sugar alcohols you may be familiar with are sorbitol, mannitol, lactitol, and maltitol. Of these, xylitol is considered the most "natural" because our body produces about 15 grams of xylitol each day as a result of normal metabolism, so it's not a strange or foreign substance to our system. It also occurs naturally in the fibers of many fruits and vegetables, and it can also be extracted from various berries, oats, and mushrooms, as well as fibrous material such as corn husks, corn cobs, the bark of birch trees, and crushed sugarcane stalks after they have been pressed to extract their juice. Erythritol is also found in our body. It occurs naturally in some fruits, in larger amounts in certain mushrooms and other fungi, and in fermented foods such as wine and soy sauce.

Sugar alcohols, as a group, are less sweet than sucrose and are incompletely absorbed into the bloodstream, resulting in lowered effects on blood sugar and insulin response. These properties make them all low-calorie and low-glycemic sweeteners. In comparison to white sugar, which has a glycemic index of 64 and contains 4 calories per gram, xylitol has a glycemic index of 13 and contains 2.4 calories per gram. Erythritol has a glycemic index of 0 and contains a mere 0.2 calories per gram. In addition, these sugar alcohols are not metabolized by cavity-causing bacteria that form in the mouth; therefore they do not contribute to tooth decay as other forms of sugar can. Xylitol is the only sugar alcohol that actually prevents tooth decay, due to the ability of its molecular structure to utilize calcium to protect tooth enamel before cavities form.

Of all the sugar alcohols, xylitol is perhaps the most popular among consumers due to its similarity to white sugar—it's a white, crystalline substance that is as sweet as sugar, and can be substituted in recipes at a 1:1 ratio. It dissolves, mixes, and behaves like sugar in many uses, but because it differs from sugar at the molecular level, xylitol does not match all the properties of sugar in all instances. For example, xylitol (and all other sugar alcohols) does not crystallize, so it cannot be used to make hard candy, and it does not brown or caramelize when heated. Because it is not a sugar, it can't perform the crucial chemical role that sugar plays in reacting with yeast in bread making, so it's not a good substitute for sugar in yeast breads. It can be added to sweeten beverages, cereals, sauces, and other foods, as desired.

Erythritol is 60 to 70 percent as sweet as sugar, so usually more is needed to obtain the same sweetness as sugar. It is often paired with small amounts of another high-intensity sweetener, such as stevia, in commercial food and beverage products. Erythritol has the same uses and limitations as xylitol, but may be preferred due to its nearly 0 calorie profile.

The one downside to xylitol (and all of the other sugar alcohols except erythritol) is the undesirable effect on the digestive tract. Xylitol is only partially absorbed into the bloodstream from the small intestine, and much of it then ends up in the large intestine (the colon). The bacteria in the colon feed on xylitol and cause it to ferment, which can cause bloating, gas, abdominal pain, and laxative effects, so it is not advisable to consume very much of it. Even small amounts of xylitol, and sugar alcohols in general, can stimulate diarrhea and exacerbate existing symptoms of irritable bowel syndrome. If you have a sensitive digestive system, I advise caution with xylitol. The one exception to these effects is erythritol. Eryrithritol has a smaller molecular structure than the other sugar alcohols, allowing nearly 90 percent of it to be absorbed into the bloodstream from the small intestine, but is then excreted in the urine. Because of this, erythritol tends to produce much less intestinal distress than do other sugar alcohols.

Xylitol and erythritol are not completely processed-free sweeteners, and I have some concerns about both of them. First, unlike the other sweeteners I've described, neither of them contains any nutrients. Second, although they do exist in nature, for most commercial purposes they are both produced through chemical means. And third, they are usually derived from corn, which has a history of being manipulated in food laboratories to make literally hundreds of food additives. Most commercial production of xylitol is derived by extracting xylose (a naturally occurring plant sugar) from corn cobs or birch trees and is then converted into xylitol through a chemical reaction. Most of the corn grown in the United States and other countries is genetically modified, which has its own set of health problems (see Chapter 8 for more details). And unfortunately, some manufacturers of corn-derived xylitol cut their xylitol with sorbitol, which looks the same and tastes very similar, but does not have the same health benefits as xylitol. For this reason, if you do use xylitol, make sure it either comes from an organic source of corn (organic foods, by law, cannot be genetically modified), or that it comes from birch. I recommend Smart Sweet, a brand of xylitol made from U.S.-grown birch trees.

Erythritol is manufactured on a commercial scale from corn syrup (also very likely from genetically modified corn). The glucose in the syrup is fermented by a natural yeastlike fungus to produce erythritol, which is then sterilized, purified, filtered, and crystallized to yield a final crystalline product that looks like sugar. The Wholesome Sweetener company produces a product called Organic Zero, which does not use corn. Instead they use organic sugarcane juice as the starting source of glucose, which is then fermented. No chemicals are used in the production of Organic Zero.

One final word: As many products contain sugar alcohols, there is no way to know whether they are from corn- or organic-derived sources. I personally feel that stevia is the superior sweetener for zero calories and zero glycemic effect, as it comes directly from the stevia leaf and is not chemically produced.

# Not-So-Skinny Sweeteners

The following sweeteners *do not* make the cut for processed free. Eating them will not make you skinny, and in fact will probably cause different but equally deadly health problems than white sugar causes.

## High-Fructose Corn Syrup

In a desperate attempt to convince consumers that high-fructose corn syrup (HFCS) is no worse for their health than refined white sugar, the Corn Refiners Association (CRA) petitioned the U.S. Food and Drug Administration (FDA) to allow it to change the name of the highly processed goopy liquid to "corn sugar." As if changing the name is going to somehow change the minds of conscious consumers and erase the scientific evidence of its insidious ramifications on the health of Americans.

Over the past decade, the controversial sweetener has been dubbed "the crack of sweeteners" and "liquid Satan" due to its addictive qualities and numerous studies showing it contributes to the development of metabolic syndrome, diabetes, heart disease, liver disease, overweight, and obesity. Since being outed as a dangerous sweetener, consumption of high fructose corn syrup is at a twenty-year low, and will likely continue to decline, despite the marketing efforts and claims by the CRA that it is the same as all other forms of sugar. It is not.

The highly processed syrup is a far cry from the natural corn it's derived from. And it's not a product that you could whip up at home from a few ears of corn. Producing the syrup involves a fifteen-step process using some pretty sophisticated laboratory equipment. It starts with corn kernels and takes place in a series of stainless-steel vats and tubes in which a dozen different mechanical processes and chemical reactions occur—including several rounds of high-velocity spinning and the introduction of three different enzymes to incite molecular rearrangements.[20]

The enzymes turn most of the natural-occurring glucose molecules in corn into fructose, which makes the substance sweeter. This 90 percent fructose mixture is then combined with regular corn syrup, which is 100 percent glucose molecules, to get the right percentage of fructose (55 percent) and glucose (42 percent). The final product is a clear, goopy liquid that is roughly as sweet as sugar.[21]

The manufacturers of HFCS still claim their product is natural because it is made from plain old corn and contains no synthetic materials or color or flavor additives.[22] They must have forgotten about those unnatural molecular rearrangements that occur during the refinement process. HFCS is *artificial* because the resulting molecular rearrangement is not found anywhere in the natural corn. This stuff still shows up on ingredient lists, so please read them carefully!

Food manufacturers are slowly beginning to replace HFCS in their products by reverting back to using "real sugar" (and proudly touting that in its advertising). The "real sugar" they are using is refined cane sugar or beet sugar, which as you've just learned has its own set of health consequences, and should not be considered healthy in any way, shape, or form.

## High Fructose Corn Syrup Leads to Fatty Liver Disease and Worse

A 2008 study out of Duke University showed that daily consumption of fructose-containing foods or drinks has been associated with a disease called nonalcoholic fatty liver disease (NAFLD). Fatty liver is a degenerative disease of the liver whereby the liver cells are literally choked to death by globules of fatty substances within them. This organ becomes enlarged and swollen with greasy deposits of fatty tissue. The term *nonalcoholic* is used because this type of liver disease is occurring in people who do not consume alcohol, such as children. Yet, in many respects, the nature of NAFLD is similar to what is seen in liver diseases of alcoholics who consume excessive amounts of alcohol.

A 2010 follow-up study, published online in *Hepatology*, goes one step further and links increased consumption of high-fructose corn syrup to the progression of liver injury, such as fibrosis (scarring in the liver), among

*continues*

## High Fructose Corn Syrup Leads to Fatty Liver Disease and Worse *continued*

people who already have nonalcoholic fatty liver disease. The concern is that continued consumption of fructose will lead to more serious liver damage. Most people with NAFLD feel well and are not aware that they have a liver problem. Nevertheless, this disease can be severe and can lead to cirrhosis, in which the liver is permanently damaged and scarred and no longer able to work properly.

Manal Abdelmalek, professor of medicine at Duke University Medical Center, who headed the study, is quoted as saying, "Non-alcoholic fatty liver disease is present in 30 percent of adults in the United States. Although only a minority of patients progress to cirrhosis, such patients are at increased risk for liver failure, liver cancer, and the need for a liver transplant." According to Abdelmalek, there is no therapy for nonalcoholic fatty liver disease. "Our findings suggest that we may need to go back to healthier diets that are more holistic," Abdelmalek said. "High fructose corn syrup, which is predominately in soft-drinks and processed foods, may not be as benign as we previously thought."[23]

## Agave Nectar

Once the darling of the natural sweetener kingdom, agave has been discovered to be a highly processed sweetener with even more fructose in it than in high-fructose corn syrup. Agave is a succulent plant, similar to aloe, which grows primarily in Mexico. Although manufacturers have claimed that the nectar is taken directly from the succulent leaves straight into the bottle, apparently that is not the truth. Most agave nectar is not made from the sap of the agave plant, but from its large root bulb. The root contains the complex carbohydrate inulin, which is made up of fructose molecules.

The process that many, if not most, agave producers use to convert this inulin into nectar is similar to that by which cornstarch is converted into high-fructose corn syrup. The agave is subject to an enzymatic and chemical process that converts the starch into a fructose-rich syrup—anywhere from 70 percent fructose and higher. For comparison, the high-fructose corn syrup used in sodas is 55 percent refined fructose.[24]

Agave nectar can contain up to 90 percent fructose—and remember all fructose gets processed in the liver, where it can be stored as fat. Too much fat in the liver leads to insulin resistance. In 2010, the Glycemic Research Institute announced that it had legally "delisted" and placed a ban on agave for use in food and beverage products, due to results of five years of clinical trials showing negative effects on diabetics. Manufacturers who use agave in products have been warned that they could be liable for any health issues related to agave consumption.

This may be very confusing and disappointing if you have been using agave under the belief that it is a healthy natural sweetener. If so, don't feel bad. For several years, I was duped right along with you.

If you do want to use agave, there is a natural unprocessed agave product that is made in Mexico. It's called *miel de agave*—a molasses-like syrup made by boiling the agave sap—but its availability is limited and it is expensive to produce. I once saw a bottle of it on the shelf at my local Whole Foods Market with a hefty price tag of twenty dollars!

You'll still see plenty of bottles of agave on the shelves of health food stores, but unless it's *miel de agave*, you should just walk on by. As for agave in "healthy foods," you should pass on those, too.

## Fructose and Crystalline Fructose

This is a substance that often shows up on the ingredient list of many foods, drinks, energy bars, and meal replacement mixes that are marketed as being "healthy." You may also see it in packages or in the bulk section of health food stores. The standard line about fructose is that it's healthy and natural because it's the same type of sugar in fruit. But the fructose in food products is *not natural*. While it is true that *small* amounts of naturally occurring fructose are found in most vegetables and fruits, that type of fructose is not what is being used in so-called health foods and drinks. Like xylitol and erythritol, crystalline fructose is produced from corn, not fruits. Sugar producers themselves on the Sugar.org website state very clearly how crystalline fructose is manufactured:

"Crystalline fructose is produced by allowing the fructose to crystallize from a fructose-enriched corn syrup. The term 'crystalline fructose' is listed in the ingredient statements of foods and beverages using this corn sweetener. It is important to understand that the 'crystalline fructose' listed as an ingredient comes from cornstarch, not fruit."[25]

Crystalline fructose is produced from processed corn in a very unnatural way. Liver damage aside, it does not qualify as processed free.

## Pink, Blue, and Yellow Packets

There has been much documentation on the ill effects of artificial sweeteners—weight gain, disruption of sleep patterns, sexual dysfunction, increases in cancer, MS, lupus, diabetes, and a list of epidemic degenerative diseases—but the companies who own their patents continue to deny any connection.

It's hard to say which of the three commonly used artificial sweeteners is the worst. They are all made in laboratories—but unlike xylitol and erythritol (which are also made in laboratories), artificial sweeteners do not exist anywhere in nature. They are completely man-made substances that the body does not recognize, thus they are more like toxins than foods. Saccharin was accidentally discovered in 1879 by a chemist named Constantin Fahlberg who was working as a research fellow at Johns Hopkins University. He was experimenting with making new compounds from toluene, a clear, colorless liquid produced in the process of making tar from coal.[26] Toluene is chemically classified as a coal tar derivative. Its sweet aroma is distinctively recognizable in gasoline, paint, and paint thinner—and it's a hazardous substance. Toluene is one of the many regulated environmental pollutants I analyzed for in my job at the lab. One day, Constantin spilled some of this new compound made from toluene onto his hand. As a chemist I can tell you that normal good laboratory protocol (and common sense) is to immediately rinse your skin when you come into contact with a chemical, especially an unknown newly created chemical. Apparently he didn't follow the protocol. Later that evening, he noticed his food at dinner tasted oddly sweet, and connected it with the new compound that he had been working on that day . . . and that is exactly how saccharin came to be invented!

Saccharin was widely used in foods and beverages throughout the United States and Europe up until 1912, when public concerns about possible health risks resulted in a ban. But the ban was short lived. In 1914, sugar rationing during World War I created a demand for saccharin, so health concerns became secondary to the need to appease the world's sweet tooth. World War II had a similar effect, and by 1945 the use of saccharin was commonplace.[27] Thirty years later, in the early 1970s, saccharin faced another ban. Studies in laboratory rats linked saccharin, later marketed as Sweet'N Low, with the development of bladder cancer. In other rodent studies, saccharin has caused cancer of the uterus, ovaries, skin, blood vessels, and other organs. Also, it has been demonstrated that saccharin increases the potency of other cancer-causing chemicals. In 1977, the results of these studies prompted the Federal Drug Administration (FDA) to propose a ban on it. Congress intervened, requiring more studies, but still permitted it to be used, provided that all foods containing saccharin bear a warning label.

Subsequent studies done by the National Cancer Institute still showed an increased incidence of urinary bladder cancer at high doses of saccharin, especially in male rats. Acknowledging these findings, in 1981 saccharin was listed by the U.S. and Canadian governments, as well as the World Health Organization, as a substance reasonably anticipated to be a human carcinogen (a substance known to cause cancer in humans). Because the evidence for bladder cancer was only seen in rats and not humans, in 2000 the U.S. Department of Health and Human Services removed saccharin from its list of cancer-causing chemicals.[28] Later that year, Congress passed a law removing the warning notice from saccharin. Despite removing the warning, the carcinogenic nature of this man-made sweetener is still highly controversial, and therefore I do not deem it a safe sweetener.

Aspartame, marketed as Equal and NutraSweet, has a very shady past. In 1965, James Schlatter, another haphazard chemist, accidentally discovered aspartame while working for G. D. Searle & Company. During one of his experiments to create a new drug to treat ulcers, his bubbling beaker spilled over onto his hand. He, too, did not follow good laboratory protocol, and later, when he licked his finger to pick up a piece of paper that had fallen to the ground, the substance was found to be sweet tasting. The company realized that the stuff in the bubbling beaker could be more lucrative as a food additive than as a limited-market ulcer drug.[29] But early testing of aspartame was fraught with results showing that it was not safe to consume, particularly that it induced brain tumors in mice. The FDA banned aspartame, based on these findings, but the president of G. D. Searle, Donald Rumsfeld (the same one who later served as secretary of state under two U.S. presidents) vowed to get it approved. Over the next five years, the evidence mounted against the safety of aspartame. After Reagan was elected president in 1980, Rumsfeld joined the transition team and told the Searle company that he would see to it that aspartame was approved within a year.[30] Indeed, it did happen.

By 1992, over ten thousand complaints had been filed with the FDA about food reactions pertaining to aspartame. The FDA once listed ninety-two different symptoms associated with the use of aspartame. Symptoms confirmed through controlled studies include headaches/migraines, weight gain, dizziness, confusion, memory loss, drowsiness, depression, irritability, anxiety attacks, tingling and numbness, convulsions, heart palpitations, shortness of breath, chest pain, nausea, diarrhea, aggravation of diabetes, menstrual problems, joint pain, decreased vision, eye pain, ear ringing, noise intolerance, hyperactivity in children, and excessive thirst.[31]

With growing public concern over the problems associated with saccharin and aspartame, the time was ripe for a new sweetener to come on the scene. In 1976, sucralose was discovered by yet another laboratory error. Shashikant Phadnis, a graduate student at Queen Elizabeth College at the University of London, was working with a team of researchers from Tate & Lyle, a British sugar company, which was seeking to use sugar (sucrose) to create a new insecticide. During one part of the experiment, Phadnis was told to "test" the new compound. However, due to difficulty interpreting English, he thought he was told to "taste" the compound.[32] Again, not a lot of common sense or good laboratory protocol being followed here. If I were working to create a new insecticide, I don't think I'd want to taste it! Nevertheless, Phadnis found the compound to be extraordinarily sweet. Although sucralose has been approved for food use, its safety remains highly controversial.

The manufacturer of Splenda markets its sucralose product as being "natural" because it comes from sugar (sucrose). They are only telling a partial truth.

Sucralose does not exist anywhere in nature. Although the starting substance is sucrose, it undergoes a complex five-step chemical process involving many caustic chemicals, which selectively substitutes three atoms of chlorine for three hydrogen-oxygen groups on the sucrose molecule (see Figure 4.1), transforming the substance into a polychlorinated compound. You may be familiar with some other polychlorinated compounds—they're called pesticides! Splenda shares many similar molecular characteristics with pesticides like DDT that can accumulate in the body's fat and tissues. It is impossible to predict the long-term consequences of ingesting this substance over many years.

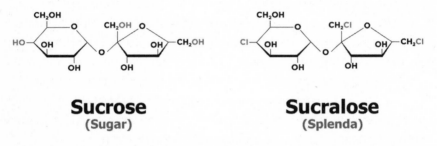

**Sucrose**
(Sugar)

**Sucralose**
(Splenda)

**Figure 4.1** Through a complex five-step chemical process, Sucralose is synthesized by adding several chlorine-containing compunds to the sugar molecule, resulting in the substitution of the hydroxyl (OH) groups with chlorine (CL) atoms.

Splenda thus contains chlorine, a known carcinogen. The sweetener's manufacturers insist that the chlorine is chemically bound to the rest of the molecule in the same way that it is bound to sodium in common table salt (sodium chloride). However, the molecular properties of the two compounds are not the same. Naturally occurring salt plays many important roles in the body. Its chlorine helps produce stomach acids and enzymes needed for digestion, and is also necessary for proper brain functioning and growth. However, man-made chlorinated carbon compounds such as sucralose are not nutritionally compatible with human metabolic functions, because the bond between carbon and chlorine is molecularly and significantly different from the bond between sodium and chlorine. Man-made chlorinated carbon compounds (pesticides, insecticides, and herbicides) have long been known to cause organ, genetic, and reproductive damage.

There have been no long-term (12–24 month) studies of sucralose's effects on humans, whereas there have been over one hundred studies on animals, many of which revealed the same disturbing problems that are caused by other polychlorinated compounds. Research on laboratory rats showed up to a 40 percent shrinkage of the thymus gland, the gland that is the very foundation of the immune system. Other animal studies showed sucralose can cause brain lesions, decreased white blood cell count, inflammation and swelling of the liver and kidneys, miscarriage, and male infertility.[33]

As there have only been a few short-term studies on humans for any of these artificial sweeteners, scientists just don't know what the long-term consumption of them can do to your health. It is best to take the precautionary approach and avoid any type of artificial sweeteners.

## Truvia and Pure Via

There were no laboratory accidents involved in the creation of the sweeteners Truvia and Pure Via. Scientists at Cargill, an international producer of food products, knew exactly what they were doing when they set out to find a way to manipulate the stevia plant to get a patent on it. In partnership with the Coca-Cola Company, they developed a new sweetener that *begins* with the leaves of the stevia plant. The end product contains a very small fraction of only one of its sweet components.

The downside of stevia, according to Cargill, is that some consumers don't like its slight (but distinct) aftertaste. To remedy this, the scientists developed a "special purification process" that does away with the "offending aftertaste," leaving nothing but "clean, pure" sweetness.

There are nine glycosides within the leaves of the stevia plant. The two sweetest are stevioside and rebaudioside A (also known as Reb A). Stevioside has the aftertaste, Reb A does not. Like the stevia leaves it is derived from, Reb A is approximately two hundred times sweeter than sugar, and contains zero calories. Cargill's "special purification process" isolates out only the Reb A and purifies it using undisclosed chemicals. The "new" purified form of Reb A is a patented compound Cargill has named Rebiana. It is important to point out here that Rebiana is not a component found in the stevia plant, nor is it found anywhere in nature. It is produced by the action of chemicals on the various stevia glycosides. By isolating only one compound, the "perfect package" that was stevia has been disassembled, leaving behind all of stevia's wonderful health benefits. Doesn't this sound very similar to how sugar is processed?

Rebiana is one of the ingredients used in the product called Truvia, marketed by the Coca-Cola Company and now used in its sugar-free colas. Pepsi developed a similar Rebiana-patented sweetener called Pure Via.

If you read the ingredient list on Truvia, you will see that it contains (in this order) erythritol, Rebiana, and the ubiquitous ingredient called "natural flavors." The ingredient list on Pure Via looks similar, but also lists isomaltose and cellulose powder (a polysaccharaide). Clearly, Truvia and Pure Via are not natural sweeteners. I recommend using real stevia, instead of these manipulated versions.

## Debbie's Story

I have always tried to eat healthy, but the ever-changing landscape of what is healthy led me to trying lots of different ideas. I never leaned toward extremes and finding this plan took all the work out of healthy eating. It is so logical, backed with Dee's simplified explanations of the science behind it that it really appealed to me. Within three months of following the plan, I lost weight (that nagging 10 pounds), and friends told me I looked great. I stopped feeling so tired and achy all the time. What I love the most is that I never feel hungry and rarely have cravings. Thanks, Dee.

—*Debbie Young, age 59, law office manager*

## Other "Natural" Sweeteners

Other types of so-called natural sugars on the market, such as muscovado, turbinado, Demerara, and organic raw sugar, and the product Sugar in the Raw, are all refined, though not as much as white sugar. They start the same way as white sugar—boiled, crystallized using seedling, then spun in a centrifuge to separate the crystals from the molasses. Then the crystals are reunited with some of the molasses in artificial proportions to produce sugars of varying colors of brown. Because of their low to nonexistent nutrient values, these types of sugars definitely do not qualify as healthy alternatives.

## Table 4.2  How Sugars Compare

|  | White Sugar | "Sugar in the Raw" | Evaporated Cane Juice | Turbinado | Organic Raw Whole Cane Sugar (Rapadura)/ Sucanat |
|---|---|---|---|---|---|
| *Carbohydrate* | | | | | |
| Sucrose (g) | 99.8 | 99.8 | 99.8 | 99.19 | 73–83 |
| Fructose (g) | 0 | 0 | 0 | 0 | 1.5–7 |
| Glucose (g) | 0 | 0 | 0 | 0 | 1.5–7 |
| | | | | | |
| *Minerals* | | | | | |
| Potassium (mg) | 0.5–1 | 15–150 | 0 | 29 | 10–13 |
| Calcium (g) | 0–5 | 75–95 | 18 | 12 | 40–100 |
| Magnesium (mg) | 0 | 13–23 | unavailable | 2 | 70–90 |
| Phosphorous (mg) | 0 | 3–4 | unavailable | 1 | 20–90 |
| Sodium (mg) | 0.6–0.9 | unavailable | unavailable | 3 | 19–30 |
| Iron (mg) | 0.5–1 | unavailable | unavailable | 0.37 | 10–13 |
| Manganese (mg) | 0 | unavailable | unavailable | 0 | 0.2–0.5 |
| Zinc (mg) | 0 | unavailable | unavailable | 0 | 0.2–0.4 |
| Fluorine (mg) | 0 | unavailable | unavailable | unavailable | 5.3–6.0 |
| Copper (mg) | 0 | unavailable | unavailable | unavailable | 0.1–0.9 |
| | | | | | |
| *Vitamins* | | | | | |
| Provitamin A (mg) | 0 | unavailable | unavailable | unavailable | 2.0 |
| A (mg) | 0 | unavailable | unavailable | unavailable | 3.80 |
| $B_1$ (mg) | 0 | 0.01 | unavailable | unavailable | 0.01 |
| $B_2$ (mg) | 0 | 0.006 | unavailable | unavailable | 0.06 |
| $B_5$ (mg) | 0 | 0.02 | 0.01–0.05 | unavailable | 0.01 |
| $B_6$ (mg) | 0 | 0.01 | unavailable | unavailable | 0.01 |
| C (mg) | 0 | unavailable | 4 | unavailable | 7.0 |
| $D_2$ (mg) | 0 | unavailable | unavailable | 5.6 | 6.50 |
| E (mg) | 0 | unavailable | unavailable | 40.0 | 111.30 |
| Bioflavonoids (mg) | unavailable | unavailable | unavailable | unavailable | 7.0 |

Amounts based on 100 grams

SOURCES: Daabon Organic Australia, www.daabon.com/australia/pdfs/Rapadura%20Specs.pdf; USDA Nutrient Database, www.nal.usda.gov/fnic/foodcomp/search/.

You should know that no sugar is completely nutritious. Unless you are eating whole, natural sugarcane or drinking its fresh, raw juice, you are not getting the full amount of nutrients.

Table 4.2 (on the previous page) compares the vitamin and mineral content of different types of sugar. What you really need to be thinking about when eating any type of sugar is how much of its vitamins and minerals have been retained in it. It is the lack of nutrients in processed sugar that makes it so detrimental to the body.

## The Truth About Grains

When I was eating compulsively, I must have eaten enough bread and pasta to feed a third-world country. In fact, sometimes, I would make a spaghetti sandwich, by putting a scoop of cold spaghetti onto a slice of white bread, folding it over, and eating it. It was like nirvana!

Today I know why I was able to eat so much bread and pasta in one sitting. Like sugar, white flour is so highly refined that the body doesn't recognize it as food. Like sugar, white flour stimulates our hunger sensation but doesn't satisfy us. As a result, even though we're filling our belly, the rest of our body isn't getting nourished, so we think we're still hungry and eat more.

### Anatomy of a Whole Grain

White sugar originates from whole, natural sugarcane, brimming with vitamins, minerals, fibers, enzymes, and phytonutrients. Similarly, white flour originates from a whole wheat kernel, brimming with vitamins, minerals, fibers, enzymes, and phytonutrients. To understand how white flour is made, you must first understand the components of a whole wheat kernel.

Figure 4.2 is a diagram of a whole wheat kernel, although you can think of it as the anatomy of all whole grains, as structurally they are all basically the same. Whole grains contain three main components: the bran, the germ, and the endosperm. The bran, located in the outer layer, contains antioxidants, B vitamins, phytochemicals, protein, fiber, and 50 to 80 percent of minerals such as iron, copper, zinc, and magnesium. The wheat germ is an inner component of the grain. It also contains fiber, B vitamins,

## THE WHOLE GRAIN

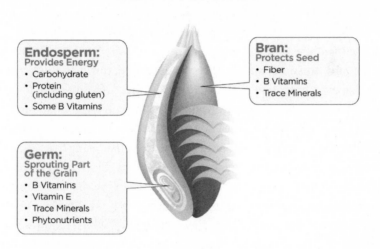

**Figure 4.2** Anatomy of a whole grain.

phytochemicals, minerals, and antioxidants such as vitamin E. Both the bran and the germ contain important fibers required by our body for the proper digestion of the grain. Additionally, the healthy fats in the germ (e.g., wheat germ oil) are required by our body to properly digest the grain. The germ also contains the embryo, or sprouting section, of the grain—the part of the grain that will form a new sprout if the kernel is placed in water or planted in the ground. In that sense, it contains the grain's Life Force.

The endosperm, which is on the inside of the kernel, contains most of the carbohydrates (starch) and proteins (including gluten) in the kernel. I call it the starchy, spongy part of the grain. It also contains small amounts of some B vitamins and minerals.

### The Refinement of Wheat

To produce white flour, the outer husk of the wheat kernel is removed, thereby stripping away all of the bran and the germ—and with them, their fiber, fats, and nutrients—leaving only the endosperm (the starchy, spongy part). The remaining endosperm is milled and bleached to remove its original brown color, and as a result, all of its nutrients and enzymes are destroyed.

As much as 75 percent of the phytonutrients in wheat are lost during refinement. As with white sugar, this process leaves a pale substance that does not resemble its original form and basically contains *no nutrition*.

We refine our wheat and other grains to give the resulting flour a longer shelf life and, to some, an attractive appearance, but it is so nutritionally empty that even bugs won't eat it! Our government doesn't seem to care that refined white flour lacks any food value, even though it is used to make thousands of foods. However, in the early 1940s, it was documented that servicemen in the British and United States military were suffering from deficiencies of B vitamins (thiamin, riboflavin, niacin) and iron. Flour was chosen for enrichment with those nutrients because everyone in the society, ranging from the rich to the poor, ate bread made from white flour. The USDA thereby enacted in 1943 what is called the "enrichment law," which requires the manufacturers of white flour to add back only five of the nutrients that were removed during refinement. Following the war, the law remained in place.

According to the enrichment law, refined flour must have the following quantities of nutrients added to each pound of flour:

2.9 milligrams of vitamin $B_1$ (thiamine)
1.8 milligrams of vitamin $B_2$ (riboflavin)
24 milligrams of vitamin $B_3$ (niacin)
0.7 milligrams of vitamin $B_9$ (folic acid)
20 milligrams of iron

Calcium may also be added (but is not required) at a minimum of 960 milligrams per pound of flour.

But flour manufacturers don't and can't possibly enrich flour enough. The original whole wheat kernel contains over one hundred vitamins, minerals, and phytochemicals, in addition to essential oils, fibers, and enzymes, all of which act together, synergistically, to assist our body in digesting the wheat. Enriched flour becomes deadly to our body because not only can we not digest it properly, but like sugar, white flour leaches calcium and other minerals from our bones, tissues, and teeth, just to be able to digest it. In fact, if you tried to live on white bread alone for sixty days, you would literally die, because there isn't enough nutrition in the flour to keep you alive for that long.

Unfortunately, the American diet is rife with products made from white flour and other refined grains. Examples include breads, crackers, pastries, baked goods, pastas, most commercial cereals, pizza dough, tortillas, fast foods, and snack foods of all types.

Excessive consumption of refined white flour has led to an epidemic of obesity and digestive illness in our country. The lack of fibers and the absence of oil from the wheat germ make it difficult to break down and utilize the proteins in the endosperm of the wheat kernel. One such protein, called gluten, has become one of the most feared food components of our time. Many people have a digestive disease called gluten intolerance or celiac disease, which causes severe inflammation of the small intestine. Such people must avoid all grains containing gluten, including wheat, rye, barley, spelt, kamut, and processed oats. Could it be that our overexposure to this protein, without the parent grain's accompanying fibers, oils, and other nutrients, has created a widespread food allergy and a change in DNA, such that this disease is now being passed down to subsequent generations?

## Skinny Grains

Refined grains are not part of a processed-free lifestyle, but skinny whole grains are! Whole grains have similar amounts and sometimes more disease-fighting phytochemicals than many typical fruits and vegetables do! There are hundreds of different phytochemicals in whole grains. They are high Life Force Energy plant foods that provide the body with energy, nutrients, and fiber for their own absorption. Fiber in itself is important because it helps our body to process waste efficiently and helps us feel full for longer periods of time.

I encourage you to expand your horizons when it comes to grains, to minimize the amount of wheat you eat, and to instead include in your meals a variety of other whole grains. These include:

Amaranth (the seed of an herb)
Barley (a cereal grass, not gluten free)
Brown rice, as well as other colored rice (e.g., red cargo rice and
    black rice)
Buckwheat or kasha (buckwheat groats)

Corn (maize), including popcorn and whole-grain cornmeal
Kamut (an ancient form of wheat, not gluten free)
Millet (a cereal grass)
Oats and oatmeal (gluten-free rolled oats and steel-cut oats)
Quinoa (the seed of an herb)
Rye (a cereal grass, light and dark, contains gluten)
Spelt (an ancient form of wheat, not gluten free)
Triticale (a hybrid of wheat and rye)
Whole wheat, including such varieties as wheat berries and cracked
    wheat (also called bulgur, often used to make tabbouleh)
Wild rice (not rice at all, but a kind of grass)

You're better off eating the cooked whole grains, rather than products made from flours that have been ground from the whole grains. The reason is that whenever a grain is ground into flour to make it into something else, such as muffins, breads, and crackers, usually other ingredients have to be added to "hold" the flour together. Most flour products are processed foods for this very reason. When we eat the whole grain, however, all that is required is some water and heat to cook it, along with some natural herbs and spices for seasoning.

But there's another important reason to avoid processed grains. All flours, including whole-grain flours, are considered potentially troublesome because research has shown that they create a brain chemical response in the form of increased serotonin levels. This is the same phenomenon that is seen with sugar addiction. This serotonin "high" may lead to cravings for more carbohydrates, which in turn may lead to overconsumption of carbohydrates in general. Also, although whole wheat flour and other whole-grain flours are absorbed more slowly than white flour, the former can still destabilize blood glucose levels by triggering the pancreas into an insulin release. Again, too much insulin creates an upsetting imbalance that affects many of our bodily functions and organs.

To avoid these problems, many people have chosen to omit all flour from their diet and just stick with grains in their whole form. (I, myself, stayed away from all flours in the first five years of my weight loss.) However, this does not mean that we can't eat whole-grain flours, just that we should be careful not to eat them at the exclusion of more grains in their whole form. We can occasionally enjoy crackers, muffins, and pastas made from whole-grain flours, such as whole wheat flour, brown rice flour, spelt flour, quinoa flour, buckwheat flour, and oat flour.

## How to Identify Whole Grain Foods When You Are Shopping

As you transition to eating more whole grains, you need to be aware of some things. First, many whole wheat breads, cereals, and whole wheat tortillas contain sugar or high-fructose corn syrup, in addition to a load of other additives or preservatives, so you need to read every ingredient list if you are purchasing these types of foods.

Also, be skeptical if you see the phrase "made with whole grain" on the front of the package. Sometimes this is a clever marketing trick to get you to buy the product. *Always* read the ingredient list and look for the word *whole* in front of the word *wheat* on any product that contains wheat. For instance, if you are considering buying a loaf of whole wheat bread, you should see the words "whole wheat flour" as the first ingredient listed.

If additional wheat flours are listed, or you do not see the word *whole* in front of the word *wheat*, then the product is not completely whole grain. For example, some products use more enriched flour than they do whole-grain flour. Beware if the label says only "wheat flour" or "enriched wheat flour" or "enriched unbleached wheat flour." These are all forms of refined white flour.

Finally, the best types of grains to eat are sprouted grains. Those will be discussed in Chapter 11.

Table 4.3 will further help you in identifying whole-grain products in the store.

## Table 4.3  Identifying Whole Grain

| Words and Phrases You May See on Packages | Do They Mean Whole Grain? |
|---|---|
| Whole grain (name of grain)<br>Whole wheat<br>Whole (name of grain) flour<br>Organic whole (name of grain)<br>Stone-ground whole (name of grain)<br>Brown rice<br>Oats, oatmeal (including old-fashioned oatmeal, instant oatmeal, rolled oats, and steel-cut oats)<br>Wheat berries<br>Sprouted [name of grain] | Yes—These phrases refer to products that contain all parts of the grain, so you know you're getting all the nutrients of the whole grain.<br><br>In nearly all cases, you will see the word "whole" in front of the name of the grain. |
| 100% wheat | Maybe—This phrase means that the only grain contained in the product is wheat, but it may not be *whole* wheat. You need to check the ingredient list to make sure it says "whole wheat." |
| Multigrain | Maybe—This phrase means that the product contains several different grains, such as wheat, corn, rye, etc. However, the grains may be whole grains or refined grains, or a mixture of both. Again, you need to check the ingredient list to make sure it contains all whole grains.<br><br>Many "multigrain" breads list the first ingredient as "enriched wheat flour." |
| Semolina<br>Durum wheat | No—These are both from varieties of wheat that have had the bran and germ removed. |
| Organic flour<br>Organic wheat flour<br>Organic unbleached wheat flour | No—Although the wheat has been grown organically, it has still been refined and thus is still just white flour. |
| Stone ground | No—This phrase refers to grain that is coarsely ground and may contain the germ, but not the bran. Often with stone-ground breads, enriched flour is the first ingredient listed, not whole-grain flour. |

*continues*

## Table 4.3 Identifying Whole Grain *continued*

| Words and Phrases You May See on Packages | Do They Mean Whole Grain? |
|---|---|
| Pumpernickel | No—This type of bread is made from refined dark rye flour and refined white flour. |
| Wheat flour<br>Enriched flour<br>Enriched bleached flour<br>Unbleached enriched flour | No—All of these phrases refer to refined flour. |
| Cornmeal (degermed) | No—Degermed cornmeal means that the germ has been removed, so it is not whole grain. |
| Rice flour | No—This phrase refers to flour made from white rice, which is not a whole grain. Only brown rice flour is whole grain. |
| Bran | No—This refers only to only the bran of the grain; it is not the whole grain. However, bran can add significant amounts of fiber and other nutrients to a diet that is rich in whole grains. |
| Wheat germ | No—This refers only to the germ of the grain; it is not the whole grain. However, wheat germ contains vitamin E, fiber, and other nutrients that can enhance a diet otherwise rich in whole grains. |

SOURCE: The Whole Grain Council, www.wholegraincouncil.org.

## Julene's Story

I'm a mother of two young children and while I wasn't really over-weight, I had been battling fatigue for years and was ready to try any-thing. After going through allergy testing, sleep apnea testing, and a full physical with my doctor, I thought to try changing my diet.

Following Dee's plan changed my life. I always knew that sugar and white flour were bad for me, but I never really understood why. Dee does a great job of thoroughly explaining it. I started with eliminating those two substances, and then over about four weeks completely moved to processed-free eating. I immediately noticed a difference in my workouts in that I had so much more energy. And almost immediately I lost the 15 pounds that I had kept (and couldn't seem to lose despite being thin most of my life) after my two pregnancies. People began complimenting me on my skin and en-ergy. It was really amazing. That was June 2010, and I'm still going strong. I can't imagine ever going back to eating like I was.

The transformation I've made has really opened my eyes to what we, as a society, put into our body—and don't really know what it is! While frus-trating and sad, it makes complete sense to me how much of our country is overweight and unhealthy.

This plan is unique in that it can help so many people—not just those trying to lose weight. I've recommended it to numerous friends, most of them frustrated at being "tired all the time."

—*Julene Montgomery, age 40, postgraduate student*

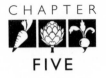
# The Scientific Skinny on Fats and Oils

*The fats and oils story may well be the biggest scandal of ignorance, disinformation and greed in the entire history of food production.*

—JOHN FINNEGAN, AUTHOR OF *THE FACTS ABOUT FATS*

There are so many myths surrounding dietary fats, and despite scientific evidence to the contrary, the underlying presumption for many people is that any fat in the diet, be it olive oil or butter, will most certainly end up on our belly, hips, and thighs. But like almost everything in nutritional biochemistry, the story is just not that simple. The role of dietary fats in the body is complex and extensive. Although some types of fat can pose serious health problems, others are absolutely vital to our survival. Most of us know this to some extent, but the problem is that nearly everything we know and believe about fat is the direct opposite of what is scientifically and historically true.

Here are some of the big "fat" lies we've come to believe:

- Eating fat makes you fat.
- Canola oil is one of the healthiest oils for cooking.

- Coconut oil is a dangerous saturated fat that should be avoided like the plague.
- Saturated fat and dietary cholesterol are the main cause of coronary heart disease.
- Real butter clogs arteries, so "healthy" margarines should be eaten in its place.
- The cholesterol in egg yolks causes high cholesterol, so we should only eat egg whites or such substitutes as Egg Beaters.

If you've been making your food choices based on these widely accepted falsehoods, you may be setting yourself up for some serious health problems. These fat myths have been perpetuated over the past few decades by the medical profession, nutritionists, and other health professionals, who themselves don't always have the most accurate information.

## Politically Correct Nutrition Leads to Poor Health

Medical misinformation dies hard, but it is time to put an end to these false "gospel" truths. It took me years to find and decipher the *real truths* about fat by becoming an astute student of cutting-edge science on the subject.

Some of that corrective research was published in the cover story of the July 7, 2002, issue of the *New York Times Magazine*. In his article "What If It's All Been a Big Fat Lie?" science writer Gary Taubes questioned the conventional wisdom handed down by the American medical establishment that obesity and heart disease are caused by the excessive consumption of fat. He boldly asserted that what most of us have believed to be true about fats and health is actually the result of an entangled web of food industry lobbying, self-promoting medical celebrities, government intervention based on unsound science, advertising, media, and our own guilt-induced desire to redeem our health by giving up "evil" fats. The proliferation of fat myths have now become so deeply entrenched in our culture that we find it difficult to believe anything else. However, when you delve into human history and the real science of fats, you cannot dispute the facts.

For example, three decades of eating reduced-fat dairy products, margarines, egg substitutes, skinless (and flavorless) chicken breasts, and about fifteen thousand low-fat and fat-free products should have rendered us a healthier and slimmer nation. In 1984, the president of the American Heart Association predicted that if everyone followed a low-fat diet, heart attacks and strokes would be rare if not eradicated by the year 2000. Because many of us jumped on the low-fat bandwagon, Americans did reduce their fat consumption from more than 40 percent of the total diet down to 34 percent by the beginning of the new millennium. However, even by 2012, the incidence of heart disease *has not declined*, and as I have already discussed, obesity is skyrocketing at an alarming rate.

Why haven't we managed to achieve the optimal state of health we were promised in exchange for giving up whole milk and real cream, eggs, real butter, tropical oils, cheese, and red meat? In his widely ignored first article on the subject, "The Soft Science of Dietary Fat," published in the prestigious journal *Science* (March 30, 2001), Taubes explains that the science proving a connection between dietary fat and heart disease simply was never there in the first place. Hundreds of millions of dollars of research later, there's no proof whatsoever that eating low-fat foods will improve your health in any way at all.[1] In fact, the research more accurately proves that eating a low-fat diet can be detrimental to your health. In an August 20, 2011, interview with Dr. Joseph Mercola, Taubes explained that even the most recent studies show the results are always the same: "There is not enough evidence to say that saturated fat is bad for you, and there has never been that evidence," Taubes said.[2] Taubes's stance, as outlined in his latest book, *Why We Get Fat and What to Do About It* (2011) is in alignment with Dr. Robert Lustig and his early predecessors Thomas Cleave (*The Saccharine Disease*) and British researcher John Yudkin (*Sweet and Dangerous*)—refined carbohydrates are the cause for heart disease.

## No Sound Science

The fat misinformation campaign is aimed at two dietary "demons"— saturated fat and cholesterol. The lies started flying in the 1950s with a faulty hypothesis proposed by a researcher named Ancel Keys. His theory suggested that there is a direct relationship between the amount of saturated fat and cholesterol in the diet and the incidence of coronary heart disease. Despite numerous subsequent studies that put his data and conclusions into question, Keys's research became the "word" and received far more media attention than any of the opposing views.

Before 1920, heart disease in America was extremely rare. By the mid-1950s when Ancel Keys was conducting his research, it was the leading cause of death among Americans.

I must admit that when it comes to heart disease, the medical establishment has made great advancements in early detection and reducing the mortality rates of people who have suffered heart attacks. In fact, my own father is still alive today because of these technological breakthroughs. But while science and technology can clear arteries once they've been severely clogged and can keep people alive once they've already suffered a heart attack, the risk and rate of our nation's leading killer continues to sharply rise. Despite the pushing of low-fat and low-cholesterol diets, blood-thinning drugs, polyunsaturated oils, and calorie counting, the twentieth century did not make a dent in the rate of heart disease. It is still the number one leading cause of death in the United States.

If, as we have been told, saturated fat and cholesterol are the leading culprits in the development of heart disease, obesity, and cancer, you would expect that during the period when the incidence of these diseases was on the rise, there would have been a correlating increase in the consumption of these dietary demons. But the exact opposite is true. From 1910 to 1970, the amount of saturated animal fat in the American diet dropped from 83 to 62 percent, and the consumption of butter in America decreased from eighteen pounds per person per year to four.[3]

You may be surprised to also discover that over the past eighty to ninety years, cholesterol intake has only increased by 1 percent. What did increase sharply, by about 400 percent, was the consumption of so-called healthy polyunsaturated vegetable oils in the form of margarine, shortening, and refined cooking oils. Also during this time, we started scarfing down more sugar and processed foods.[4]

One of the most famous research studies conducted on heart disease in America is the Framingham Heart Study. This study is often cited as "proof" of the correlation between the amount of saturated fat and cholesterol in the diet and the incidence of coronary heart disease. Begun in 1948 in Framingham, Massachusetts, researchers studied and evaluated different groups of six thousand participants who consumed either high or low levels of saturated fat. For forty years, participants were tested and evaluated at five-year intervals. Although the study did show that those who weighed more and had abnormally high blood cholesterol levels were slightly more at risk for future heart disease, it was not due to their fat and cholesterol intake.

At the end of the forty years, the director of the study had to readily admit, "In Framingham, Massachusetts we found that the more saturated fat one ate, the more cholesterol one ate, the more calories one ate, the lower the person's serum cholesterol." The study also showed that the people who ate the most cholesterol and saturated fat also weighed the least and were the most physically active.[5]

Another study performed in Britain, involving several thousand men, asked half of them to reduce their saturated fat intake, stop smoking, and increase the amount of "good" fats such as margarine and polyunsaturated cooking oils. The other half did not make any changes to their diet but were also asked to stop smoking. After just one year, those on the "good fat" diet had twice the number of deaths as did those eating saturated fats, even though some of the men eating saturated fat continued to smoke! However, when the results were presented to the public, the study's author ignored these results in favor of the politically correct conclusion: "The implication for public health policy in the U.K. is that a preventive program such as we evaluated in this trial is probably effective."[6]

## Disproving the Link

Many other studies have shown similar biased and falsely presented data. And although it has been proven in laboratories that heart disease can be induced in animals if they are given massive amounts of oxidized and rancid cholesterol (about ten times the amount in any normal human diet), there are many more compelling human studies disproving the link between saturated fat, cholesterol, and heart disease.

Michael DeBakey, the famous heart surgeon, conducted a study of 1,700 patients with hardening of the arteries and found no relationship between the level of cholesterol in the blood and the incidence of atherosclerosis. The Medical Research Council found that men eating butter (a traditional whole food) ran half the risk of developing heart disease as did those eating margarine.[7]

Studies of people in northern and southern India, the Inuit in Alaska, Mediterranean societies, and Soviet Georgia all reveal a similar pattern: the lowest rates of heart disease are found among those eating the highest amounts of animal fats.

Modern Japanese, Swiss, and French populations also eat diets high in saturated fat and have lower rates of coronary heart disease than many other Western countries. Unfortunately these societies suffer from other degenerative diseases owing to their ever-increasing consumption of refined sugar and flour and other processed foods.

## Saturated Fats Are Crucial for Health

The reason for the correlation between high saturated fat intake and healthy people is that saturated fats play a crucial role in body chemistry. You may be surprised to learn just how important they are. In their best-selling book *Nourishing Traditions*, Dr. Mary Enig, a nutritionist and biochemist of international renown for her research on the nutritional aspects of fats and oils, and Sally Fallon, a journalist and nutrition researcher, listed some key roles of saturated fats:

- Saturated fatty acids constitute at least 50 percent of all cell membranes. They are what sustain the integrity of the entire cell, providing necessary stiffness and stability.
- At least 50 percent of the dietary fat we eat should be saturated, otherwise calcium cannot be effectively incorporated into the skeletal structure. In other words, a lack of an adequate amount of saturated fat in the diet can lead to bone density problems such as osteoporosis.
- Contrary to the fat myths, saturated fats actually lower lipoprotein (a), a key substance in the blood that indicates proneness to heart disease.
- Saturated fats protect the liver from alcohol and other common toxins, such as those contained in nonsteroidal anti-inflammatory drugs (NSAIDs), for instance, Tylenol.
- Saturated fats, especially the type found in coconut oil, enhance the immune system.

- Our body needs saturated fats to properly utilize the other fats in our diet, especially the all-important omega-3 fats from fish oil and flax-seed oil. Omega-3 fats are better retained in the tissues when the diet is rich in saturated fats. This means that your omega-3 supplement may not be providing its full health benefit if you are restricting your saturated fat intake too severely.
- While foods high in saturated fat are widely blamed for causing heart disease, they are actually the preferred fuel for the heart, meaning the heart works best when it is fueled by saturated fats. This is why the fat around the heart muscle is highly saturated. During times of stress, the heart draws on this reserve of saturated fat. If there isn't enough, the heart cannot function properly.
- Short- and medium-chain saturated fatty acids found in coconut oil, palm oil, and butter have important antimicrobial properties. They protect us against harmful microorganisms in the digestive tract.

Enig and Fallon sum up their study of saturated fats with this profound statement: "The scientific evidence, honestly evaluated, does not support the assertion that 'artery-clogging' saturated fats cause heart disease. Actually, evaluation of the fat found in clogged arteries reveals that only about 26 percent is saturated. The rest is unsaturated, of which more than half is polyunsaturated."[8]

## The Big Fat Canola Lie

If you are like most Americans, you believe canola oil is the best oil to use for cooking. Restaurants proudly tout they only use "healthy" canola oil. Nearly every cookbook on the market includes canola oil in its recipes. Check the ingredients of packaged foods, and you will probably find canola oil ranking high on the list. The marketers of canola oil have claimed that it is the perfect oil, owing to its low saturated fat content, high monoun-saturated fat content, and a bonus omega-3 content, making it particularly beneficial for the prevention of heart disease. Sadly, once again, we have been subjected to a twisted truth.

Canola oil has a hidden history. As mentioned earlier, the incidence of heart disease rose sharply from the 1930s on. By the mid-1980s, the high mortality rates from heart attacks had the medical community in a tizzy, and the media was having a field day. Since the 1930s, the food industry, in collusion with the American Heart Association, numerous government agencies, and departments of nutrition at major universities, had been promoting polyunsaturated oils as a heart-healthy alternative to "artery-clogging" saturated fats. Unfortunately, it had become increasingly clear that polyunsaturated oils, particularly corn oil and soybean oil, cause numerous health problems, including and especially cancer.[9]

The food industry was in a quandary. In the face of mounting evidence of the dangers of polyunsaturated oils, it was becoming hard to convince the public that these oils were safe to eat. The industry couldn't go back to using traditional fats such as butter and tropical oils without also causing a public scare. Besides, traditional fats are way too expensive to allow for the huge profit margins the industry had been enjoying thus far. Food manufacturers were losing lots of money and needed to come up with a new plan.

Their plan was to convince the public to use a "new" monounsaturated oil. Studies had shown that olive oil, a monounsaturated oil, has a "better" effect than polyunsaturated oils on cholesterol levels and other blood parameters. Besides, Ancel Keys and others had popularized the notion that the Mediterranean diet—rich in olive oil—protected against heart disease and ensured a long and healthy life.[10]

Promotion of olive oil, with its long history of food use, seemed more scientifically sound to health-conscious consumers than the promotion of corn and soy oils, which had never been used in the history of humanity and could only be extracted with modern stainless-steel presses and chemical processing. The problem for the industry was that there was not enough olive oil in the world to meet its needs. And, like butter and other traditional fats, olive oil was too expensive to use in most processed foods. Manufacturers needed to find a less expensive monounsaturated oil. That's when the new wonder oil—canola oil—stepped onto the scene.[11]

## There's No Such Thing As a Canola

The real name of canola oil is rapeseed oil. The natural, untainted rapeseed is high in heart-healthy monounsaturated fats and also contains omega-3 fats. The problem is that about two-thirds of the monounsaturated fat in natural, untainted rapeseed is a type called erucic acid, which has been associated with heart lesions and other ailments. To remove the erucic acid, Canadian plant breeders had to genetically engineer the rapeseed using a seed-splitting technique, to create a mutation called low erucic acid rapeseed (a.k.a. lear).

The new oil, called lear oil, was slow to catch on in the United States. To be marketable, it had to be renamed. Neither *lear oil* or *rape oil* were very enticing terms, so the industry settled on *canola,* for "Canadian oil," because most of the engineered rapeseed at that time was grown in Canada.

## Twisted Science

Via genetic engineering, the industry had managed to manipulate rapeseed to make a perfect oil—very low in saturated fat and rich in monounsaturated fat. As a bonus, canola oil contains about 10 percent omega-3 fatty acids, which had been shown to be beneficial for the heart and immune system. Since most Americans are deficient in omega-3 fats, the oil was a dream come true for health-conscious consumers. But how healthy is it really?

Although rapeseed has been used as a source of oil since ancient times in China and India, the way it was historically obtained, using small stone presses to press out the oil at low temperatures, rendered a fresh, healthy oil that was consumed immediately. It has even been proven by recent studies that the erucic acid in rapeseed oil does not create heart lesions, as long as a significant amount of saturated fat is also part of the diet. In fact, erucic acid is helpful in the treatment of the wasting disease adrenoleukodystrophy and was the magic ingredient in Lorenzo's oil (a combination of olive and rapeseed oils).[12]

However, the way we now process canola oil, and most other oils for that matter, is a different thing entirely, rendering them very unhealthy. Because canola oil, and all modern vegetable and seed oils (e.g., soybean oil and corn oil), are so unstable, it is nearly impossible to keep them from turning rancid. So they have to be highly processed and refined at high heat (400 to 500 degrees Fahrenheit) and treated with chemical solvents such as hexane, a fluid also used in dry cleaning. Traces of hexane remain in the oil, even after considerable refining. The refinement process involves bleaching and degumming, which require the use of additional chemicals of questionable safety.

Canola oil contains a good amount of omega-3 fats, which easily become rancid and foul smelling when subjected to oxygen and high heat, so the oil also has to be deodorized. The deodorization process converts a large portion of the healthy omega-3 fats into very unhealthy trans fats. Trans fats are formed at 320 degrees Fahrenheit, so imagine how much damage is done at 400 to 500 degrees. Although the Canadian government lists the trans-fat content of canola oil at a minimal 0.2 percent, research at the University of Florida at Gainesville found trans-fat levels as high as 4.6 percent in commercial liquid canola oil. The consumer has no clue about the presence of trans fats in canola oil because they are not listed on the label.[13] Trans fats will be discussed in the next chapter.

## Oil Refinement Destroys Any Original Health Benefits

Similar to the refinement of sugar and flour, anything good that was in the original oil, such as vitamins, antioxidants, and other nutrients are all destroyed in the oil-refinement process. The remaining "pure" oil is tasteless, and by the time that bottle of oil ends up on your supermarket shelf, it's full of trans fats and free radicals (the dangers of the latter are discussed later in this chapter). The kicker is that once you buy this oil and take it home, you also heat it very high when you cook or bake, destroying it even further!

Liquid canola oil is easily changed by a chemical reaction into partially hydrogenated canola oil (a dangerous trans fat), which is the type of canola oil used in processed foods. This canola oil contains up to 40 percent trans fats. Almost all restaurants use the partially hydrogenated form of canola oil, so don't be fooled by those "We only use canola oil" claims. These high levels of trans fats allow for a longer shelf life for processed foods, a crispier texture in cookies and crackers—and more dangers of chronic disease for anyone who eats those foods.[14]

The widespread acceptance of canola oil and its "heart-healthy" claims come at a high price. Even those newfangled "improved" margarines made with canola oil and soybean oil are a lie. They're highly processed fake foods that have lost whatever claim they originally had to any health properties. Do yourself a favor: avoid canola oil at all costs. Eat real butter, cook with extra-virgin coconut oil, and use extra-virgin olive oil for salad dressings.

# The Fourth Law of Skinny Science: You Must Eat Fat to Lose Fat

Even when you are a chemist as I am, the world of fats can be confusing. However, I am going to do my best to explain it, because it is important for you to understand the essential role fats play in achieving and maintaining a healthy, slim body.

Before I delve into the chemistry, first let me say that you must eat fat to lose fat. And you must eat more of it than you probably realize, with one caveat—it must be the right type of fat. If you have been a low-fat dieter, you've been depriving yourself of the delicious and satisfying tastes of the good fats our ancestors ate, as are found in avocado, olives, butter, coconut, meat, fish, nuts, and seeds. These fats are startlingly health protective and provide many other benefits for a beautiful, well-functioning body, such as glowing skin, shiny and supple hair, a good sex life, fertility, a strong and vital immune system, enough vitamin E for your heart, balanced hormones, and antiaging properties.

Vitamins A, D, E, and K (found in many foods) are called fat-soluble vitamins, because they can only be absorbed into the body through fat. Fat also aids in the absorption of beta-carotene, lycopene, and many other micronutrients. This is one reason why low-fat diets are dangerous. Without adequate amounts of dietary fat, you can become deficient in these important nutrients, which can then have a cascading effect. For instance, if your body does not have enough vitamin D, calcium cannot be absorbed, which could then lead to poor bone health. Aside from fat-soluble vitamins, we need fat to properly assimilate protein and minerals. Many people do not realize that proteins and fats are packaged together in nature for a reason— because we need the fat to utilize the protein!

Your hormones, which control every cell in your body, don't work properly without adequate fat, and neither does your immune system. Every one of the 60 trillion cells in your body relies on fat—to keep its membranes flexible so that nutrients can enter and toxins can exit, and so it can communicate with the other cells in the body.[15]

Fat is important for proper growth and development and provides insulation for our internal organs and nerves. Fat provides taste, consistency, and stability in our foods. Because of its high energy content, fat quickly satisfies hunger, so you will tend to eat less when you have enough fat in your diet.

According to Dr. Ron Rosedale of the Colorado Center for Metabolic Medicine, fat, not sugar, is the body's preferred fuel. He points out that when the body stores excess sugar, it's stored as fat, in a good usable form. Fats not only don't make you fat (unless you eat them to huge excess—and even then, only if you also ingest enough sugars and starches to stimulate your fat-storage system), they're good weapons against obesity.[16]

## The World of Fats "Dee-Mystified"

I put together this section for those who want to know the science behind healthy and unhealthy fats. You don't absolutely have to know all of this information to be skinny, but if you're interested in how it all works, I think it will help clear up some of the mystery shrouding the world of fats. If it's too technical for you, you can skip it, but make sure you read the next chapter on trans fats, because you do need to know about those to save yourself from serious health problems.

You already know a little of the chemistry: in general, fats do not dissolve in water. This is why your oil-and-vinegar salad dressing separates. But what will concern us here is the composition of the fats themselves.

Chemists have a whole language of their own to describe molecules and their structures. This language is called nomenclature. In recent years, some of this nomenclature has trickled out to the public by way of food descriptions, particularly fats. In chemistry, fats are classified according to their molecular structures and physical properties. *Saturated, trans fat, omega-3, fatty acid, free radical, monounsaturated,* and *polyunsaturated* are all chemical terms that describe how the carbon atoms and hydrogen atoms within the fat molecules are attached to one another other and how they react with other substances.

In simple terms, fat molecules look like chains with two little balls attached to one end. The chains are made up of strings of carbon (C) atoms bonded, or linked, together. Each carbon atom has four bonding sites. Two of the bonding sites are linked to another carbon atom, and the other two bonding sites are linked to hydrogen (H) atoms, with the exception of the carbon atom at the very beginning of the chain, which is bonded to three hydrogen atoms (see Figure 5.1). This is often referred to as a hydrocarbon chain.

The balls at the end of the chain are actually a group of atoms called a carboxyl group. It consists of one carbon atom, two oxygen (O) atoms, and one hydrogen atom (COOH). In chemistry, the carboxyl group functions as an acid; therefore, fats are interchangeably called fatty acids. Figure 5.1 is a simple depiction of a fatty acid:

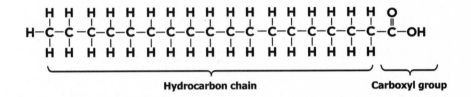

**Figure 5.1** A simple chemical structure of a fatty acid chain. Carbon atoms are linked together with hydrogen atoms filling in the bonding sites.

Most fats are very long chains (containing anywhere from 14 to 24 carbon atoms linked together), some are medium-length chains (8 to 12 carbon atoms), and some are short chains (4 to 6 carbon atoms). Some fat chains are straight, whereas others are bent. Their length and their shape determine their physical and chemical properties.

As mentioned before, each carbon atom in the chain has bonding sites where hydrogen atoms are attached. The bonding sites can either be all filled with hydrogen atoms or some of the sites can remain empty. When all the bonding sites are filled with hydrogen atoms, the fat is termed saturated. If some of the bonding sites are empty, or missing hydrogen atoms, the fat is called unsaturated. The fat in Figure 5.1 is an example of a saturated fat because all the bonding sites are filled.

## Saturated Fats

The Webster's dictionary definition of the word saturated is "to treat, furnish, or charge with something to the point where no more can be absorbed, dissolved, or retained." Think of a towel that has soaked up all the water it can, to the point where it is sopping wet and cannot absorb any more water.

In the chemistry of fats, all the bonding sites of a saturated fat molecule are filled with hydrogen atoms and nothing else can attach to it. Because of this saturation, the fat molecule is highly stable. This means that saturated fats do not normally go rancid, even when heated for cooking purposes. All of the carbon bonds within the fat chain are single bonds, giving the molecule a straight shape; therefore they pack together easily, so that they form a solid or semisolid fat at room temperature.

The most common saturated fats are found in butter, mother's milk, coconut oil, palm oil, cocoa butter, goat's milk, cow's milk and dairy products, and meat. Typically, the saturated fats in animals are made up of long-chain saturated fats, whereas the saturated fats in plants such as coconuts and palm fruit are made up of medium-chain or short-chain saturated fats. An exception to this is one of the fats in butter, which is a short-chain saturated fat called butyric acid, responsible for its yummy butter flavor. Our body can also make saturated fats from carbohydrates, which is why you store lots of fat if you eat too many carbohydrates. Figure 5.2 shows a molecular structure of a saturated fat.

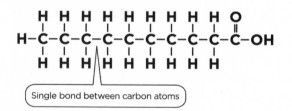

Single bond between carbon atoms

**Figure 5.2** Molecular structure of a saturated fat

## Unsaturated Fats

The other types of fats are called unsaturated, meaning that binding sites on two adjacent carbon atoms are not filled. Each adjacent carbon atom is missing one hydrogen atom, which causes them to form a double bond to each other, but this double bond is not as stable as the single bonds in saturated fats. Therefore, unsaturated fats are more reactive and susceptible to being changed by heat, oxygen, and light—meaning they go rancid more easily. Figure 5.3 is a molecular structure of an unsaturated fat.

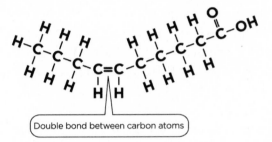

Figure 5.3  Molecular structure of an unsaturated fat

There are two types of unsaturated fats: monounsaturated and polyunsaturated.

Monounsaturated:  The prefix *mono* means "one," hence monounsaturated fats have one empty bonding site (one double bond). Monounsaturated fats have a kink or bend at the place in the molecule where the double bond occurs, making them V shaped (see Figure 5.4). This V shape prevents them from packing together as easily as the saturated fats do, so monounsaturated fats tend to be liquid at room temperature but can turn solid, like butter, if refrigerated (this is why your olive oil salad dressing solidifies when you put it in the refrigerator).

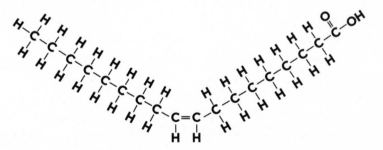

Figure 5.4  Molecular structure of oleic acid, an 18-carbon monounsaturated fat with one double bond. Two adjacent carbon atoms are each missing one hydrogen atom, so they have formed a double bond (=) with each other and the molecule has a V shape.

Like saturated fats, monounsaturated fats are relatively stable. They do not go rancid easily and therefore they can be used in low-heat cooking. The most common monounsaturated fat found in our food is called oleic acid. It is the main component of olive oil and the fat found in avocados, almonds, pecans, cashews, and peanuts. Our body can make monounsaturated fats from saturated fats and uses them in a number of ways. Monounsaturated fat, if it has not been heated too hot, is known to protect against heart disease.

Polyunsaturated: The prefix *poly* means "many, or more than one," hence polyunsaturated fats have more than one empty bonding site (two or more double bonds). They have kinks or turns at the positions of each double bond, making them V shaped or U shaped; therefore, they do not pack together easily. They are liquid even when refrigerated.

Our body cannot make polyunsaturated fats; hence they are called essential fats, or essential fatty acids (EFAs). We must obtain these essential fats from the foods we eat. The two polyunsaturated fats found in many of our foods are linoleic acid—also called omega-6, which has two double bonds; and linolenic acid—also called omega-3, which has three double bonds. (If you count the carbon atoms in the chain from left to right, the omega number refers to the position on the carbon chain where the first double bond occurs.)

Polyunsaturated fats (both omega-3 and omega-6) are found in such foods as fish, whole grains, nuts, seeds, eggs, and vegetables.

The double bonds in these fat molecules make them extremely fragile and susceptible to becoming rancid, especially the omega-3s. They must be treated with great care so as not to expose them to oxygen, heat, and light for too long. Because of this, *polyunsaturated fats should never be heated or used in cooking.*[17]

This may confuse you because the supermarket shelves are full of polyunsaturated cooking oils. They are derived mostly from soy, as well as from corn, safflower, and rapeseed (canola oil). They are also widely used in restaurants and food production (either soybean or canola oil appears on the ingredient list of nearly every packaged food). While polyunsaturated oils contain essential omega-6 and omega-3 fats that are crucial to our health, these fats are only healthy for us when we eat them in their natural state, not as oils that have been extracted from the foods and then highly processed. In other words, we need to obtain these oils by eating raw nuts and seeds, whole grains, and fish, not from processed oils. An exception to that is the omega-3 oils that are cold pressed from flaxseeds, hemp seeds, and fish. Flaxseed oil and fish oil are pressed from the foods and stored in such a way as to not destroy their fragile omega-3 fat.

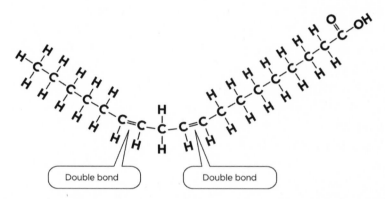

Double bond

Double bond

**Figure 5.5** Molecular structure of linoleic acid, an 18-carbon polyunsaturated fat with two double bonds commonly found in vegetable oils, whole grains, nuts, and seeds. Two double bonds (=) in the molecule give it a bent U shape.

## Dangers Associated with Polyunsaturated Oils

Polyunsaturated vegetable oils were never part of the human diet prior to the 1930s. Today, the Western diet can contain up to 30 percent of calories from these oils, derived mainly from soy, corn, safflower, and rapeseed (canola oil). But scientific research indicates that this amount is way too high.[18]

In native populations, the intake of polyunsaturated oils comes from the small amounts found in legumes, grains, nuts, green vegetables, fish, olive oil, and animal fats, but not from commercial vegetable oils. As I described earlier, the processing of these oils is extremely damaging to the healthful qualities found in the natural plants. For instance, if you eat raw sunflower seeds, you get healthy, unadulterated polyunsaturated oil. But if you eat a tortilla chip that has been deep-fried in processed sunflower oil, you get nothing but poor health.

Overconsumption of polyunsaturated oils has been shown to contribute to a large number of diseases, including cancer and heart disease; a compromised immune system; liver damage; digestive disorders; diseases of the reproductive organs and lungs; and weight gain.[19]

## A Free Radical Is Not a Hippie Dude from the '60s

There is a reason why polyunsaturated oils cause so many health problems. The double bonds in unsaturated fats are sites on the fat molecules where a pair of electrons is being shared between two adjacent carbon atoms. When subjected to heat, oxygen, and moisture, as in cooking and processing, the bond becomes unstable and loses one of its electrons, leaving a carbon atom with an unpaired electron. In simple terms, one of the chain links has been broken open, leaving a gap or loose link. In chemical terms, this is called a free radical. Free radicals are basically rancid, or oxidized, molecules, also known as oxidants.

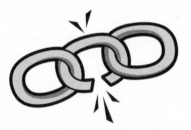

**Figure 5.6**  A free radical is like a broken chain link

A free radical is an unstable molecule with an unpaired electron that is highly reactive. It wants to become stable again, and so it will try to steal an electron from another molecule to close up the chain. The problem is that when we ingest a free radical, it acts like a little terrorist Pac-Man racing through our body looking to replace its missing electron by gobbling up an electron from a healthy cell, which then in turn becomes a free radical itself. This cascading effect can do a huge amount of damage.

Because we typically don't ingest just one free radical—we ingest an army of them—the result is an exponential amount of altered cells. And remember, polyunsaturated fat molecules have two or more double bonds, so it is possible there are two or more free radical sites acting from just one fat molecule. There are literally *millions* of fat molecules in just one tablespoon of oil! This is why French fries are so bad for you—just one French fry can potentially contain millions of free radicals.

Free radicals not only attack cell membranes, they can also damage the cell's DNA—the basic building block of cells—thus triggering mutations in tissue, blood vessels, and skin. When a free radical steals an electron from a cholesterol molecule, the cholesterol becomes oxidized, which is another word for "bad cholesterol." Oxidized cholesterol is stickier than normal cholesterol, so it clings to blood vessel walls, where it builds up plaque that clogs the arteries. Free radicals can add to the severity of asthma attacks by causing airways to clamp down and close. Free radical damage to the skin causes wrinkles and premature aging; it also increases the inflammation and joint damage that occurs in osteoarthritis and rheumatoid arthritis. Free radical damage to the tissues and internal organs is the precursor for cancer.

It should not be any surprise that numerous studies have repeatedly shown a high correlation between cancer and heart disease with the consumption of polyunsaturated oils. Evidence now links free radical damage with premature aging, autoimmune diseases, Parkinson's, amyotrophic lateral sclerosis (ALS, or Lou Gehrig's disease), Alzheimer's, and cataracts.[20]

## Antioxidants Are the Only Defense

Food is not our only means of exposure to free radicals, but it is certainly one of the most prevalent in modern times. Free radicals also come from pollution and other sources. Throughout human history, we have always been exposed to free radicals. However, that exposure was quite low because we did not eat processed oils, and environmental pollution was minimal. Our body was able to deal with free radicals easily because our traditional diet contained significant amounts of antioxidants. Today, we are exposed to millions of free radicals without also supplying our body with sufficient amounts of antioxidants. As a result, free radicals multiply to a point called oxidative stress, a point beyond the body's ability to neutralize them. When this occurs, premature aging and disease take over.

Antioxidants are the body's only defense against free radicals. Antioxidants are special types of phytochemicals found in plants—yes, that's right, from fruits, vegetables, legumes, and whole grains. Antioxidants stop free radicals (oxidants) in their tracks, before they can do serious damage. They are like the ghosts in the Pac-Man game, swallowing up and stopping the hungry Pac-Man from stealing any electrons from healthy cells. They do this in a philanthropic way: by simply donating one of their own electrons. In fact, this is an antioxidant's sole purpose; it doesn't need its extra electron and so it doesn't even miss it. Another way of looking at it is to think of a philanthropist who has an abundance of money, donating just one dollar to someone who has no money and who would otherwise have to steal that dollar from someone else to survive. The philanthropist donating the dollar never misses it, and the donation stops the recipient from stealing.

The philanthropists of the antioxidant world are vitamins A (as beta-carotene and other carotenoids), C, and E; the minerals selenium and zinc; the phytonutrients lycopene and squalene (found in olive oil); and alpha-lipoic acid. With the exception of alpha-lipoic acid (an important compound found in every cell of the body that helps turn glucose into energy), our body cannot make these antioxidants; they all need to come from foods. This is why it is so important to eat plenty of vegetables, fruits, and other foods that contain these antioxidants (see the sidebar for a list of antioxidant-rich food sources).

## The Essential Fats

In my initial stages of weight loss in the early 1990s, I bought in to the "fat" lies. I reduced my fat intake to 10 percent of my calories, using all the wrong fats. Like most Americans, I ate salad dressings made from soybean and canola oils and used margarine instead of butter. Although I did lose weight (mainly from a reduction of overall calories and the elimination of sugar and flour), a few years after my weight loss, my joints were stiff and I was very cold all the time. I hadn't yet learned about the essential fats, which keep our joints lubricated and regulate our body temperature. Essential fats are now recognized as crucial to our good health, but we also have to be aware of the important delicate balance of these fats in our foods and in our diet.

As mentioned earlier, polyunsaturated fats are considered essential because our body cannot make them but we must have them, therefore we

# Food Sources of Antioxidants

Vitamin A (beta-carotene and other carotenoids): dark- and vividly colored vegetables such as asparagus, beets, bell peppers, broccoli, carrots, collard and turnip greens, corn, kale, pumpkin, squash, spinach, and sweet potato; and fruits such as apricots, cantaloupe, dates, grapes, mangoes, nectarines, peaches, pink grapefruit, tangerines, tomatoes, and watermelon.

Vitamin C: bell peppers, berries, broccoli, Brussels sprouts, cantaloupe, cauliflower, grapefruit, honeydew, kale, kiwi, mangoes, nectarines, oranges, papaya, snow peas, sweet potato, strawberries, and tomatoes.

Vitamin E: bell peppers, broccoli, carrots, chard, mangoes, mustard and turnip greens, nuts, papaya, pumpkin, spinach, and sunflower seeds.

Alpha-lipoic acid: A healthy body makes enough alpha-lipoic acid, however, it is also found in red meat, organ meats (such as liver), and yeast (particularly Brewer's yeast), as well as dietary supplements.

Flavonoids: fruits, particularly darker fruits such as berries, cherries, citrus fruits, and red grapes; also beans, eggplant, greens onions, peppers, and tomatoes.

Lignans: flaxseeds and flaxseed oil, nuts and seeds, and whole grains.

Lycopene: grapefruit, red bell peppers, tomatoes, and watermelon. Lycopene in tomatoes is better absorbed into the body when it has been heated, as in cooked tomato products such as stewed tomatoes, tomato sauce, and tomato paste, which can be used to make sauces, soups, and chili.

Polyphenols: apples, cacao (chocolate), green tea, plums, prunes, popcorn, raisins, raw sugarcane, red grapes, and red wine.

Selenium: Brazil nuts, beef, poultry, tuna, and whole grains.

Squalene: amaranth seeds, olive oil, rice bran, and wheat germ.

have to get them from our food. And while we must avoid processed polyunsaturated vegetable oils at all costs, we absolutely must eat real, whole foods that contain these essential fats. Without them, we literally begin to die; virtually every cell function in the body shuts down and degenerative disease takes over.[21]

There are two essential fat groups in the polyunsaturated family: omega-3 and omega-6. It is the omega-3s that are truly the miracle workers. They are found in cold-water fish such as salmon, tuna, mackerel, and sardines; as well as walnuts, meat, and leafy green vegetables (once again, those leafy greens are loaded with nutrients). Of the meats, lamb has the most omega-3s. Flaxseeds, hemp seeds, and chia seeds also contain a high amount of omega-3s. Likewise, flaxseed oil and hemp seed oil are also excellent sources of omega-3s.

## The Amazing Health Benefits of Omega-3s

Omega-3s provide us with some amazing health benefits. They reduce plaque buildup in arteries, increase levels of HDL (the good cholesterol), and drastically reduce triglycerides. According to a study published in the medical journal *The Lancet,* researchers at Southampton University found that omega-3s stop the buildup of fatty deposits in arteries.[22] It has been said that omega-3s act like a Teflon coating in the blood vessels, preventing other fats from sticking. Omega-3s also keep our cell membranes fluid for optimum functioning, protect against stroke by preventing platelets from sticking together to form blood clots, lower blood pressure, inhibit erratic heartbeat (a primary factor in fatal heart attacks), allay the effects of attention-deficit disorder (ADD), eliminate osteoporosis, keep joints lubricated, discourage gout and arthritis, facilitate weight loss, and protect memory and brain function. A daily dose of omega-3 fats have also been shown to correct mood disorders such as depression and bipolar disease better than any known medication. Omega-3s have anti-inflammatory properties; in fact, all of my arthritic clients experience a relief in symptoms after adding the right amount of omega-3 fats to their overall healthy diet.

At this point, the classification of omega-3s gets a little confusing. Some omega-3s are short-chain fats and some are long-chain fats. The short-chain kind are found in plant foods such as flaxseeds, hemp seeds, and some green leafy vegetables. The long-chain ones are found in marine algae and in fish that eat the algae. When we eat short-chain omega-3s, they have to be converted in our body to the long-chain omega-3s for us to experience their amazing health benefits.

Long-chain omega-3s come in two forms: EPA (eicosapentaenoic acid) and DHA (docosahexaenoic acid). EPA is more involved in the functioning of the heart, whereas DHA is associated with brain function, but we need both. Fatty fish contain both EPA and DHA (though only about 20 percent of the fish's fat contains these two oils; the rest is saturated fat—another example of the perfection of whole foods. Remember, our body needs saturated fats to properly utilize the other fats in our diet, especially the all-important omega-3s. Omega-3 fats are better retained in the tissues when the diet is rich in saturated fats).

The neurological significance of omega-3s can hardly be overestimated. Omega-3s are one of the few substances that can cross the blood-brain barrier. The brain is close to 70 percent fat, so we're literally fatheads, and although it's in every cell in the body, most of the omega-3s are concentrated in the brain and the retina. To promote optimal brain function and visual acuity, we need a steady supply of omega-3s, which also increases blood flow (the brain gets 25 percent of the body's blood). Omega-3s have a profound role to play in Alzheimer's, dementia, memory loss, mood disorders, and a healthy nervous system.

## Woefully Deficient in Omega-3s, Grossly Abundant in Omega-6s

Most Americans are deficient in omega-3 fat, mainly because fish and leafy greens are no longer the staple foods they once were. Historically, humans obtained adequate amounts of omega-3 fats from eating cold-water fish and dark green, leafy vegetables on a regular basis. Today we get only about 125 milligrams of omega-3 fat per day, whereas our grandparents got 2,500 milligrams by taking a daily spoonful of cod liver oil (sometimes your grandmother made you take it, too!), a traditional practice that is nearly extinct in our modern times. For some reason back then, everyone knew it was good for us. The Japanese, who eat lots of fish and seaweed, have omega-3 levels about ten times higher than do most Americans.

## Table 5.1  Types of Fats

| Saturated | Monounsaturated | Polyunsaturated |
|---|---|---|
| **Animal Sources** | **Omega-9s** | **Omega-3s** |
| Beef, bison, wild game Lamb | Olives, extra-virgin olive oil Avocados | Fatty cold-water fish: salmon, mackerel, tuna, sardines |
| Pork (ham, bacon, sausage) | Almonds, almond butter Cashews | Fish oil |
| Milk | | Eggs (enriched) |
| Butter | Sesame seeds, unrefined sesame oil | Purslane (dark, leafy green used throughout Mediterranean countries) |
| Cheese | Peanuts, natural peanut butter, unrefined peanut oil | |
| Yogurt | | Pumpkin seeds (pepitas) |
| | Rice bran oil | Hemp seeds, hemp seed oil |
| **Plant Sources** | Hazelnuts | Flaxseeds, flaxseed oil |
| Coconut oil | Macadamia nuts | Chia seeds |
| Palm oil | Cocoa butter | Wheat germ (oil) |
| Cocoa butter | Rapeseeds, canola oil* | |
| | | **Omega-6s** |
| | | Black currant seed oil |
| | | Borage seed oil |
| | | Corn, corn oil* |
| | | Cottonseed oil* |
| | | Eggs (yolks) |
| | | Evening primrose oil |
| | | Grapeseed oil |
| | | Partially hydrogenated oil or hydrogenated oil (trans fats)* |
| | | Pine nuts (raw) |
| | | Pistachios (raw) |
| | | Poultry |
| | | Safflower oil* |
| | | Soybean oil* |
| | | Sunflower oil* |
| | | Sunflower seeds (raw) |
| | | Vegetable oil or shortening (usually a blend of soybean oil and canola oil)* |

*Typically sold or found in foods in a refined, nutrient-deficient form.

We usually get plenty of omega-6 fats; in fact, we get too many of them (mainly from those nasty processed vegetable oils found in most of our processed, fast, and restaurant foods). Omega-6 fats are also found in smaller amounts in whole foods such as eggs, whole grains, sunflower seeds, pumpkin seeds, sesame seeds, corn, soybeans, and other plant sources. Eating these foods in their natural form ensures that the oils contained within them are not oxidized.

Other not-so-well-known sources of omega-6 fats are evening primrose oil, black currant seed oil, and borage seed oil—usually only available in supplement form. These oils provide a good source of a type of omega-6 fat called gamma-linolenic acid (GLA), which has been used to help treat arthritis, allergies, multiple sclerosis, cancer, and PMS.

When we have too many omega-6s in our body, they have the opposite effect as the omega-3s. Research shows that an excess of omega-6 creates a disruption in the body that results in an increased tendency to blood clots, inflammation, high blood pressure, irritation of the digestive tract, depressed immune function, sterility, cancer, and weight gain.[23] Yet omega-6s are still essential; without them we die. As with the helpful qualities of GLA, omega-6s in general have some important functions in the body (such as blood clotting for wounds), but we have to make sure that we keep them in an ideal ratio with omega-3s.

## The Ideal Ratio of Omega-3s to Omega-6s

Good health requires the right ratio of omega-3 fats to omega-6 fats in the overall diet. The ideal ratio is about 1:1 omega-3 to omega-6, or the Japanese ratio of 2:1. However, the modern American eats a ratio of about 1:20 or 1:50, with way too much omega-6s and not enough omega-3s.[24]

Recent statistics indicate that nearly 99 percent of people in the United States do not eat enough omega-3 fat.[25] However, the symptoms of omega-3 deficiency are very vague, and can often be attributed to some other health conditions or nutrient deficiencies. The symptoms of omega-3 deficiency include fatigue, dry and/or itchy skin, brittle hair and nails, constipation, frequent colds, depression, poor concentration, lack of physical endurance, and/or joint pain. Chronic deficiency leads to more serious symptoms such as cancer, arthritis, heart disease, artherosclerosis, and type 2 diabetes. Studies have shown that consuming enough omega-3s and reducing consumption of omega-6s could prevent, treat, or reverse all of these health conditions.

Even if a person is taking in sufficient or even some omega-3s, sugar consumption, trans fats, and alcohol can interfere with the enzymes that convert the short-chain omega-3s into the useable long-chain omega-3s, creating an even greater deficiency. The recommended intake of omega-3s is 3,000 milligrams per day (the average American intake is 125 milligrams!). You can increase your intake of omega-3s by eating some of the recipes in this book, by eating cold-water fish several times each week, and through supplementation.

I recommend taking a high-quality supplement in addition to dietary sources of omega-3, to make sure you are getting enough. The absolute best source of omega-3 fat is fish or a pharmaceutical-grade fish oil or cod liver oil (it will say "pharmaceutical grade" on the label, meaning all toxins, such as heavy metals, have been safely removed from the oil without destroying the oil's healthful qualities). The second-best source is organic flaxseed oil with lignans (phytochemical compounds found in the fiber of flaxseeds that are effective in fighting breast cancer), about one tablespoon for every 100 pounds of body weight. Flaxseeds are also a good source, but it takes about ¼ cup of ground seeds to get the equivalent amount of omega-3 fat in one tablespoon of flaxseed oil or a piece of fish. I recommend a combination of oil and ground seeds.

## The Role of Omega-3s in Weight Loss

Omega-3 fats play an integral role in weight loss. At the very least, eating foods that contain omega-3 fat creates a feeling of satiety, meaning you feel full and satisfied for a longer period of time. A tablespoon of flaxseed oil or a capsule of fish oil will keep you feeling satiated for three to four hours. When you feel full, you don't snack between meals. However, more important, omega-3s work in a very unique way in regard to the effect on weight loss. Studies have shown that omega-3s burn fat even without a reduction in caloric intake.[26] Omega-3s promote circulation, so your fat-burning ability is enhanced because of increased blood flow to your muscles. Omega-3s also assist fat-transporting enzymes, enabling fat to be better used for energy. This is especially beneficial for liquefying and eliminating the stored hard fats often found in overweight people.

## Expeller-Pressed and Cold-Pressed Oils

It would seem that because polyunsaturated oils go rancid so quickly, they wouldn't be able to be pressed and bottled. However, some types of bottled oils are extracted from plants in ways that protect them. Natural oils are crushed from seeds or grains, using the hydraulic action of an expeller press. No heat is involved in the pressing and no chemical antioxidants are added to preserve the oils. The label will say "expeller pressed" on the front of the bottle.

Expeller pressing yields less oil than solvent extraction, usually 50 to 70 percent of the oil, so expeller-pressed oils are usually more expensive than conventionally processed oils. Because they are not preserved, they will have a shorter shelf life, but they are much healthier than commercially refined oils. The best oils are those made with health in mind. They come from organically grown seeds, are expeller pressed under protection from heat, light, and oxygen (i.e., cold pressed), and are packaged in tightly sealed glass bottles. Oils such as flaxseed oil, hemp seed oil, and wheat germ oil are packaged in this way, shipped in light-excluding boxes, and stored refrigerated. Oils made with this care are mostly found in health food stores. They should never be used for cooking.

I hope that this chapter has given you a true understanding of the important role fats play in your overall health and well-being. The Processed-Free Eating Plan will ensure that you are getting the right types of fat in the proper amounts. In addition to enjoying the wonderful flavor and satiety that fats provide, you will also experience glowing skin, pain-free joints, and loads of energy.

There is one type of fat I didn't include in this chapter because I felt it required separate mention. In the next chapter you will learn why trans fats are the real dietary demons and should never have been approved for human consumption.

## Ted's Story

In 2006 I was 15 pounds overweight and had developed high blood pressure. I was so upset at being put on several blood pressure medicines, because I knew of the potential negative effects they might have on my kidneys. I resolved to find a way to naturally lower my blood pressure and get off the medicine.

That was when I found out about Dee McCaffrey's Processed-Free Eating Plan. She laid out the science in layman's terms, and taught me how the food choices that I make impact not just my blood pressure, but also my metabolism. In fact, her plan is the only one that I have tried that got my metabolism working right.

Within three months of eliminating processed foods, my energy level increased and my blood pressure naturally decreased. I lost 15 pounds, and was able to go off all but one of the medications, which I now only take a very low dose for maintenance.

I've been on this plan for five years, and still have tons of energy—I am 67 years old and can still put in a twelve-hour workday. This is a plan that I take with me wherever I go, including bringing my own salad dressing to restaurants. My motto is, "Cook my own, carry my own." This plan is the kingpin for all of my food choices and food decisions. It is a program that works, no questions asked. Thank you, Dee, for my life-changing experience.

*—Ted Alber, age 67, carpet cleaner*

# The Worst Nutritional Disaster in History

*No problem can be solved in the same level of consciousness that created it.*

—ALBERT EINSTEIN

In the last chapter I discussed how the public scare over polyunsaturated corn and soy oils forced the food industry to come up with canola oil. Prior to the engineering of canola oil, the same type of twisted science led to the discovery of the first man-made solid fat—trans fat. Even though we got the bad news about this processed, artery-clogging stabilizer some time ago, it is still very prevalent in pantries all across the country. How have we allowed the worst nutritional disaster in history to happen?

Trans fats have been around since the turn of the twentieth century. In 1901, Wilhelm Norman, a German chemist, patented the process for changing a liquid oil into a solid fat. Thus was born the trans fat—a cheap and stable, chemically altered oil that provides yummy flavor and long shelf life to food products. The first trans-fat product, Crisco, was introduced in grocery stores in 1911. During the Second World War, butter rationing created a demand for margarine made from trans fats. As saturated fats were becoming unpopular, due to the "fat lies" surrounding them, the soy oil industry saw a chance to seize this strong market for itself. By the late 1980s, nearly all saturated fats in commercial food products had been replaced by trans fats made from soybean oil. The problem is, like high-fructose corn syrup and artificial sweeteners (and most everything else that food scientists come up with), trans fat is an artificial oil that our body doesn't recognize as food.[1]

## Quintessential Twisted Science

The method by which trans fats are created in a laboratory may seem like chemistry mumbo-jumbo, but here's the real skinny on why they're so bad for your body. Many of my clients and students have found the science very interesting and helpful as they've transitioned to a new way of eating.

Trans fats are made through a process called hydrogenation. Hydrogenation turns a polyunsaturated natural oil, which is normally liquid and fragile at room temperature, into a fat that is more solid and stable at room temperature. The result is an unnatural fat that looks, tastes, and behaves like the saturated fats—butter and tropical oils—it was designed to replace. Like saturated fats, trans fats will keep for a very long time, which is why cookies and baked goods such as Twinkies have such a long shelf life!

To produce trans fats, manufacturers begin with the cheapest oils—soy, corn, cottonseed, or canola, already rancid from the extraction process—and mix them with a metal catalyst, usually tiny metal particles of nickel oxide. This oil-nickel mixture is then subjected to hydrogen gas in a high-pressure, high-temperature reactor. Next, soaplike substances, called emulsifiers, and starch are squeezed into the mixture to give it a better consistency. The oil is yet again subjected to high temperatures, when it is steam-cleaned to remove its unpleasant odor. At this point, the color of the oil is an unappetizing gray (unbecoming of anything we'd want to spread on our toast), so the gray color is bleached away. Dyes and strong artificial flavors must then be added to the oil to make it look and taste like butter (they do such a good job of it that manufacturers were able to come up with such gimmicky names as I Can't Believe It's Not Butter!). Finally, the mixture is compressed and packaged in blocks or tubs, and for many years was sold as a healthy alternative to real butter![2]

## Choosy Mothers Should Not Choose Trans Fats

If you read the ingredient list of any packaged food, you won't see the term *trans fat*. Because the process of creating trans fats is called hydrogenation, the fats themselves are called hydrogenated oils, or partially hydrogenated oils. The most common phrases you'll see in ingredient lists are *partially hydrogenated soybean oil* and *partially hydrogenated cottonseed oil or safflower oil*. Vegetable shortenings and margarines are hydrogenated, so virtually all commercial baked goods such as cookies, crackers, breads, pastries, cake mixes, pancake mixes, dough mixes such as pizza dough and piecrusts, biscuits and rolls, and tortillas (even the whole wheat versions) contain trans fats. According to Dr. Mary Enig, a leading American lipid researcher, extensive studies of the food supply have found that the most trans fats turn up in sandwich cookies, vanilla wafers, animal crackers, and honey graham crackers—favorite treats for kids. Almost all frozen food includes partially hydrogenated oils, and microwave popcorn and movie popcorn are popped in trans fats. Even peanut butter, unless it is completely natural, contains trans fats.[3]

In her book *The Good Fat Cookbook*, an extensive exposé of the good and bad fats, Fran McCullough details the extent and pervasiveness of trans fats:

> Virtually all fake fat, from margarine and Olestra, to imitation cheese (processed cheese) to anything labeled "lite" or "fat-free," is loaded with trans fats. Powdered fats, such as the powdered milk that gets added back into skim and low-fat milk (to give it better color and flavor), or the powdered eggs that go into baked goods, belong in this category too. Another great source of trans fats are the artificial creamers that everyone adds to their coffee, the powdered ones and the liquid ones. The great irony, of course, is that we choose these products to protect our health, while the very act of consuming them jeopardizes it more than any other food we could eat, including pure sugar and pure natural fat. Dr. Mary Enig reports a claim that birds will not eat margarine; they're apparently much better at spotting potential toxins than we are, good canaries in the coal mine. Or possibly margarine just doesn't please the avian palate, as it shouldn't please ours.[4]

Prior to the 2006 FDA ruling that trans-fat counts be listed on nutrition fact panels, Americans were consuming 2,500 percent more of them than we did seventy-five years ago—a whopping statistic that applies to no other food, even sugar. Some researchers believe this fact alone accounts for the skyrocketing rates of heart disease and cancer.[5]

## It's Not Nice to Fool Mother Nature

Trans fats are even worse for you than the highly refined polyunsaturated vegetable oils from which they are made. The reason has to do with the chemical changes that occur during the hydrogenation process. As noted in the previous chapter, unsaturated fats have one or more double bonds. Before hydrogenation, at the site of the double bond, a pair of hydrogen atoms occur together on the same side of the double bond, causing the molecule to bend slightly. This is called the cis configuration.

The Latin prefixes *cis* and *trans* describe the orientation of the hydrogen atoms with respect to the double bond. *Cis* means "on the same side" and *trans* means "across" or "on the other side." The cis configuration is the one that generally occurs in nature and makes oils liquid at room temperature. The cis configuration can only be changed through a forced chemical reaction that breaks the double bond and rearranges the hydrogen atoms.

This forced chemical reaction is called hydrogenation. Under high temperatures, the nickel catalyst causes the hydrogen atoms to change position at the double bond: one hydrogen atom of the pair is moved to the other side so that the molecule straightens. This is called the trans configuration, a molecular structure rarely found in nature. Because of this change in configuration, the chemical properties of the trans fat are quite different from the chemical properties of the naturally occurring cis fat.

Trans fats resemble saturated fats because of their straight molecular shape and their being solid at room temperature. But that's about all that's similar about these two fats. First of all, a trans fat is *not* a saturated fat. Remember, saturated fats do not contain double bonds, whereas trans fats do. Second, saturated fats, though solid at room temperature, get broken down easily by body heat and do not stay hard at body temperature. They do not oxidize in the body and are not easily susceptible to becoming free radicals.

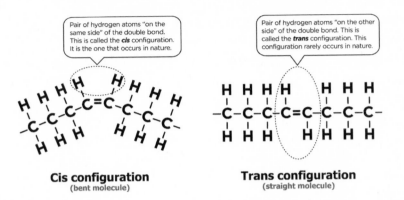

**Figure 6.1** Through the process of hydrogenation, the V shape of the naturally occurring cis fat is converted to a straight shaped trans fat. This changes the oil from a liquid to a solid and changes how it behaves in the body.

Trans fats, on the other hand, are so solid they can't be broken down by body heat, thus they stay very solid and hard once they get into our body. Our system doesn't quite know what to do with these fats, because it doesn't recognize their altered structure. They therefore become toxins to the body, but unfortunately our digestive system invites them in as if they were real fats. Instead of being rejected as toxins, trans fats are incorporated into our cell membranes as if they were natural cis fats. Because of their solid nature, trans fats make our cell membranes stiff and hard, whereas genuine cis fats allow our cell membranes to be supple and pliable.

## Wolves in Sheep's Clothing

Trans fats are like wolves in sheep's clothing because our cell membranes have V-shaped receptor sites that are specifically designed to accept the bent V shape of natural cis fats. When we eat natural cis fats, they fit nicely into those perfectly designed receptors. Once there, the cis fats act as conduits for nutrients and other substances to move into the cell for important biochemical reactions to occur. For example, glucose (blood sugar) is converted to energy on the inside of our cells. But the sugar has to be transported into the cell by way of the conduit—the cis fat. This occurs easily when natural cis fats occupy the receptor sites. When sugar is converted to energy inside the cell, it does not build up outside of the cell in the bloodstream, thus preventing high blood sugar that leads to diabetes.

However, because our body thinks the trans fats are real fats, these straight fats can actually force their way into the bent V-shaped receptor sites. But trans fats do not act like conduits; once they are incorporated into the cell membrane, they get stuck there because they don't fit properly. Unlike natural cis fats that allow nutrients to freely flow in and out of the cell, trans fats just block the receptor sites and nothing can get in, not even the good fats. It's kind of like when you have a key that looks like it's the right key for your keyhole. You can actually fit the key into your keyhole, but once you turn the key, it breaks off in the lock. Now you can't even get the right key into the keyhole because it is completely jammed up. That's what trans fats do to our cell membranes: they jam up the receptor sites and important body chemistry is completely disrupted. Glucose cannot be converted to energy, so it builds up in the bloodstream and eventually becomes diabetes. LDL cholesterol cannot get into the cells, so it builds up in the bloodstream and leads to high cholesterol levels and heart attacks. What's worse is that even when we are eating the good essential fats, they don't get utilized properly because the trans fats block them from being incorporated into the cells.

The blockage of cell receptor sites leads to many problems. Trans fats have now been implicated in cancer, heart disease, multiple sclerosis, and diverticulitis, among other diseases. Trans fats also interfere with the reproductive system, producing abnormal sperm and decreasing the amount of cream in human milk. They weaken the immune system and inhibit enzymes that metabolize toxic chemicals, carcinogens, and medications. They decrease the response of cells to insulin, setting the stage for insulin resistance and all the terrible things it brings in its wake, from obesity and diabetes (which are now epidemic in our country) to heart disease.[6]

There are a host of other problems with trans fats. When our body tries to metabolize them, our normal biochemistry is blocked and enzymes are inhibited from the natural production of our body's own fatty acids (remember, our body can produce its own saturated and monounsaturated fats).

Trans fats also affect our body's electrical circuitry. The cis fats are necessary for electrical and energy exchanges that involve proteins, oxygen, and light. These electrical currents are responsible for all body functions, from the way our mind works to our heartbeat, cell division, muscle coordination, and energy levels. Trans fats are not suitable for these processes and jam the route needed by the cis fats.

Trans fats are stickier than cis fats, increasing the likelihood of a clot in a small blood vessel—causing strokes, heart attacks, or circulatory occlusions in other organs, such as lungs, extremities, and sense organs. Our heart uses fatty acids as its main fuel source. Trans fats are less easily broken down by enzymes and have slower use as an energy source, which could have serious consequences in a high-stress situation. Trans fats also interfere with our liver's detoxification pathways. They're just bad news all around!

## Zero Grams Trans Fat Not Necessarily True

To escape the havoc trans fats play in our body, our best defense is to avoid them like the plague. We need to eliminate them as much as possible from our diet by avoiding margarines, vegetable shortening, fried foods (especially French fries), and other obvious sources such as commercially popped popcorn and foods cooked in oil. *You must read every ingredient label,* looking for "hydrogenated oil," "partially hydrogenated oil," "soybean oil," and "canola oil" (remember that even liquid canola oil contains trans fats). Never buy anything labeled "lite," "low calorie," or "fat free."

In 2006, the FDA tried to help us out by making it mandatory for food manufacturers to list on their nutrition fact panel the amount of trans fat in their products. As usual the FDA didn't go far enough. A manufacturer is only required to list trans fats if the food contains 0.5 gram (half a gram) or more per serving. Therefore, if a serving contains 0.4 grams, it does not have to be listed on the nutrition fact panel. This misleads the unsuspecting consumer into thinking that the product does not contain trans fats. The tricky food industry even boasts claims on the front of the packaging of "0 grams trans fat," but if you read the ingredients and still see "hydrogenated oil" listed, the product is not trans fat free.

Before the FDA approved the requirement of listing trans fats on nutrition fact panels, it asked the Institute of Medicine (a branch of the National Academy of Sciences) to prepare a report. Three years later, in July 2002, the institute declared that *there is no safe level of trans fats in the diet.* You have to realize that trans fats act on a cellular level and are harmful even in tiny amounts, even less than 0.5 gram per serving (most people eat more than one serving of processed foods anyway, so those partial grams of trans fats can add up to anywhere from 1 to 5 grams). Any amount of trans fat, no matter how minute, will jam up the receptor sites in our cell membranes, making our cells hard and stiff. Dr. Walter Willett, professor of epidemiology at Harvard School of Public Health, has called the introduction of trans fats into the food supply "the worst food-processing disaster in human history."

The good news is that by eating processed-free you can completely eliminate trans fats from your life. No recipe or food product recommended in this book contains trans fats!

## 0 Grams Trans-Fat Crisco?

When the J. M. Smucker Co. bought the Crisco brand in 2002, its scientists went to work on finding a way to convert the original product to one with zero trans fat. In 2004, the company produced a limited-edition zero trans product, but wasn't able to produce it in quantities that would meet customer demands. Most important, the reformulated shortening didn't provide the same qualities of tenderness and flakiness in baked goods as the original.

After tinkering with the kinds of soy oil and cottonseed oil that wouldn't raise saturated fat levels, Crisco with zero trans fat is now available in supermarkets. Just as with the original, the reformulated Crisco is marketed in butter flavor, sticks, and 1- and 2-pound cans. The ingredient list on the reformulated Crisco reads as follows: Soybean oil, *fully hydrogenated palm oil, partially hydrogenated palm and soybean oils,* mono and diglycerides, THBQ and citric acid. Apparently the amount of hydrogenated oil is less than 0.5 grams of trans fat per serving, which is allowed under FDA guidelines. The serving size on the nutrition fact panel indicates that one tablespoon constitutes a serving. Although it will never be revealed, I would be willing to bet that each tablespoon contains 0.499 grams of trans fat.

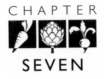
# Food Chemistry Gone Mad

*Fake food—I mean those patented substances chemically flavored and mechanically bulked out to kill the appetite and deceive the gut—is unnatural, almost immoral, a bane to good eating and good cooking.*

—JULIA CHILD

The discovery of sodium lauryl sulfate in my angel food cake mix back in 1989 set me on a path to find out what else is in the foods most Americans eat each day, and the effect they have on our health. As an environmental chemist, I was unaware that there was a whole other world of chemistry devoted entirely to making food additives. In fact, a food chemist's main job responsibility is to concoct new chemicals for the purpose of preserving, developing, or improving foods and beverages. Going by the average salary of a food chemist these days ($71,000 per year in 2011, according to simply hired.com), I would say that the food additive industry is a very big business. Even in my long career as a chemist working to clean up the environment, my salary never reached such a comfortable level.

The more I learn about food additives and their effects on human health, the harder it is for me to wrap my brain around how this kind of science even exists. It's one thing to use the principles of chemistry to preserve foods

131

the way our not-so-distant ancestors did, by pickling with vinegar, using salt to preserve meats and fish, adding herbs and spices to improve flavor, or culturing, as with yogurt and buttermilk. But what we do to our foods these days is food chemistry gone mad. With the proliferation of processed foods in the second half of the twentieth century, thousands of synthetic additives have been introduced into our foods. The FDA maintains a list of over three thousand ingredients in its database titled "Everything Added to Food in the United States." Some of these items are recognizable ingredients such as sugar, baking soda, and spices, but the majority of them are synthetic chemical concoctions.

The testing for the safety of these chemicals is usually funded or performed by the company that wants to produce the chemicals or to use the chemical additives in the foods they produce. This is why the studies on chemical additives are often biased and unchallenged. Back in 1958, food additive laws prohibited any additives (including pesticides) that were proven to cause cancer in humans or animals from being added to our food. However, economic pressure from industries caused the FDA to relax these standards and now allows some cancer-causing and otherwise harmful substances through. For instance, pesticides are no longer subject to food additive laws and may be used on foods without undergoing the same type of testing required for other food additives.

You may find the information in this chapter disturbing, and I hope you do. The subject of food additives and their effects on human health is one of the most disturbing things I deal with every day in my work as a food educator. Knowing what's in your food and how it affects your body is the single most important factor in getting and staying skinny. Our fifth Law of Skinny Science states that food additives don't honor how our body is designed; they are catalysts for poor health and should be avoided. To avoid the most harmful food additives, you need to be educated and aware of what's in your food, and stop relying on the government to keep you safe.

## Generally Regarded as Safe?

It seems that every week we're hearing about the dangers of food additives or chemicals found in other products such as sunscreens and cosmetics. In March 2011, the FDA held hearings on the safety of artificial food colorings

(Blue 1, Blue 2, Green 3, Orange B, Red 3, Red 40, Yellow 5, and Yellow 6), after the Center for Science in the Public Interest (CSPI) petitioned to have them removed from the nation's food supply. They were banned in the United Kingdom in 2008 after researchers at the University of Southampton concluded that specific mixtures of artificial colors increase hyperactivity in children. Other studies have shown that they are carcinogenic and contribute to visual disorders and nerve damage. But the FDA failed to make a definitive ruling—stating that there was not enough evidence to ban the additives. This was a huge blow to CSPI, and to the thousands of parents, consumers, and advocates who signed the petition.

The FDA has taken a similar ambiguous stance on Bisphenol-A (BPA), a chemical that is often used in clear, shatterproof plastics, such as baby bottles and food-storage containers, as well as the liners of metal food cans. Studies have shown BPA can leach from plastic and cans into food, and according to the U.S. Centers for Disease Control, 93 percent of Americans have detectable levels of BPA in their body. Dozens of laboratory studies have also linked BPA exposure to breast and prostate cancer, infertility, early puberty in girls, obesity, and attention deficit hyperactivity disorder.[1]

Despite this mounting evidence, these chemicals, and hundreds of others, remain on the FDA's Generally Regarded as Safe (GRAS) list, the system that the agency uses to regulate food additives. However, this system is not effective. Just because an additive makes it onto this elite list, *it is not a guarantee that the additive is safe.* According to Dr. Michael Hansen, a senior scientist at Consumers Union, many additives in our food supply are never even tested. That's because the GRAS designation is a voluntary process—instead of being required to register food additives, companies may notify the FDA about their product, but only if they so choose. He states that even for those additives considered GRAS, he doesn't have much faith in the designation.[2] Neither does the Government Accountability Office (GAO). In February 2010, the GAO released a scathing report that the FDA is not systematically ensuring the continued safety of current GRAS substances.[3]

The FDA evaluates additives based on only whether they cause cancer and harmful reproductive effects. The FDA *does not* evaluate other harmful reactions or outcomes from ingesting a food additive, such as migraines, weight gain, or neurological disorders such as attention deficit disorder. A number of additives that were once on the GRAS list have been removed *after they were found to be harmful.* Due to the fact that most additives are toxic, it is a virtual certainty that some additives that are now being commonly used in foods and are considered to be safe will be taken off the GRAS list at some point in the future. Furthermore, additives that are individually safe may be harmful in combination with other additives. Testing for additive safety is performed for individual additives only, not for combinations of additives. However, this is an antiquated system of regulation, as it is rare that any food has only one additive in it. The effects on human health of the many different additives used in the thousands of different combinations are unknown. As yet, no study has determined this number nor has looked at what the effects of the various combinations might be.

In 2007, the International Food Additives Council estimated that each person consumes 14 pounds of food additives per year.[4] If you include sugar and salt—the food-processing industry's most used additives—the number jumps to over 160 pounds a year, with some people possibly eating considerably more.[5]

There have been many adverse effects attributed to the consumption of food additives, from minor complaints such as sleepiness, lethargy, eczema, dermatitis, nausea, vomiting, diarrhea, allergies, and migraines, to more serious conditions such as irritable bowel syndrome, hyperactivity and other behavioral disorders, lupus, MS, Parkinson's, Alzheimer's, and cancer.

Just how many chemicals do you think people are exposed to every day? I've got some numbers for you. Based on what I've seen in my client's food journals, people eating processed and packaged foods are unknowingly consuming high amounts. A client will typically report eating cereal with fat-free milk for breakfast, yogurt for a snack, and a sandwich from a deli for lunch. While this might seem fairly harmless, here's what it really looks like based on the ingredients found in some popular "healthy" versions of these items:

One serving of Kellogg's Fiber Plus Antioxidants Berry Yogurt Crunch contains more than thirteen different additives, preservatives, and food dyes, including Red 40 and Blue 1, which are known to cause allergic reactions in some people and mutations leading to cancer in lab animals. It also contains BHT, monoglycerides, and cellulose gum. In addition, conventional milk often contains residues of artificial bovine growth hormones, which are known endocrine disruptors, as well as antibiotics used in industrial milk production.

Dannon Light & Fit fruit-flavored yogurt contains more than eleven different additives, including Red 40, aspartame, potassium sorbate, sucralose, and acesulfame potassium.

A deli sandwich of turkey and cheese on nine-grain bread with fat-free honey mustard, peppers, and pickles contains more than forty different additives, preservatives, and dyes. The pickles and peppers have Yellow 5 and polysorbate 80; the bread has ten different additives, including dough conditioners, DATEM (diacetyl tartaric [acid] ester of monoglyceride), and sodium stearoyl lactylate; and the turkey contains ten additives as well.

The person in this example has consumed more than sixty food additives by eating breakfast, a small snack, and lunch alone, to say nothing of dinner, dessert, further snacking, and drinks. Based on other food records I've analyzed, it is not uncommon that people are consuming up to one hundred or more food additives a day.[6]

If this looks like a typical day for you, you'll want to start paying attention to the ingredient lists on the foods you're eating. The lists may look surreal. Have you ever seen "diacetyl tartaric (acid) ester of monoglyceride" on the label of *your* loaf of bread? Sounds like something you'd find in a degreaser, not food. It's an emulsifier primarily used in baking to strengthen the dough. It is used in crusty breads, such as rye bread with a springy, chewy texture, as well as biscuits, jars of salsa con queso, and dressings. I don't know about you, but when I make my own bread and salad dressings, I don't add DATEM.

## The Most Egregious Food Additives

While it's not realistic to think that you can lead a completely preservative and additive-free life, you can certainly avoid the most egregious ones that have been found to cause some very serious health issues. You should become familiar with the names of some of the most common food additives and their documented health effects on humans. In her book *Food Additives: A Shopper's Guide to What's Safe & What's Not*, author Christine Hoza Farlow classifies over a thousand commonly used food additives according to safety, whether they may cause allergic reactions, and if they are Generally Regarded as Safe (GRAS) by the FDA.

In addition to the sweeteners mentioned in Chapter 4, and the partially hydrogenated oils (trans fats) mentioned in Chapter 6, the following is a short list of some of the ingredients you need to look out for.

## Artificial Flavorings

The Food and Drug Administration does not require the companies that carefully manufacture flavor additives to disclose the ingredients that are in their product, as long as the chemicals used are "generally regarded as safe." There are often more ingredients in the artificial flavoring than in the processed food that it is made for! I suppose it's an easy way for the food manufacturers to save space on the packaging. If they had to list all the chemicals in a typical artificial flavoring, they wouldn't have enough room! Here's what's in "artificial strawberry flavoring," something you might find in a strawberry-flavored Pop-Tart or milkshake:

amyl acetate, amyl butyrate, amyl valerate, anethol, anisyl formate, benzyl acetate, benzyl isobutyrate, butyric acid, cinnamyl isobutyrate, cinnamyl valerate, cognac essential oil, diacetyl, dipropyl ketone, ethyl acetate, ethyl amyl ketone, ethyl butyrate, ethyl cinnamate, ethyl heptanoate, ethyl heptylate, ethyl lactate, ethyl methylphenyglycidate, ethyl nitrate, ethyl propionate, ethyl valerate, heliotropin, hydroxy-phenyl-2-butanone (10 percent solution in alcohol), a-ionone, isobutyl anthranilate, isobutyl butyrate, lemon essential oil, maltol, 4-methylacetophenone, methyl anthranilate, methyl benzoate, methyl cinnamate, methyl heptine carbonate, methyl maphthyl ketone, methyl salicylate, mint essential oil, neroli essential oil, nerolin, neryl isobutyrate, orris butter, phenethyl alcohol, rose, rum ether, g-undecalactone, vanillin and solvent. [7]

Yep, we call the fruits of this mad science *food*. Something's not right here.

## Monosodium Glutamate (MSG)

One of the most common and harmful food additives is monosodium glutamate (MSG). It has been called the nicotine of food additives because, in addition to its harmful effects on the body, it is highly addictive. Comprised of sodium and glutamic acid, MSG is a flavor enhancer that triggers our taste buds and makes us eat more and eat faster. Nearly every fast-food and chain restaurant uses MSG in some form, and it is added to thousands of prepared and processed foods. The foods that contain the most MSG are processed fat free and sugar free, mainly because when fat and sugar are absent, the food is nearly flavorless, so MSG is added to enhance its flavor.

Use of MSG has doubled every decade since it was first introduced to the United States in the 1940s, and in 2001, 3 billion pounds were manufactured. It is used in hospitals, nursing homes, school cafeterias, and everywhere else food is served. MSG is found in everything from ketchup, soups, and mashed potatoes to chips and ice cream. Most sauces, dressings, canned soups, and seasoning products such as bouillon and broth contain MSG or free glutamic acid, a similar product. It is the main ingredient in additives clumped under the term *seasonings* on food labels.[8]

MSG belongs to a class of compounds called excito-toxins, meaning it upsets the delicate balance of various chemicals in the brain that help regulate many functions. Specifically, it affects the normal appetite mechanism that controls how much we eat. It excites and stimulates our taste buds, fooling our brain to think the food tastes better than it actually does. This allows food manufacturers to use cheaper ingredients while helping the lower-quality food seem to taste good. Because MSG affects the mechanism in our brain that tells us to stop eating, we eat far beyond our normal stopping point. The substance is also known to be toxic.

The effects of MSG were first documented in 1968 when a Chinese doctor developed numbness, tingling, and tightness in his chest after eating in certain Chinese restaurants. This is why so many Chinese and other restaurants now boast that they don't use MSG. But don't be fooled by those claims. While the restaurant may not *add* any MSG to their food, if it is using prepared items (as most restaurants do) such as sauces, egg rolls, dressings, and broths, then its food will still contain plenty of MSG.

## MSG Causes Headaches and Obesity

Another common MSG-related symptom is a headache that feels like a tight band around the head. But the most alarming effect of MSG is its link to obesity. Scientists have observed that animals fed glutamic acid become grotesquely obese.[9] No strain of rat or mice is naturally obese, so in laboratories scientists feed MSG to them to induce obesity and prediabetes. The MSG triples the amount of insulin the pancreas creates, causing rats to become obese; the researchers even have a title for the race of fat rodents they create: MSG-Treated Rats.

When the rats eat foods containing MSG, they eat more than they need to. If the lab rats are getting grotesquely obese from eating MSG, doesn't it make sense that humans are too?

## Hidden MSG

The real scary thing about MSG is that it can be hidden in nearly forty other food additives. When food chemists make their concoctions to enhance flavors and textures, MSG is one of the ingredients they use to make new compounds. If an additive contains less than 79 percent MSG, the FDA does not require food manufacturers to list it as an ingredient—they only need to list the name of the "new" ingredient that contains MSG. So, for example, an additive could contain up to 78 percent MSG, and you would never know there was MSG in the food. But smart scientists and other food detectives have caught on to this, and have figured out which additives contain high percentages of MSG. Following is a list of other additives that contain plenty of MSG:

| | |
|---|---|
| "Anything" hydrolyzed | Isolated soy protein |
| Autolyzed yeast | Maltodextrin |
| Bouillon, stocks, and broths | Natural flavorings |
| Calcium caseinate | Seasonings |
| Gelatin | Sodium caseinate |
| Hydrolyzed soy protein | Textured soy protein |
| Hydrolyzed yeast | Yeast extract |

It's important to point out here that there is no strict regulation on the word *natural,* and food manufacturers use it liberally, especially on patented ingredients such as "natural flavorings" (see next section).

## Natural Flavors vs. Natural Flavorings

When reading an ingredient list, you may see the words "natural flavors" or "natural flavorings." What's the difference between the two? The term *natural flavors* is often used interchangeably with the term *extract*. A natural flavor or extract is generally made from a natural ingredient; for example, natural lemon flavor or lemon extract is made from lemon oil, and natural vanilla flavor or pure vanilla extract is made from real vanilla beans. The term *natural flavoring* refers to substances that are made in a laboratory that have the same or similar chemical formulas and flavors as a natural food, but are not derived from real foods as extracts are. They cannot contain any substances that are also contained in artificial flavorings.

The way natural flavorings are made reminds me of my first-year college chemistry course where we "made" aspirin in the laboratory. By our mixing different chemicals together, the end product after the chemical reaction was a white crystalline compound called acetylsalicylic acid (aspirin), which is chemically similar to salicylic acid, a compound found in the bark of white willow trees. So basically, it doesn't actually come from a natural source, it just looks and tastes as if it did. Our not-so-distant ancestors would brew the bark of the white willow tree to make a tea that could be drunk to relieve pain, the same way we take aspirin today. Aspirin is the "natural flavoring" version of the compound naturally found in the white willow bark.

## Sodium Benzoate

Derived from benzoic acid, sodium benzoate is used as a preservative by the carbonated drinks industry to prevent mold in soft drinks. Peter Piper, a professor of molecular biology and biotechnology at Sheffield University who is considered an expert in aging, conducted research to examine the effect of sodium benzoate on the mitochondria DNA in cells. After testing the effect of sodium benzoate on living yeast cells in his laboratory, Professor Piper reported,

> These chemicals have the ability to cause severe damage to DNA in the mitochondria to the point that they totally inactivate it: they knock it out altogether. The mitochondria consumes the oxygen needed to produce energy

and if it is damaged—as happens in a number of diseased states—then the cell starts to malfunction very seriously. There are now a whole array of diseases that are being tied to this type of damaged DNA—Parkinson's and a host of neurodegenerative diseases, but above all the whole process of aging.[10]

## Sodium Nitrates and Sodium Nitrites

Nitrates and nitrites are found mainly in processed meats such as hot dogs, bacon, bologna, salami, and other packaged or canned meats such as SPAM and corned beef hash. Their primary purpose is to prevent botulism and to improve color and flavor.

Unfortunately, these additives have been shown to cause cancer. In 1995, a petition was brought before the FDA requesting the agency to require a cancer risk warning on packages of hot dogs that contain nitrites. The grounds for this petition were alarming: scientific information on excess risks of childhood brain tumors and leukemia have been linked to the consumption of hot dogs—specifically hot dogs containing nitrite preservatives.

Recent case-control studies have confirmed the risks of cancer from consumption of hot dogs. Eating many hot dogs, as well as maternal hot-dog consumption while the children were in utero, has been shown to be associated with brain cancer and leukemia in children. The Cancer Research Center of Hawaii and the University of Southern California reported in the *Journal of the National Cancer Institute* that they studied 190,000 people, aged 45 to 75, for seven years. Those who ate the most processed meat (bacon, ham, cold cuts) had a 68 percent higher risk of pancreatic cancer than did those who ate the least. More recently nitrites have been linked to lung disease.

The USDA tried to ban sodium nitrite in the 1970s, but was preempted by the meat processing industry, which relies on the ingredient as a color fixer to make foods look more visually appealing. Sodium nitrite is found everywhere, in foods served at school and hospital cafeterias to literally thousands of different menu items at fast-food restaurants and dining establishments. The use of this ingredient is widespread and it's part of the reason we're seeing skyrocketing rates of cancer in every society that consumes large quantities of processed meats.

When you are in the store, look for nitrite- and nitrate-free hot dogs and meat products, which are far healthier alternatives. The other alternative is to cook your own chicken and turkey to use for lunchmeats. When you make it yourself, you are guaranteed that it isn't prepared with sodium nitrite.

## Acesulfame K (Acesulfame Potassium)

This additive is a high-potency artificial sweetener. It is about two hundred times sweeter than sugar, and is typically used together in products with sucralose (another toxic additive). Even when compared to aspartame and saccharin (which are afflicted with their own safety problems), acesulfame K is the worst. In the 1970s, the FDA based its approval on tests of acesulfame K that fell short of the agency's own standards. Two studies carried out in rats and one in mice indicated that the additive might cause cancer in lab animals, which means it may increase cancer risk in humans. It may also cause blood sugar attacks and has been shown to elevate cholesterol in lab animals. In addition, large doses of acetoacetamide, a breakdown product, have been shown to affect the thyroid in rats, rabbits, and dogs.[11]

In 1996, the CSPI urged the FDA to require better testing before permitting acesulfame K in soft drinks. That request was not followed. In July 1998, the FDA allowed this chemical to be used in soft drinks and supplements such as protein powders, thereby greatly increasing consumer exposure.

## Artificial Colorings

Most artificial colorings are synthetic chemicals that do not occur in nature. They are used almost exclusively in processed foods, particularly candy, soda pop, breakfast cereals, gelatin desserts, and others. Studies show that artificial colors may be carcinogenic and may contribute to learning disorders, visual disorders, and nerve damage. In addition to the dyes' causing other problems, recent studies show colorings cause hyperactivity in some sensitive children.[12]

The following health risks are associated with the following artificial colors. The CSPI's 2011 petition to remove them from the nation's food supply was rejected by the FDA in March of that same year.

Blue 1 (FD&C Blue No. 1): One (unpublished) animal test suggested a small cancer risk, and a test-tube study indicated the dye might affect neurons. It also causes occasional allergic reactions (itching) and low blood pressure. The additive has not been adequately tested.[13]

Blue 2 (FD&C Blue No. 2): Animal studies found some—but not conclusive—evidence that Blue 2 causes brain cancer in male rats, but the FDA concluded that there is "reasonable certainty of no harm."[14]

Green 3 (FD&C Green No. 3): A 1981 industry-sponsored study gave hints of bladder and testes tumors in male rats, but the FDA reanalyzed the data, using other statistical tests, and concluded that this dye was safe. Fortunately, this possibly carcinogenic dye is not widely used.[15]

Orange B: This artificial food dye was approved only for use in sausage casings. Studies show that high doses of this dye are harmful to the liver and bile duct. Thankfully Orange B has not been used for many years, but consumption of it in the past may still have lingering effects in the body.[16]

Red 3 (FD&C Red No. 3): According to a 1983 review committee report requested by the FDA, there is "convincing" evidence that this dye caused thyroid tumors in rats. The agency recommended banning the dye, but that recommendation was overruled. Red 3 was formerly used as the red color in maraschino cherries, but it has been replaced by the Red 40 dye. It is still used in a small selection of foods ranging from frostings to fruit roll-ups and chewing gum.[17]

Red 40 (FD&C Red No. 40): Although Red 40 is one of the most-tested food dyes, the key mouse tests were flawed and inconclusive. An FDA review committee acknowledged problems, but said evidence of harm was not "consistent" or "substantial."[18]

Yellow 5 (FD&C Yellow No. 5): This is the second-most widely used food dye. It causes hay fever reactions, primarily in aspirin-sensitive persons, gastrointestinal upset, and skin rashes. It has also been shown to trigger hyperactivity in some children. It may be contaminated with such cancer-causing substances as benzidine and 4-aminobiphenyl (or chemicals that the body converts to those substances).[19]

Yellow 6 (FD&C Yellow No. 6): This is the third-most widely used food dye. Animal tests indicated that this dye causes tumors of the adrenal glands and kidneys. It, too, may be contaminated with such cancer-causing substances as benzidine and 4-aminobiphenyl (or chemicals that the body converts to those substances). The FDA reviewed those data and found reasons to conclude that Yellow 6 does not pose a significant cancer risk to humans. Yellow 6 may cause occasional, but sometimes-severe hyper-sensitivity reactions. The CSPI still petitioned to have it banned from the food supply.[20]

Authorities in the United Kingdom banned six of these eight artificial colors, in response to research linking the consumption of those additives and hyperactive behavior. Since the ban was enacted, the food industry has responded positively, replacing banned colors with natural pigments in products. However, many of these same products are still sold in the United States using the original artificial food colors.

You can buy natural food dyes in health food stores to use in your recipes. India Tree Natural makes food coloring from highly concentrated vegetable pigments.

## BHA, BHT, and TBHQ (Fake Antioxidants)

BHA stands for butylated hydroxyanisole; and BHT, for the related compound butylated hydroxytoluene. Both are synthetic (man-made) compounds that are often added to foods to preserve fats and prolong shelf life. They are called antioxidants because they retard the chemical reaction that occurs when fats, oils, and oil-containing foods are exposed to air. That chemical reaction is called oxidation.

It would be one thing to add chemicals into foods for the sole purpose of prolonging shelf life—but now food manufacturers are taking advantage of the good reputation the term *antioxidant* has earned in recent years by making claims on their packaging that target and fool unsuspecting consumers into thinking these foods actually contain healthy antioxidants. This is a prime example of how food manufacturers twist the definition of chemistry terms and present these wolves in sheep's clothing to the public.

BHA and BHT are used in bacon, baked goods, breakfast bars, candy, canned fruits and vegetables, cream and creamers, fried foods, gelatin desserts, margarine, roasted nuts, peanut butter, powdered soups, salad dressings, shortening, spices, whipped topping, chewing gum, potato chips, the ubiquitous ingredient "vegetable oil," and foods containing artificial color or flavor. These fake antioxidants prevent the color, flavor, or texture changes that occur when foods are exposed to air. You may also find it disturbing (I know I did) that these same chemicals are also used for the same purposes in cosmetics, pharmaceutical drugs, rubber and petroleum products, jet fuels, and embalming fluids.

TBHQ stands for tert-butylhydroquinone. It's a white, crystalline solid used as a general-purpose chemical to preserve various oils, fats, and food items by retarding their oxidative deterioration. It is also used in formulating varnish, lacquer, resins and oil field additives, and is used as a fixative in perfumes to reduce the evaporation rate and improve stability.

Wow, with so many uses, one must wonder how safe any of these three substances are for human consumption!

What these food additives *do not* do is act like the antioxidants that come from real, whole plant foods. In fact, they do the exact opposite. The International Agency for Research on Cancer considers BHA and BHT carcinogenic (cancer causing). Repeated studies agree, as well as demonstrate that BHA and BHT accumulate in body tissue, cause liver enlargement, and retard cell development.[21] They may also cause hives and other skin reactions. TBHQ has not been adequately tested, yet has still been approved for food use.

Some experts believe that consumption of BHT can cause metabolism problems leading to behavioral changes. Dr. Benjamin Feingold, a diet specialist in the 1970s, stated from his studies that BHT could produce hyperactivity in children. In light of this, isn't it interesting that many of the foods that are mainly consumed by children, including breakfast cereals, convenient lunchbox meals, and snack foods, all contain BHA and BHT?

Author and doctor Christine Hoza Farlow states in her book *Food Additives: A Shopper's Guide to What's Safe & What's Not*, that BHA and BHT can cause liver and kidney damage, behavioral problems, infertility, weakened immune system, birth defects, and cancer. Infants, young children, pregnant women, and those sensitive to aspirin should avoid them. My opinion is that everyone should avoid them.

BHT has been banned in England. It has also been banned in Romania, Sweden, Australia, and nearly every other country except for the United States. This makes one wonder why, if a substance is questionable enough to be banned in other countries, is it still used by most major cereal companies in America and why it also shows up in many other processed foods, especially those that are marketed to children?

## Sodium Lauryl Sulfate

I couldn't end this section without telling you what I learned about the chemical I used in my lab and that also showed up in my angel food cake mix. Sodium lauryl sulfate (SLS) is a detergent. Like BHA, BHT, and TBHQ, sodium lauryl sulfate has many different uses, mainly in products that require nice, foaming suds. It is found in cosmetics, shampoos, bubble baths, shaving creams, toothpastes, soaps, dish and laundry detergents, and cleaning products. In higher concentrations it is found in engine degreasers, garage floor cleaners, and car-wash soaps. In foods, it is used as a thickener and a whipping aid in powdered eggs, liquid egg whites, frozen egg whites, and egg white solids (hence, it shows up on the ingredient lists of angel food cake mixes); it's also in the gelatin that is used to make marshmallows.

You may have heard that sodium lauryl sulfate is natural because it is derived from coconut oil. That is like saying Splenda is natural because it comes from sugar. The lauric acid in coconut oil is only a starting point for a multistep chemical process using many caustic chemicals. Although sodium lauryl sulfate has been deemed safe by the FDA, studies have shown that it has harmful effects on the body and is a potential cancer risk. However, most of the studies have been done on its use in personal care products, rather than as a food additive.

A report in the *Journal of the American College of Toxicology* (ACT)[22] listed many concerns about sodium lauryl sulfate, namely that cancer-causing compounds called nitrosamines can form during its manufacture. Nitrosamines can also be formed when sodium lauryl sulfate reacts with other compounds being used in the same product containing it. Although sodium lauryl sulfate is not carcinogenic in experimental studies, it has been shown that it causes severe changes in the area of the skin where it is applied, indicating a need for more testing. Other studies have indicated that once sodium lauryl sulfate is absorbed through the skin, it enters the cells of the heart, liver, lungs and brain, and remains there for long periods of time. The ACT report questions whether sodium lauryl sulfate poses a serious potential health threat from its use in cleansers, shampoos, and toothpastes.[23]

Because of these concerns and the lack of adequate research, many personal care product companies are choosing not to use sodium lauryl sulfate, and health-conscious consumers are seeking out this safer merchandise.

## Additives with No Known Toxicity

Learning about all the nasty food additives may seem overwhelming, but there is some good news: not all food additives are dangerous. Aside from acceptable ingredients such as sea salt, baking soda, vinegar, and spices, here are a few of the good ones.

### Annatto

Annatto is produced from the reddish pulp which surrounds the seed of the achiote and is used to produce a red food coloring. It is used in cheese (Cheddar and Red Leicester), margarine, butter, rice, smoked fish, and custard powder. Annatto is commonly found in Latin American and Caribbean cuisines as both a coloring agent and for flavoring. Central and South American natives used the seeds to make a body paint, and it is used as a lipstick. For this reason, the achiote is sometimes called the lipstick tree. In Venezuela, annatto (locally called *onoto*) is used in the preparation of *hallacas, perico,* and other traditional dishes.

### Arrowroot

Derived from the root of a South American plant, arrowroot can be used as a thickener in place of cornstarch (a processed refined carbohydrate).

### Beta-carotene—Vitamin A

Beta-carotene is used as a coloring and a nutrient supplement. The body converts it to vitamin A, which aids in the light-detection mechanism of the eye and helps maintain the normal condition of mucous membranes. Large amounts of beta-carotene in supplements have posed risks to some people, but small amounts used as food additives are safe.

## Coconut Oil, Nonhydrogenated Palm Oil

These are excellent stable oils that help extend the shelf life of foods and also help the body metabolize fatty acids. They've historically been used in the food industry with no known toxicity prior to their replacement by trans fats. Make sure only nonhydrogenated forms of these oils are listed on ingredient lists.

## Oligofructose (Fructooligosaccharide, or FOS)

This is a soluble fiber found in a variety of common plants, fruits, and vegetables. Although it may be extracted from any of these sources, the most common source used in supplements is derived from chicory root, due to its naturally high FOS concentration. This ingredient is commonly used as an "artificial" sweetener because FOS is sweet to the taste but the body cannot utilize its calorie content.

## Inulin

This is a fructooligosaccharide derived from chicory roots and is used as a fiber and bulking agent As a prebiotic, inulin stimulates the growth of friendly and healthy intestinal bacteria, which supports good colon health. As it also has a very low glycemic index, it is suitable for many people who are on restricted diets. Its taste is comparable to sugar. Inulin is often blended with the powdered forms of stevia.

## Stevia

This natural herbal sweetener is one to two hundred times sweeter than sugar but does not affect blood sugar levels. You'll find it in supplements and some natural sodas. This is an excellent sweetening agent in foods that are safe for those with candida, diabetes, and hypoglycemia.

A lot of this information may seem overwhelming and downright daunting. It may seem as if the commercial food suppliers are only trying to poison us, and that there's nothing safe to eat! I've felt that way myself sometimes, but with just a little time and extra effort, you'll soon know what to put in your shopping cart and what should stay on the shelf.

One final word of caution: Just because a packaged food is sold in a natural food market doesn't mean that it is free of harmful additives. Cereals, crackers, cookies, sauces, salad dressings, and other packaged foods can still contain maltodextrin, hydrogenated oils, sugars, and MSG. So whether Newman-O's are really better for you than Oreos comes from your ability to interpret their respective ingredient list.

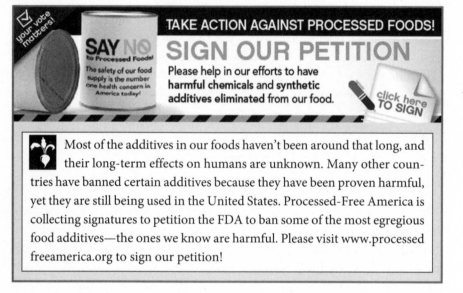

TAKE ACTION AGAINST PROCESSED FOODS!

SAY NO to Processed Foods!

SIGN OUR PETITION

The safety of our food supply is the number one health concern in America today!

Please help in our efforts to have harmful chemicals and synthetic additives eliminated from our food.

click here TO SIGN

Most of the additives in our foods haven't been around that long, and their long-term effects on humans are unknown. Many other countries have banned certain additives because they have been proven harmful, yet they are still being used in the United States. Processed-Free America is collecting signatures to petition the FDA to ban some of the most egregious food additives—the ones we know are harmful. Please visit www.processed freeamerica.org to sign our petition!

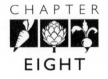
# Living Processed Free in an Overprocessed-Food World

*Eat close to the source; if I can't pronounce it, or don't know what it is, it's not going in to my body. Beware of any "food" that has been created by humans rather than nature.*

—LAIRD HAMILTON, CHAMPION SURFER,
AUTHOR OF *FORCE OF NATURE*

You're now aware that a good majority of the food available to us—mainly sugars, flours, and oils—has been processed in some way. So how are we supposed to live processed free in a world that hardly supports our doing so?

We have to become conscious and aware shoppers and diners, and take responsibility for everything we put into our body. Until the food industry catches up to our high level of awareness, we have to be our own advocates.

The first step in making sure we are getting the best food available is to learn how to shop. And while there may be some items that you'll want to go to the health food store to get, you can still buy healthy foods in a mainstream grocery store. Besides, just because an item is sold in a store named Whole Foods, it doesn't mean that it's a whole food! Health food stores also contain many items that are not necessarily healthy. This chapter will help you live processed free in a processed-food world.

## Shop the Perimeter

The most common mistakes people make when trying to shop healthily at the grocery store is that they scour the packaged food aisles looking for supposedly healthy options. Usually they wind up with way too much junk in their carts. You will do far better avoiding the store's central aisles altogether. That's where all the processed-food temptations hang out.

Shopping the perimeter of the grocery store is a much better strategy. The perimeter is where all the perishable food is—fruits and vegetables, fish and chicken, eggs and dairy, and bulk foods such as nuts, seeds, and whole grains.

## Avoid Low-Fat, Fat-Free, Sugar-Free, and Low-Carb Items

Butter is better for you than margarine. Real eggs are better for you than egg substitutes. Whole grains are better for you than low-carb items with added artificial sweeteners. For the most part, products claiming to be fat free or sugar free are designed to mislead people and give them a false sense of security. They're attention getting, but they rarely tell the whole story.

For example, a fat-free product may not have any fat in it, but it will probably have more sugar in it than the regular version of that item. This is particularly true of salad dressings. Sugar is converted into fat in your body, so the claim "fat free" is very misleading.

A soda might have "no fat" on the label, but that doesn't make it good. Foods that say "low carb" could be full of trans fats and other processed chemicals that work against you. Most foods that have marketing claims on them are loaded with chemical ingredients.

## Beware of Foods Containing Soy

Even if you don't eat edamame, tofu, veggie burgers, or soy milk doesn't mean you're not eating soy. Nearly every processed food and many health foods contain one or more forms of soy. Unfortunately, soy can carry some hefty negative health effects. You may be wondering how this can be—isn't soy a health food? The answer is no, and yes. Let me explain.

Soybeans are a cheap source of polyunsaturated vegetable oil, used to make hydrogenated oil (trans fats)—namely margarine and shortening. After the outer hull of the soybean is stripped off, the oil is extracted and highly refined—leaving hulled, defatted soybean meal. This meal was traditionally used for animal feed, until companies seeking to profit from the alleged health benefits of soy started looking for more lucrative uses. In the 1950s, methods were developed to process the hulled and defatted soybeans into three kinds of high-protein commercial food products: soy flour, soy protein concentrates, and soy protein isolates. Next came an increasing trend of adding these products to everything under the sun, from bread and breakfast cereals to ice cream and salad dressings. Today you'll find some form of processed soy in soups, imitation meats such as bacon bits and imitation crab, protein bars, nondairy creamer, frozen desserts, frozen dinners, whipped topping, infant formula, pastas, and pet foods, not to mention the endless vegetarian products resembling traditional animal foods—soy milk, yogurt, ice cream, and cheese; soy burgers, sausage, and hot dogs; soy protein powder, soy crumbles, and Tofurky (that last one just plain sounds wrong!).

But how healthy can this really be—adding highly processed proteins to nearly every food we eat? Not very. Dismantling the soybean and processing the heck out of its individual parts, and then expecting those products to bestow fabulous health benefits are where we go wrong. As with sugar and flour, any highly processed food just isn't what nature intended and contributes to a host of diseases.

But even in their whole raw state, soybeans are not healthy—so if you're a fan of edamame, read on. The only soybean with any health value is one that has been fermented.

## Unfermented Soybeans Contain Toxins

In their raw whole form, soybeans contain high amounts of natural toxins, also known as antinutrients. The three major antinutrients are phytates, enzyme inhibitors, and goitrogens, which function as the immune system of the plant, offering protection from the radiation of the sun and from invasion by bacteria, viruses, or fungi. All plants have some antinutrient properties, but the soybean plant is especially rich in these chemicals, which unlike the phytonutrients in other beans, have detrimental effects on the human body.[1] Although soybeans do contain compounds that can be healthful to humans, such as cancer-fighting antioxidants called isoflavones, they are not available to the human body from unfermented soybeans or processed soy products.

Thousands of years ago, around 1000 BC, the Chinese discovered that a mold, when allowed to grow on soybeans, destroyed the toxins present. This process, known as fermentation, is a natural chemical reaction that activates enzymes in the soybeans that release the isoflavones and make them available for use by the human body. Therefore, only fermented forms of soy are healthy for people to consume. These include tempeh, miso, soy sauce, tamari sauce, and natto.

A few centuries later, a simpler process was developed to prepare soybeans for consumption. After lengthy soaking and cooking, the beans were treated with nigari, a substance found in seawater. The end product was tofu. During the Ming dynasty, *fermented soy* appeared in the Chinese *Materia Medica* (the most complete and comprehensive medical book ever written in the history of traditional Chinese medicine) as a nutritionally important food and an effective remedy for diseases.[2] This is how soy became known as a health food, but unfortunately the vast amount of soy that Americans are eating is not the healthy type.

## Other Concerns with Soybeans

Nonabsorbable minerals:  Due to their high concentration of phytate (also known as phytic acid), soybeans render minerals (such as calcium, copper, iron, magnesium, and zinc) nonabsorbable. As phytate content is still quite high in tofu, only very small quantities of tofu should be consumed. In addition, eating meat or fish with soy foods (such as miso soup with some chicken, tofu in a fish broth, meat with tofu) also reduces the phytates and allows our body to absorb the essential minerals.

Interference with digestion of protein:  The high content of enzyme inhibitors in unfermented soybeans interferes with the process that helps nutrients assimilate into the body, ultimately making carbohydrates and proteins from soybeans impossible to completely digest.

Blocked production of thyroid hormone:  Unfermented soybeans are also loaded with compounds called goitrogens, substances that can block the production of thyroid hormone as well as cause goiter formation.

## Only Organic, Fermented Forms of Soy Are Healthy

Another growing concern about soy is that a large percentage of soybeans grown in the United States are from genetically modified (GM) seeds. GM soybeans have only been in the food supply since the early 1990s, suggesting that genetic modification may be the reason for the growing number of soy allergies among children and adults. Organic soybeans are not genetically modified. See the sidebar on page 165 for more information on genetically modified foods.

For these reasons, only organic forms of fermented soy foods are recommended. The nutrients found in miso, tempeh, and natto can be beneficial in the moderate amounts found in the typical Asian diet. Small amounts (about an ounce) of organic tofu can also be part of a healthy diet if consumed with other protein foods. Traditional Asian diets do not include foods with processed soy ingredients, and neither should yours.

# Read Ingredient Lists

The single most important tool you have for going processed free is the ability to read and decipher ingredient lists. It's important to do this carefully. This may take you longer the first few times you go shopping, but once you know what you're looking for, you'll be zipping through the store with your newfound ability to analyze the terminology.

The basic rule of thumb is this: If you have to buy something with a label, make sure you know what all the ingredients are and that you're comfortable putting them in your body. If the ingredient list includes chemical names you can't pronounce, it's a pretty sure bet that the product isn't real or healthy. For the most part, unless you know what every ingredient is, you should avoid foods with more than five or six ingredients.

Package labels may make such declarations in large type as "natural fruit flavors," "made with real fruit juice," "all natural ingredients," and "no pre-servatives added." These statements do not mean that there are no harmful chemicals in the product. Manufacturers bank on the hope that you'll read only the large print and think these are healthy, natural products. Remember, there is little regulation on the word *natural*. Manufacturers are really stretching it these days, trying to convince the public that their product is natural just because it was *derived from* a real food. For instance, the Splenda company claims its product is more natural than other artificial sweeteners, just because sucrose is the starting ingredient.

Ingredients are listed in order of the weight of the ingredient in the product's recipe. Therefore, the ingredient that weighs the most is listed first; the ingredient that weighs the least is listed last. Take note: you will often see the statement, "Contains less than 2% of the following ingredients." Do not be fooled by this. If a food contains less than 2 percent of arsenic or another poisonous substance, it is still a poison—and it's in your food!

As a general rule, even if the ingredient list is short, it may or may not still have harmful additives in it, so read the ingredients carefully before you decide to purchase the product.

The top ingredients to avoid are:

- Acesulfame K (also called acesulfame potassium)
- Anything with a number after it (e.g., Red 40, polysorbate 80, etc.)
- Artificial colors
- Artificial flavors (remember how many chemicals are in artificial strawberry flavoring!)
- Aspartame (Equal)
- BHA, BHT, and TBHQ
- Canola oil (contains trans fats)
- Enriched wheat flour
- High-fructose corn syrup
- Hydrogenated oil (also known as trans fats)
- Isolated soy protein, hydrolyzed soy protein, or any other soy protein
- Maltodextrin

- Mono- and diglycerides (these are similar to trans fats and have many harmful effects)
- Monosodium glutamate (MSG)
- Partially hydrogenated oil (usually soybean oil, also known as trans fats)
- Saccharine
- Sodium nitrate and sodium nitrite
- Soybean oil
- Sucralose (Splenda)
- Sugar
- Unbleached enriched wheat flour
- Wheat flour

## Choose Local, Fresh, and as Close to Natural as Possible

Local foods, meaning foods that are grown in the proximity to where you live, will have the highest Life Force Energy and the highest level of nutrients. Shop farmers' markets or grocery stores that carry locally grown produce.

Eat loads of fresh fruits and vegetables, whole grains, and high-quality fresh meats and poultry. Following the Processed-Free Eating Plan will help you do this. That doesn't mean that there aren't *any* good foods in the canned, boxed, or frozen-food aisle; it just means they're few and far between. Things like frozen fruits and canned beans can still be good for you, as long as they don't contain a bunch of unhealthy and unnecessary ingredients. Many healthy organic and frozen food items are now available in natural food markets, but it's still better to eat more of your foods fresh.

I realize that it is not always realistic to eat everything fresh all of the time. We need to have convenience foods, and we need to eat out sometimes. The way to do this processed free is to read every label and to be very picky about what and where you eat. Choose packaged foods that are made with real food ingredients over those with factory-created components. Be a smart consumer and look for things that are going to help your body thrive. When you pick something up, ask yourself the question, "Is this something my great-grandmother would have eaten?" If the answer is no, you should probably put it back.

# Choose Organic When Possible

There's an old saying, "You are what you eat," which is true; but in today's world, we now have to say, "You are what *they* ate." So, if your apple soaked up pesticides, or your chicken ate hormones, *you* ingest what *they* ate. I didn't start out my weight-loss journey eating organic, but I have since converted as much as I can. You will do well to start eating more organic food as you adopt a processed-free lifestyle. Even small doses of chemicals can cause lasting damage to human health. Pesticides have been linked to various disorders and diseases, including cancers of the reproductive, endocrine, and immune systems. Pregnant women and children are especially vulnerable, as pesticides have also been linked to developmental and behavioral disabilities and impairment.

The specific effects of many pesticides are unknown. Pesticide manufacturers claim their products are safe, but the studies on these products are usually done with high doses, rather than testing the chronic low doses that people typically experience. Companies used to claim that DDT (a classic example of an endocrine-disrupting pesticide) was safe, right up to the day it was banned!

This reason alone should convince you to eat organic food; however, most of us have budgets that dictate our food choices. A common misperception is that organic food is so expensive that it is out of range for the average family or even for the average single consumer. It is also commonly perceived that the average grocery purchase of processed foods at a neighborhood supermarket, using manufacturers' coupons or store discounts, makes a processed-food diet inexpensive. If you go along with those hypotheses, you may be surprised to learn how you can eat a mainly organic diet for about the same amount of money as a typical processed-food diet. The key is to learn how to shop and what foods to choose.

## How to Eat Organic on a Budget

Here are some tips and resources I have found to help make eating organic a healthy and affordable choice (for more information, see "The Most Important Foods to Buy Organic," page 158).

Decide which foods you consume the most, then prioritize. For instance, if you eat yogurt on a daily or regular basis, you should buy it organic. If you eat radishes only every once in a while, then you don't have to worry so much about buying those organically grown.

Once you've decided on your core items, try these ideas:

Buy in season and be flexible. Purchase what is in season and you can save big on your produce purchases. Find your local farmers' market, which is a great source for in-season, fresh produce that, if not certified organic, may still be pesticide free. Many cities have farmers' markets year-round, rain or shine. Also, I just want to point out that organic produce doesn't always look "perfect" because it's not sprayed, waxed, or engineered to look pretty. But it sure does taste better than conventional produce.

Join a local food co-op. You can become a member for very little money and you then have access to all types of organic foods at great prices. Many times, if you can find about eight hours a month to donate to the co-op, you can save an additional 10 to 12 percent off your purchases. To find a local co-op or learn how to organize one, contact the co-op directory service at www.coop directory.org. (Note: Co-ops often still let you shop there without taking a membership; you just won't receive some of the same perks as members.)

Be on the lookout for coupons. Many natural products have coupons right on the package to be redeemed at checkout. Company websites for healthy products may offer coupons online or in circulars or magazines, and incentives to try their products.

Keep an eye out for sales. Yep, organic products go on sale the same as anything else. This is where you can scoop up some great deals, especially if you bring your coupons! Don't forget to watch for these at mainstream supermarkets that may also carry their own house line of organic products.

Buy in bulk. This is one area that many people ignore yet can save you quite a bit of money. You can purchase nearly all of your grains, pastas, dried fruits, and nuts from the bulk bins. You can buy organic brown rice or fresh shelled almonds for anywhere from fifty cents to a dollar less than the pack-aged versions, and in whatever quantity you need. The difference is that you are not paying for packaging. Your local grocery store and natural foods stores have bulk aisles where you simply fill a bag, write the price on the twist tie, and the cashier will weigh it at the register. Reuse your plastic bags and you'll help preserve the environment and natural resources, too.

Shop online. If you can't find a local source for the organic food you want, don't give up. Hop online. One of my favorite online stores in Tropical Tra-ditions.com, which e-mails out weekly sales and always offers two-for-the-price-of-one deals. Check it out at www.tropicaltraditions.com.

Rearrange your food budget. Free up more dollars for organic food by trimming the fat from your conventional food budget. Add up all the dol-lars you spend every month on food, including fast-food meals, morning cups of coffee, bagels, and even trips to vending machines. A small change in your eating habits could mean large change by freeing up the money you need to buy the organic foods that you really want.

Ease into organic. Begin the transition to eating organic with some of your favorite foods. Pick a product or two that you decide you really notice a difference in taste and that really excites you. If you have young children, you may want to start by buying organic baby food and dairy products. Whatever your kids eat the most of is where you start.

Get into the kitchen. Preparing your own healthy food is more economical than buying preprepared health foods. Not only do you have more control over your ingredients, but you can also make larger quantities that will stretch over several days. Learning to cook your own meals is a true invest-ment in your health and one that will last a lifetime.

## The Most Important Foods to Buy Organic

### Milk, Cheese, Yogurt, and Butter

Milk that is conventionally produced often comes from cows that are raised under disturbing farm conditions. They may graze on pastures that have been treated with pesticides, herbicides, and sewage sludge. When the cattle are not let outside, they feed on less nutritious dried grass and hay, grains that may be genetically modified, and fish meal that may contain PCBs and mercury. Eating grains, instead of grass, dramatically alters the nutritional content of the milk. Also, cows on conventional farms are often given antibiotics—even when they are healthy—to prevent their getting sick. In some factory farms, thousands of cows are crammed inside barns to allow easy access for milking. Their milk production can be forced beyond normal capacity through injections of a synthetic growth hormone called rbST (also called rbGH). The rbST affects natural hormones that are transferred from the cow into the milk. One of these, called insulin-like growth factor 1 (IGF-1) has been associated with an increased risk of breast, colon, prostate, and lung cancers in humans.[3] Because of this, rbST has been banned in Canada, Japan, New Zealand, Australia, and the entire European Union, but here in the good old USA we still allow it.

Organic milk has none of these toxins, because their use is forbidden in USDA-certified dairy cows, which are fed only certified organic feed. And in 2010, the USDA changed its organic regulations to require that organic dairy cattle must spend much of the year grazing in open pastures. What a cow eats is very important, because research shows that the more a cow feeds on grass, the higher the level of a special type of essential fatty acid called conjugated linoleic acid (CLA). This very special fat, found mainly in the meats and milkfat of cows, goats, and other grazing farm animals, has strong anticancer properties and can also protect against heart disease and diabetes. According to a 1999 study published in the *Journal of Dairy Science*, meat and full-fat dairy products from grass-fed animals can produce 300 to 500 percent more CLA than do cows fed the usual grain diet.[4]

CLA also has a significant effect on weight loss, lowering the body's ability to store fat and mobilizing stored fat to be burned for energy. CLA also helps convert fat to lean muscle tissue; the more muscle you have, the higher your metabolism. Imagine that—you can actually lose weight by consuming full-fat, whole milk!

So, while this may fly in the face of conventional wisdom, *I recommend only whole milk and whole-milk products*. Reduced-fat milks are relatively new processed foods. I don't know of any cows that deliver reduced-fat or fat-free milk out of their udders. Removing fat from milk makes the milk less nutritious and less digestible. The skim milk of yesteryear was very thin and had a kind of blue color to it, which looked somewhat weird and unappealing to most consumers. Now it's artificially colored. Low-fat milks, 1 percent and 2 percent, have dried milk powder added to bulk them up. This milk powder contains rancid fats, oxidized cholesterol, and lots of nitrites. A few ethical dairy farms do not do this to their milk, but they are few and far between.[5]

Pasteurization and homogenization are also damaging to milk. The pasteurization process, which entails heating the milk to a temperature of 145 to 150 degrees Fahrenheit and keeping it there for at least half an hour, then reducing the temperature to not more than 55 degrees Fahrenheit, completely changes the structure of the milk proteins (known as denaturization) into something far less than healthy. While the process certainly destroys germs and bad bacteria, it also destroys enzymes, diminishes vitamins, destroys vitamin $B_{12}$, and vitamin $B_6$, and kills beneficial bacteria. One reason so many people are lactose or dairy intolerant is that pasteurized milk lacks the enzymes to help us digest it.[6] Whole milk, like sugarcane and whole grains, is a perfect package food. It contains all of the nutrients that are required by our body to properly digest it. When we take it apart (as in removing the fat), or when we alter it (as in pasteurization) that's when we start to experience problems.

The homogenization process may be even more dangerous, as it alters the fat globules and creates a compound known as XO, or xanthine oxidase, which is believed by some to cause damage to the arterial walls and may lead to an increased risk for cardiovascular disease.[7]

For these reasons, I highly recommend consuming milk and milk products in the form that humans have enjoyed them for thousands of years, prior to the advent of pasteurization—*raw*. Raw milk is a supremely healthy food, as are raw cheese and raw butter. There's a raw milk revolution going on in this country right now, as more than half a million Americans have returned to drinking their milk the way nature intended. Many who are lactose or dairy intolerant to pasteurized milk are able to consume raw milk and raw milk products. The reason is that the milk is in its whole form and contains all the nutrients for its digestion.

Unfortunately, raw milk is not available in many states. If you don't have access to raw milk, the next best thing will be organic whole milk and such products as organic whole-milk yogurt, cheeses, and butter. Raw cheese is more widely available than raw milk, and you can find it in most health food stores.

For sources of raw milk in your area, go to www.realmilk.com. For more information on raw milk, log on to www.raw-milk-facts.com.

I know for some of you it may take some getting used to, but whole-milk dairy products are much healthier for you than low- or nonfat versions. Think of it as a liberation!

## Produce

According to a January 2005 report in *The Organic Center State of Science Review*, organic produce has about 30 percent greater antioxidants than do conventionally grown fruits and vegetables. On an organic farm, the fruits and vegetables must work hard to stay alive by fighting off pests. Doing so triggers their innate defense mechanisms (similar to human antibodies), building a diverse array of natural chemicals called secondary plant metabolites (SPMs). SPMs are responsible for flavor, color, and antioxidant density. Along with increased nutrient density and flavor, organic produce is free from potentially harmful pesticides, fungicides, and herbicides that are detrimental to the soil, the water supply, and the health of farmers.

If you cannot afford to buy all of your produce organic, there are some general guidelines to help you select the least contaminated produce. First, if it grows below the ground (e.g., potatoes, carrots, beets, parsnips, rutabagas, and radishes), you should buy organic, because foods that grow below the ground absorb more toxins. If it has an outer protective peel or shell, it is likely less contaminated and okay to eat conventionally grown—unless you are eating the peels. (Examples of above-ground fruits are bananas, coconuts, avocados, pineapples, and citrus.)

Second, you can use the Environmental Working Group's (EWG) Shopper's Guide to Pesticides in Produce. The EWG, a nonprofit advocacy group, has domestic and imported produce tested for residues of pesticides and herbicides. Each year the EWG publishes an extensive list of the most contaminated produce, dubbed "The Dirty Dozen." The group's studies show that we can lower our pesticide exposure by 90 percent if we avoid the twelve most contaminated conventionally grown fruits and vegetables and substitute organic produce instead.

According to EWG's 2011 Guide, the "Dirty Dozen" are the most contaminated conventionally grown produce. You should eat these organically grown:

- Apples
- Celery
- Strawberries
- Peaches
- Spinach
- Nectarines
- Grapes
- Sweet bell peppers
- Potatoes
- Blueberries
- Lettuce
- Kale/collard greens

According to EWG's 2011 Guide, the "Clean 15" have the least amount of pesticide residue. It is okay to eat the following conventionally grown fruits and vegetables:

- Onions
- Corn
- Pineapples
- Avocados
- Asparagus
- Sweet peas
- Mangoes
- Eggplant
- Cantaloupes
- Kiwifruit
- Cabbage
- Watermelons
- Sweet potatoes
- Grapefruit
- Mushrooms

You can download this list on a nice a wallet-size guide by logging on to www.foodnews.org. Take it with you to the market to help you select produce wisely.

## How to Identify Organic Produce

Grocery stores are required by law to keep the organic produce separate from the conventionally grown produce; you can tell if the produce you are buying is organic by looking at those annoying little stickers, which are part of an international PLU (price look-up) system grocers use to make checkout and inventory control easier. If the item does not have a sticker on it, just look at the sign for a four- or five-digit PLU number.

If the item is conventionally grown, the number has four digits (for example, 4060 stands for broccoli). If the item is organically grown, the number has five digits starting with a 9 (so it's 94060 for organic broccoli).

There's also a third PLU option: a five-digit number beginning with an 8, which indicates that the produce you are holding has been genetically modified. If you're eating nonorganically grown food, you're probably eating some genetically modified items without even knowing it. Genetically modified food has been in the food supply for many years now (the rapeseeds used to make canola oil are genetically modified). Unfortunately, at this time, there is no way of knowing if the ingredients in packaged or canned foods have been genetically modified, unless they are organic. Organically grown foods are *not* genetically modified. See the sidebar on page 165 for more information on GMOs.

## Meats, Poultry, Fish, and Eggs

The disturbing farm conditions for dairy cows is just as bad for cows that are raised for beef, maybe even worse. Prior to World War II, all beef cattle were raised on grass. And because eating grass makes a lean steer, it could take up to four years to get a steer fat enough for slaughter. But after the war, beef farmers switched to feeding cows corn, molasses, sugar beet waste, soybean meal, protein supplements, antibiotics, and growth hormones to speed up their weight gain. And it worked. Today, cattle are fat enough for slaughter after only fourteen or sixteen months.

Because of their unnatural diet, the meat of grain-fed beef has fat marbled all throughout it. There's no way to trim it off the sides. Beef from organic grass-fed cows is very lean. As a result, a 6-ounce steak from a corn-fed cow has 100 more calories and twice the saturated fat than one from a grass-fed cow. Beef from grass-fed cows has two to six times more omega-3 fats than grain-fed beef. Grass-fed beef is also much higher in vitamin E, vitamin C, beta-carotene, and conjugated linoleic acid (CLA).[8]

Conventionally raised poultry is also fed grains and antibiotics, which are not a normal diet. As you might expect, the same health hazards are associated with eating such birds. Chickens that are allowed to graze on their natural diet have 21 percent less total fat, 30 percent less saturated fat, 28 percent fewer calories, and 100 percent more omega-3 fats than do chickens given high-energy specialty feeds. The eggs of the naturally fed chickens have 400 percent more omega-3 fats.[9] You will notice the difference in the taste, as well as the difference in the color of the yolk. Organic eggs from naturally fed chickens have a nice, brightly colored yolk that is brimming with nutrients.

Unfortunately organic meats, poultry, and eggs are much more expensive than their conventionally raised counterparts. For this reason alone, it is best to consume meats occasionally rather than often, and when you do eat them, enjoy smaller quantities than what you may be accustomed to. The Processed-Free Eating Plan recommends 3- to 4-ounce portions of meats and poultry (roughly palm sized), quite a stark difference to the 6- to 8-ounce portions you get in restaurants.

With the rising popularity of eating fish, grocery stores and food establishments have turned to farm-raised fish to meet the demand. Farm-raised fish are not fed their natural diet, either. Like cows and poultry, they are also fed grains that upset the ratio of their fat content. Research has shown that farm-raised fish contain higher ratios of omega-6 fats, which create a harmful imbalance for our body.[10] Wild-caught fish eat their natural diet of smaller fish and sea creatures, making them leaner with higher levels of the healthy omega-3s. According to Vital Choice Wild Seafood and Organics Company, the best wild fish are wild sockeye salmon, wild king salmon, wild silver coho salmon, Alaskan cod, albacore tuna, Alaskan halibut, and Alaskan sablefish ("black cod").

## Coffee

Coffee is one of the most heavily chemically treated crops of any agricultural commodity in the world. Over two hundred pesticides are used on coffee crops.[11] To mass-produce coffee, traditional growers often clear wide swaths of land, predominantly in the rainforest, where the plants receive direct sunlight all day. This incessant exposure to the sun weakens the immune system of the coffee crops and makes them more vulnerable to pests and insects. This is one of the reasons that conventional coffee-growing requires such large amounts of pesticides and insecticides. Many of these pesticides and insecticides sprayed directly on the crops end up in the beverage that people drink on a daily basis and are harmful to the body. These chemicals also cause damage to the soil and pollute the local water supply.

# Just Say No to GMOs

In 1996, the first genetically modified organisms (GMOs), also said to be "genetically engineered," entered our food supply. Today, it is estimated that genetically modified ingredients are found in the majority of processed foods. Is it a coincidence, or a direct correlation, that in the years since GMOs use became commonplace, the number of Americans suffering from three or more chronic diseases nearly doubled—from 7 to 13 percent?[12] Have GMOs been contributing to the dramatic rise of obesity, diabetes, asthma, allergies, and other food-related illnesses?

Environmental organizations and public interest groups have been actively protesting against genetically modified foods for years. The results of the few studies that have been conducted have raised grave concerns about the health effects of GMOs on the animals, insects, and humans that eat them.[13]

## What Is a GMO?

GMOs are plants, animals, or microorganisms whose genetic code has been altered to give it characteristics that it does not have naturally. Genetic engineering of food involves the laboratory process of artificially inserting genes into the DNA of food crops or animals.

Although there have been some attempts to increase nutritional benefits or productivity, currently food crops are genetically modified to enhance two main traits: to increase tolerance to herbicides and to insects.

If they grow herbicide-tolerant GMO crops, farmers can spray large amounts of weed killer directly on the plants without the risk of also killing the crops. This practice leads to more chemicals in your food.

Insect-resistant GMO crops produce pesticides inside the plant, enabling the crops to produce their own pesticides against insects, killing or deterring them, saving the farmer from having to spray the crops with pesticides. The problem is that the plants themselves are toxic, and not just to insects. When you eat insect-resistant GMO plants, it may be like eating pesticides.[14]

## Early Warnings About GMOs

In 1991, there was overwhelming consensus among scientists at the FDA that GM foods were substantially different and could create unpredictable,

*continues*

# Just Say No to GMOs *continued*

unsafe, and hard-to-detect allergens, toxins, diseases, and nutritional problems. The scientists urged the agency to require long-term safety studies, including human studies, to protect the public.

But in spite of the protests, the warnings were not heeded by the FDA, which was under orders by the White House administration at the time to promote biotechnology. As a result, GMOs—such as soybeans, corn, cottonseed, and rapeseed (canola) that have had bacterial genes forced into their DNA—entered our foods without any required safety evaluations.

As crazy as it sounds, there have never been any human clinical trials on the effects of GMOs on our health, and not many long-term animal-feeding studies, either, so we are largely in the dark about their effect on living creatures. In 2009, the American Academy of Environmental Medicine (AAEM) stated, "Several animal studies indicate serious health risks associated with genetically modified (GM) food," including infertility, immune problems, accelerated aging, faulty insulin regulation, and changes in major organs and the gastrointestinal system. The AAEM has asked physicians to advise all patients to avoid GM foods.

## How to Avoid GMOs in Your Food

Aside from PLU numbers on produce, the United States does not require labeling of GM foods. However, many manufacturers are now voluntarily choosing not to use GM ingredients. Those who participate in the non-GMO project typically carry a label on the packaging, or list ingredients as non-GMO. For instance, you may see non-GMO soy or non-GMO corn on ingredient lists.

The best way to avoid GMOs is to avoid the five major GMO crops (also called "at risk" ingredients): soybeans, canola (rapeseed), corn, cottonseed, and sugar made from sugar beets, all of which are typically used in processed foods. Unless these foods are grown organically, a large percentage of them are GMO.

Soybeans. About 93 percent of the soybeans grown in the United States are GMO. The most common uses of GMO soybeans are soybean oil, hy-

*continues*

## Just Say No to GMOs *continued*

drogenated soybean oil, and soy proteins (see page 150). Examples of products containing GMO soy are salad dressings made with soybean oil, breads and snacks containing soy flour, frozen foods and snacks containing soy protein isolates, protein shakes and nearly every protein bar on the market that contains soy protein concentrate, and anything containing soy isoflavones. Vegetable oils and vegetable proteins are typically from GMO soybeans; however, they may also be derived from other sources.

Cotton:  About 93 percent of the cotton grown in the United States is genetically modified. The most common food use is cottonseed oil, which may be found in fried snack foods such as chips, and in roasted nuts, trail mixes, and other snack foods.

Canola (rapeseed oil):  Most of the rapeseeds used to make canola oil are grown in Canada, of which about 90 percent of them are GMO. Most fried foods and baked goods contain canola oil, as do most salad dressings. Many "healthy" foods contain canola oil and nearly every restaurant and fast-food chain uses it. You will be hard pressed to find a processed food that does not contain canola oil.

Corn:  About 90 percent of the corn grown in the United States is genetically modified. One of the most common uses of GMO corn is high-fructose corn syrup, which is used to sweeten sodas, cereals, cookies, candy, salad dressings, soups, spaghetti sauces, and about a thousand other products.

Baked goods use cornstarch, vegetable oils contain corn oil, and breads such as corn bread use corn flour. Other ingredients include cornmeal, corn syrup and corn syrup solids, modified food starch (often found in yogurt and other thickened products), and sweeteners such as fructose, dextrose, and glucose.

There is no GM popcorn on the market, nor is there any GM blue corn or GM white corn. However, as conventionally grown corn is heavily sprayed with pesticides, you should take care to eat organic corn, organic popcorn, and organic versions of any other corn products.

*continues*

## Just Say No to GMOs *continued*

Sugar beets: About 90 percent of sugar beets grown in the United States are genetically modified. They are mainly used to make refined beet sugar, which can be found in many processed foods.

The three minor GMO crops are Hawaiian papaya, and a small amount of zucchini and yellow crookneck squash.

By reading the numbers on the little stickers (or the price sign, if the stickers are missing), you can determine if produce is genetically modified. If the number is a five-digit number beginning with an 8, then the item you are holding is GMO. Put it back and buy something else!

## How to Read USDA Organic Labels

The U.S. Department of Agriculture (USDA) has approved four categories of organic labels, based on the percentage of organic content. The organic labels began to appear on store shelves on October 21, 2002:

1. 100 Percent Organic—Must contain 100 percent organically produced ingredients, not counting added water and salt. (May carry the USDA Organic seal.)
2. Organic—At least 95 percent of content is organic by weight (excluding water and salt) and cannot contain added sulfites. (May carry the USDA Organic seal.)
3. Made with Organic Ingredients—At least 70 percent of content is organic and the front product panel may display the phrase "made with organic" followed by up to three specific ingredients. Cannot contain added sulfites, with the exception of wine, which may contain a certain level of added sulfur dioxide. (May *not* display the new USDA Organic seal.)
4. Other: Less than 70 percent of content is organic and may list only those ingredients that are organic on the ingredient panel with no mention of organic on the main panel. (May *not* display the new USDA Organic seal.)

# The Case for Organic Popcorn

Popcorn is a food that most people consider to be relatively harmless and safe during dieting. Its high-fiber and low-calorie content are espoused on websites and diet books galore. But dieters take note: popcorn has a darker side.

If you eat popcorn that is not organically grown, you could be eating yourself sick.

The 2011 Agri-Chemical Handbook of the Popcorn Board (yes, there is such a thing) lists 38 insecticides (including malathion), 53 herbicides, 6 fumigants, 19 fungicides, and 9 "miscellaneous" chemicals that are approved for use on nonorganic popcorn crops.[15]

Furthermore, the corn grown for popcorn use is among the food crops that are routinely tested for residues of persistent organic pollutants (POPs). These pollutants are approved for use by the FDA and are commonly used in agriculture, electronics manufacturing, water treatment, exhaust from the combustion of fossil fuels, and many other industrial purposes.

To top it off, popcorn was among the top ten foods most contaminated with pesticides and other toxic organic chemicals in the FDA's 2003 Total Diet Study (TDS). Nonorganic popcorn—one of America's most beloved snack foods—was found to contain thirty-three toxic organic compounds, including some that have been linked to serious health consequences. Even when exposure is extremely low, these chemicals are known to cause cancer, reproductive disorders, birth defects, lower IQ in children, and the decline of bird and aquatic species.[16]

Perhaps now you'll think twice the next time you cuddle up with a bag of popcorn at the movies. As for me, I make mine organic.

# Alkalize and Liver-ize

## The Secrets to a Clean and Balanced Body Chemistry

The first time I heard the term *pH* was on a TV commercial for Wella Balsam shampoo. As Farrah Fawcett was tossing around her gorgeous mane, the announcer said the shampoo was "pH balanced for beautiful hair." Therefore, I thought pH had something to do with hair.

Some years later, in the early 1980s, I read Richard Simmons's inspirational book *Never Say Diet*, which emphasized drinking a glass of warm water every morning with fresh squeezed lemon juice added to it. Following Richard's wise eating and exercise guidelines, I lost 40 pounds. But, as you know, I didn't stick with the plan and gained the weight back. The warm lemon water in the morning did stick with me, but I never understood its important role in weight loss until many years later.

My first-year college chemistry class cleared up my confusion about pH—the term refers to the relative proportions of acidity and alkalinity—and I came to understand that not only beautiful hair needs a balanced pH, but every living system on Earth. Maintaining the proper pH in our body is one of the basic necessities for good health—*our life literally depends on it*. When our pH is balanced, we should lose weight easily. But if our main fat-burning organ (our liver) is clogged with toxins and fat (which is very common, considering the extensive exposure to sugar and food additives these days), it will not be able to burn fat efficiently, and we may have difficulty losing weight despite a balanced pH. To maximize our body's ability to get skinny, we need to alkalize and liver-ize. *Alkalizing* means that we consume foods and beverages that balance our pH; *liver-izing* means that we consume foods and beverages that cleanse our liver. Not surprisingly, water with lemon juice can do both. As you will learn, there are many other delicious foods that powerfully serve this dual purpose, and they are highly emphasized in the Processed-Free Eating Plan. This chapter is mostly about the science, so let's dive in.

## Life and Death in a Very Narrow Range

Every living organism either thrives or dies, depending on the pH of the environment in which it has been designed to live. It is well understood that trees, crops, and other plants can only grow in soil that has the right pH, which specifically affects a plant's ability to derive nutrients from the soil. If the soil's pH is out of range (either too acidic or too alkaline), new plants will not grow, and existing plants will die. Marine life can only survive if the pH of the water the creatures swim in is kept in a range that their body is designed for (try putting a freshwater fish into a saltwater aquarium and see what happens). Swimming pools and hot tubs will turn a yucky green if the pH goes out of range (this happened to me once when I added too much of the wrong chemical to my hot tub—not a pretty sight and a real mess to clean up).

Likewise, if your internal pH goes out of balance, your health deteriorates. Your body is only able to assimilate minerals and nutrients properly *when its pH is balanced.* Therefore, it's quite possible for you to be taking vitamin, mineral, or nutritional supplements and yet be unable to absorb or use them. This relates to how sugar upsets the body chemistry and negates an otherwise healthy diet. If you are not getting the results you expected from your nutritional supplements, especially a calcium supplement, pH imbalance could be the reason.

So what the heck are pH, acidity, and alkalinity, and what do they have to do with getting and staying skinny? These are concepts that can get a bit heady, so the best way for me to explain them is to give you some background, and then some simple examples. If you find yourself getting confused or lost while reading this next section, take a few deep breaths, put the book down for a minute, and then come back to it, because this could be some of the most valuable information regarding your health you will ever read.

## Defining pH

To begin, *pH* is a chemistry term that stands for potential hydrogen. It is always written with a lowercase *p* and an uppercase *H* (the chemical symbol for the element hydrogen). A layman explanation is that pH is what determines whether a solution is acidic or alkaline. A more scientific definition is that pH is a logarithm for an aqueous (water-based) solution's ability to attract hydrogen ions. An aqueous solution can be anything from the moisture in agricultural soil; to the water in oceans, lakes, and hot tubs; to the blood running through your veins and the fluids in your tissues.

Similar to how the Richter scale is used to measure the energy contained in an earthquake, the pH scale measures the amount of hydrogen in aqueous solutions. The pH scale ranges from 0 to 14. Solutions with a pH below 7 are acidic; solutions with a pH above 7 are alkaline. Acidity increases in strength as the number decreases from 7 down to 0; in other words, the closer the pH number is to 0, the more acidic the solution. On the other hand, alkalinity increases in strength as the number increases from 7 to 14; the closer the pH number is to 14, the more alkaline the solution. A solution with a pH of 7, which is in the middle of the scale, is considered neutral (neither acidic nor alkaline). There is really only one solution with a pH of 7, and that is pure distilled water.

The Richter scale uses a logarithmic scale (where each successive unit of measurement is ten times greater than the one before it). For example, an earthquake that measures 5.0 on the Richter scale has a magnitude ten times larger than one that measures 4.0. Likewise, an acidic solution with a pH of 5 is ten times more acidic than one with a pH of 6 (because acidity increases as you go *down* the scale). An alkaline solution with a pH of 9 is ten times more alkaline than a solution with a pH of 8 (because alkalinity increases as you go *up* the scale). Measurements of pH can also fall between the whole numbers; for instance, a solution can have a pH of 6.2 or 8.4. In

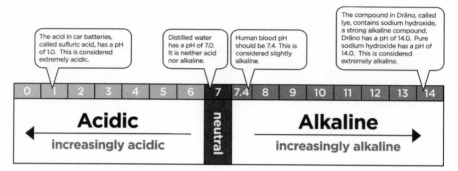

**Figure 9.1** The pH Scale

fact, in many instances, a change in a fraction of a pH measurement can greatly impact the health of a living organism.

Keep following me; I promise this is all going to make sense soon. But before I can talk about food, I need to tell you a little more about water, acidity, and alkalinity.

## How Acidic and Alkaline Solutions Are Formed

In the seventeenth century, an amateur chemist named Robert Boyle first observed that an acidic solution will become less acidic when mixed with an alkaline solution, and vice versa. In other words, acidic and alkaline solutions counteract each other. This phenomenon is called neutralization.

As you can see in Figure 9.1, the battery acid in your car is very acidic, and Drāno is very alkaline. If you were to add enough Drāno (pH 14) to a glassful of car battery acid (pH 1), eventually the acid would be neutralized to a pH of 7. So instead of a glass of very corrosive hydrochloric acid, you would have a glass of neutral water. And if you added a little more Drāno the pH would become slightly alkaline, let's say a pH of 7.4.

How would you know how much Drāno to add to the battery acid to completely neutralize it into water? One way is to use a special type of indicator called litmus, which changes colors according to the pH of the solution. The most common type of litmus will be red in acid solutions, blue in alkaline solutions, and clear when the solution is neutral.

For instance, if you add a drop of litmus into a glass of hydrochloric acid before adding any Drāno, the solution will turn red. As you add Drāno to the acid, the red color will get lighter and lighter as the pH gets closer to 7. Once the pH reaches 7, the solution in the glass will turn clear, as it should because it is a glass of water! If you were to continue adding Drāno past the point of neutrality, the color of the solution would turn blue because the excess Drāno shifts the water to an alkaline solution. You would easily be able to shift the solution back to neutral simply by adding enough acid to turn it clear again. I hope you're still with me, because now I'm going to bring this all together and tell you how the pH of your body is the most important factor in your health—and how it all depends on what foods you choose, or don't choose, to eat.

## Your Body's pH

As mentioned earlier, nature has defined pH ranges for all living things. For example, most freshwater fish can only survive in waters that range in pH from 6.0 to 7.0, but as values dip below 6.0, problems abound. As the water's acidity increases (due to pollution or other contamination), the fishes' food base dwindles, and their eggs cannot survive—ultimately affecting their ability to reproduce. In fact, if the pH of the water goes below 5.0, just about all species of freshwater aquatic plants and animals die.

Whereas fishes' ability to survive depends upon the pH of the fluids *outside* their body, our ability as humans to survive and be skinny is dependent upon the pH of the fluids *inside* our body—namely, our blood and the other bodily fluids that fill our cells as well as the spaces between our cells. Our body has been designed by nature to optimally function when the pH of our blood is 7.4 (slightly alkaline). This specific pH controls the activity of every metabolic function happening within us. Therefore, if this pH is shifted even slightly—if our blood becomes too acidic—we die, just like the fish.

To keep us alive, our body is designed to maintain the alkaline pH of our blood at 7.4. The way it does this is through neutralization. Similar to the Drāno example, our body has a way of neutralizing too much acidity in our system. Our body's "Drāno" is our alkaline reserve, which consists of certain minerals that are stored in our bones, tissues, and teeth. These minerals are drawn upon every time our body needs to neutralize acid. A healthy body maintains adequate alkaline reserves to meet the demands of acidity created by normal body functions. For instance, the muscles create lactic acid during exercise. Breathing, cell building, and burning calories to fuel the metabolism are also normal functions of the body that create acid. But the minerals in our alkaline reserve are not infinite, so it is up to us to replenish them regularly by eating a varied diet.

Our pH is determined mostly by what we eat and drink, but it can also be affected by stress, worry, anger, and even by how much sleep (or lack of it) and exercise (or lack of it) we get. Therefore, what we eat and drink is very important in maintaining our alkaline pH, as well as getting enough sleep and exercise and managing our stress.

As you may have guessed, certain foods will create alkalinity in our body and replenish our alkaline reserve, whereas some foods create acidity. All foods, after they are digested and metabolized, will leave either acid- or alkaline-forming minerals in our body. The alkaline-forming foods are those that predominantly supply calcium, sodium, magnesium, potassium, iron, and manganese. The acid-forming foods are those that predominantly supply copper, bromine, fluorine, chlorine, iodine, phosphorus, sulfur, and silicon.

To maintain our proper body pH, the majority of our foods should be alkaline forming, and the acid-forming foods should be minimized. However, the typical diet of most Americans is the exact opposite. Most fruits and vegetables are alkaline forming, whereas meats, grains, most fats, dairy products, and all the junk foods are acid forming. The most acid-forming foods are refined carbohydrates—white sugar and white flour—in addition to sodas (especially diet sodas), artificial sweeteners, alcohol, coffee, and prescription drugs.

Eating too many of the acid-forming foods and not enough of the alkaline-forming ones results in excess acidity, which overwhelms the body's alkaline reserve. It's like continuing to draw money out of a dwindling savings account without replacing it. Ideally, you should have more than you need to ensure you have enough in case of an emergency. The alkaline reserve consists mainly of calcium, which is drawn from the bones, tissues, and teeth. When calcium is continually removed from the bones, without adequate replacement, you end up with a calcium deficiency, which leads to osteoporosis.[1] Calcium deficiency, which is also known as hypocalcaemia, is responsible for approximately 150 different degenerative diseases and conditions, including arthritis, heart disease, gout, high cholesterol, cancer, acid reflux, high blood pressure, overweight, and obesity.

When your alkaline reserve becomes chronically low, your body is less able to neutralize additional acid coming in. As a result, other defense mechanisms are employed to protect your blood and organs from getting overly acidic. This may sound like a good thing, that your body is working hard to keep you alive despite your poor diet, but this is how many health problems begin.

One way that your body keeps acid from entering your vital organs is to store the acid in your fat cells, leading to weight gain and obesity. Your body then holds on to this fat as a way to continue protecting the organs. Hence, when your body is acidic, you gain weight that is very difficult to lose. Another place your body stores acid is in your muscles. Acidic muscles lead to low energy, muscle cramps, and chronic fatigue syndrome. Your body may also try to expel acid through the skin, causing hot flashes, strong perspiration, psoriasis and rashes. Frequent colds and other immune responses are other ways the body works to expel acid.[2]

Because of this strain, the body can suffer severe and prolonged damage due to chronic high acidity—a condition known as acidosis, that may go undetected for years.

Acidosis can cause other problems such as:

- Acceleration of free radical damage
- Acne
- Cancer (see sidebar)
- Diabetes
- Headaches
- High blood pressure
- Hormone imbalances
- Joint pain
- Lack of focus
- Premature aging
- Sleep problems
- Slow digestion and elimination
- Yeast/fungal overgrowth[3]

## Acidity, Alkalinity, Sugar, and Cancer

In 1931, Dr. Otto Warburg, a medical doctor and one of the twentieth century's leading biochemists, was awarded the Nobel Prize in medicine for his discovery that cancer cells thrive when the bodily fluids surrounding them are acidic, but they die when the bodily fluids are alkaline. The opposite is true for healthy cells—they thrive in an alkaline body, but die when the body becomes too acidic.

Healthy cells and cancer cells can be compared to humans and fish. Healthy cells are like humans. They need air (oxygen) to breathe—to function and survive. If the oxygen supply is diminished or cut off, they die. Excess acid depletes oxygen from the bodily fluids, which kills healthy cells.

Cancer cells are kind of like fish. They require a different environment to survive, and breathe through a different mechanism. Cancer cells "breathe" by fermenting glucose (sugar). Fermentation of sugar creates more acidity in the body, leading to more of the perfect environment for cancer. But, when you take a fish out of water, it cannot breathe air, so it dies. Similarly, cancer cells cannot "breathe" oxygen and will die when subjected to a high-oxygen environment.

What is a high-oxygen environment? An alkaline environment! Alkaline bodily fluids create high levels of oxygen in the cells. Cancer cells become dormant and will die when the body fluids are alkaline. In other words, regardless of the causative factors that lead to its formation, *cancer cannot survive in an alkaline body.*[4]

This is why maintaining an alkaline pH is so vital in preventing and treating cancer.

Acidosis is common in our society mostly due to the typical American diet, which is far too high in acid-producing animal products (e.g., meat, eggs, and dairy), and far too low in alkaline-producing foods (e.g., fresh vegetables). Additionally, we eat acid-producing processed foods (e.g., white flour and sugar) and drink acid-producing beverages (e.g., coffee and soft drinks).

We use too many drugs, which are acid forming; and, we use artificial chemical sweeteners that are extremely acid forming. The increasing number of food additives and pesticide residues are putting so much strain on our body, it is no wonder we have so many sick people in our country.

What most people don't realize is that diseases thrive in an acid environment, but cannot survive in an alkaline environment.[5] When you alkalize your body, you turn it into a healthy environment. This is our sixth Law of Skinny Science: A body can only be skinny when its alkalinity is balanced.

## A Note About Calcium: Why We're Deficient

One very serious effect of overacidity is calcium depletion. Contrary to what most doctors will tell you, in many instances, it is not a lack of calcium in your diet that is responsible for a deficiency, but the over-consumption of acid-forming foods that leads to poor bone health and eventually osteoporosis. Aside from sugar, sodas (especially diet sodas) are the largest contributor to calcium loss.

Colas have a pH of approximately 2.5, and almost no soda has a pH higher than 3.0. When you drink a soda, your body draws large amounts of calcium from your bones, to raise your pH to a livable level of alkalinity. For instance, if we were to perform the same neutralization experiment that we did with the car battery acid and the Drāno, instead using a soda and alkaline water at a pH of 9, it would take thirty-two glasses of the alkaline water to neutralize the acid from one 12-ounce can of soda! That's an enormous amount of alkaline reserve required, which translates to an enormous amount of calcium being drawn out of your bones!

One of the best things we can do to correct an overly acidic body is to clean up the diet and lifestyle, drink plenty of water, and begin to eat more calcium-containing foods. Dark green leafy vegetables, such as collard greens, mustard greens, turnip greens, kale, cabbage, and broccoli, are high in calcium. Other food sources for calcium are almonds, asparagus, blackstrap molasses, buttermilk, carob, organic raw cheese, figs, filberts, goat's milk, kelp, oats, prunes, sesame seeds, tofu (in moderation), watercress, whey, and organic yogurt.

## Maintaining Proper pH Balance

To maintain the proper pH, your diet should consist mainly of alkaline-forming foods—fruits and vegetables. If you need to lose weight and restore your health, the goal for your daily food intake is to eat 80 percent alkaline-forming foods and 20 percent acid-forming foods. Don't worry about trying to figure it out; the Processed-Free Eating Plan is designed to help you achieve this. Once you've achieved your optimal health, your diet should consist of 60 percent alkaline-forming foods and 40 percent acid-forming foods.

Table 9.1 outlines which foods are the most alkaline forming and which foods are the most acid forming.

Note that a food's acid- or alkaline-forming tendency in the body has nothing to do with the actual pH of the food itself. For example, lemons are very acidic outside the body; however, the end products after digestion and assimilation are very alkaline, so lemons are alkaline forming in the body. Likewise, meat will test alkaline outside of the body, before digestion, but it leaves an acidic residue in the body, so, like nearly all animal products, meat is very acid forming.

A common misconception is that you should not eat any of the foods on the acid-forming side of the chart. This is not the case. While it is true that many of those foods you should definitely avoid (e.g., white sugar) are acid forming, you cannot completely eliminate acid-forming foods. Excessive alkalinity is worse than excessive acidity, because your body only has an alkaline reserve to neutralize acid, but it doesn't have the ability to automatically decrease alkalinity. Your meals should consist mainly of alkaline-forming foods, but you still must eat some of the healthy acid-forming foods.

Your body requires a certain amount of high-quality protein and fat every day for cellular maintenance and metabolic function. For instance, a pH-balanced meal for an omnivore would look something like this:

A large salad with dark green lettuces, carrot, cucumber, celery, tomato
Olive oil and apple cider vinegar dressing
Baked potato (with skin) with small amount of organic butter
Chicken, fish, or beef

## Table 9.1 Chart of Alkaline-Forming and Acid-Forming Foods

| Alkaline-Forming Foods | Acid-Forming Foods |
|---|---|
| **FRUITS AND VEGETABLES** | |
| Most vegetables and fruits are alkaline forming. Lemons, dates, figs, cantaloupe, watermelon, parsley, asparagus, avocados, endive, escarole, watercress, kelp, and other seaweeds are extremely alkaline forming. | Blueberries, cranberries, plums, prunes, black and green olives (processed), pickles, white potatoes without skin, jams and preserves with sugar, and canned fruits. |
| **GRAINS AND LEGUMES** | |
| Amaranth, quinoa, millet, wild rice, brown rice, and buckwheat. Acid-forming grains and dried beans become alkaline when sprouted; therefore, sprouted-grain bread products are alkaline forming. Tempeh and miso are alkaline forming if they are made from organic fermented soybeans. | Most grains (even whole grains), and grain products (breads, cereals, pastas, muffins, tortillas, etc.), beans, peas, lentils, oat bran, wheat bran, wheat germ, corn, popcorn, spelt, kamut. Processed soy foods, tofu, and foods made from nonorganic soybeans are acid forming. White rice and refined grains (white flour products) are extremely acid forming. |
| **NUTS AND SEEDS** | |
| Almonds, chestnuts (dry roasted), chia seeds, fresh coconut, coconut butter, flaxseeds, hemp seeds, hemp seed butter, pine nuts, sesame seeds, tahini. Nuts should be consumed raw. Soaking nuts increases their digestibility and alkalinity. | Dried coconut, most nuts, and seeds (and their nut or seed butters) are acid forming. With the exception of dried coconut, cooking, smoking, or roasting destroys their healthful oils and vitamins, and increases their acidity. |
| **MEATS, POULTRY, FISH, SEAFOOD** | |
| There are no alkaline-forming foods in this category. | All meats, poultry, fish, and shellfish are acid forming. Processed, cured, and preservative-laden meats and poultry (such as lunchmeats, bacon, hot dogs, and SPAM) are extremely acid forming. |
| **EGGS AND DAIRY** | |
| Raw cow and goat milk and products made from them—raw cream, raw butter, raw ghee, raw buttermilk, raw cheese, fresh kefir and yogurt made from raw milk. Whey protein powder—cold-processed whey concentrate from pesticide-free, hormone-free, grass-fed goats or cows. | Eggs, pasteurized cow or goat milk and products made from this milk (both organic and conventional) including cream, half and half, butter, ghee, cheese, buttermilk, kefir, and yogurt. Whey protein powder from pasteurized milk—contains whey protein from grain-fed cows, and typically contains artificial sweeteners and soy lecithin. Processed cheese, ice cream, puddings, custards, and flavored yogurts are extremely acid forming. |

*continues*

## Table 9.1  Chart of Alkaline-Forming and Acid-Forming Foods *continued*

| Alkaline-Forming Foods | Acid-Forming Foods |
| --- | --- |
| **ALTERNATIVE DAIRY PRODUCTS** | |
| Freshly made milks from coconuts, coconut cream, and almonds are alkaline forming.<br><br>Ice creams made from fresh coconut milk and almond milk, using alkaline forming sweeteners, are alkaline forming. | Most commercial alternative dairy products are acid forming due to additives, sweeteners, and synthetic vitamins added to them—milks, cheeses, yogurts, ice creams and other products made from soy milk, rice milk, hemp milk, almond milk, and coconut milk. |
| **FATS AND OILS** | |
| Extra-virgin coconut oil, extra virgin palm oil, extra-virgin olive oil, unrefined avocado oil, flaxseed oil, hemp seed oil, unrefined sesame oil, pharmaceutical-grade fish oil supplements, evening primrose oil, borage oil, black currant seed oil, Udo's Oil. | Most refined cooking oils and vegetable oils (canola oil, corn oil, safflower oil, soybean oil, sunflower oil, hydrogenated oils, etc.), margarines, shortenings, mayonnaise, commercial salad dressings, animal fats, and lard are extremely acid forming. |
| **SWEETENERS** | |
| Stevia, coconut nectar, raw honey, brown rice syrup, sprouted barley malt, coconut crystals, date sugar, organic whole cane raw sugar (rapadura), Sucanat, *luo han guo,* unsulfured blackstrap molasses. | Artificial sweeteners (saccharine, aspartame, sucralose, acesulfame K) are extremely acid forming. These should be avoided.<br><br>Refined white sugar (both cane and beet sugars), brown sugar, high-fructose corn syrup, corn syrup, corn syrup solids, and processed, pasteurized honey are extremely acid forming. These should be avoided.<br><br>Agave, barley malt syrup, erythritol (Zero), Truvia, Pure Via, xylitol, mannitol, sorbitol, fructose, crystalline fructose, evaporated cane juice, turbinado, Demarara, muscovado, Sugar in the Raw, processed sulfured molasses. |
| **BEVERAGES** | |
| Freshly juiced fruits and vegetables are extremely alkaline forming and can reverse many illnesses, including obesity.<br><br>Lemon water and vitality vinegar tonic are also extremely alkaline forming.<br><br>Alkaline water, spring water (Fuji, Evian), mineral water (still), coconut water (plain, unsweetened), green drinks, green tea, herbal teas, kombucha tea. | Sodas, both regular and diet, are extremely acid forming. These should be avoided.<br><br>Hard liquor, beer, and wine should be occasional. If overindulged in, they become extremely acid forming.<br><br>Coffee, black tea, tap water, sparkling water, club soda, coconut water (sweetened), energy drinks, sports drinks, pasteurized fruit juices, herbal coffee substitutes such as Teeccino. |

*continues*

## Table 9.1 Chart of Alkaline-Forming and Acid-Forming Foods *continued*

| Alkaline-Forming Foods | Acid-Forming Foods |
|---|---|
| **HERBS, SPICES, CONDIMENTS** | |
| Agar-agar, cayenne, garlic, and ginger are all extremely alkaline forming.<br><br>Raw (unpasteurized) apple cider vinegar, brown rice vinegar, coconut vinegar, arrow-root, Bragg Aminos, coconut aminos, carob, chili pepper, herbs and spices (all), sea salt, Himalayan salt, Bio-salt, Herbamare, wheat-free tamari sauce, ketchup (natural and home-made from alkaline ingredients), mayonnaise (natural and homemade from alkaline ingredients), pure vanilla bean extract, salad dressings (natural and homemade from alkaline ingredients), gelatin from home-cooked poultry. | Prepared mustards, dried mustard, nutmeg, ketchup (refined, sugared), mayonnaise (made from acid-forming oils, sugared), iodized salt (refined table salt), seasoning salts, seasoning packets, black pepper, soy sauce, tamari sauce (wheat-containing), most commercial salad dressings, boxed gelatin mix and Jell-O.<br><br>Distilled vinegars are extremely acid forming. Avoid these and the foods that contain them (salad dressings, condiments, etc.). |
| **CHOCOLATE AND CACAO** | |
| Raw forms of unsweetened cacao—cacao nibs, cacao powder, cacao butter—are the most alkaline-forming types of cacao.<br><br>Other forms of cacao—unsweetened organic cacao powder, 100% cacao content unsweetened organic baking chocolate, and organic dark chocolate bars with 70% or higher cacao content—are slightly alkaline forming. The higher the cacao content, the more alkaline forming it is. Make sure the chocolate is not treated with "alkali" (Dutched). | Any chocolate (even organic dark chocolate) that is less than 70% cacao content.<br><br>Milk chocolate and white chocolate are acid forming.<br><br>Chocolate and cocoa powder treated with "alkali" (Dutch process) are actually acid forming. |
| **OTHER** | |
| Bee pollen, royal jelly, chlorella, spirulina, and chlorophyll are all extremely alkaline forming.<br><br>Nutritional yeast, probiotics, whole food vitamin and mineral supplements, green superfood powders, most naturally prepared whole food supplements. | Synthetic vitamin and mineral supplements, aspirin, Tylenol, over-the-counter drugs, prescription drugs, recreational drugs, tobacco, food additives, preservatives, pesticides, hormones, chewing gum, breath mints, candy, chips, junk foods, protein bars. |

For a vegetarian, it would look like this:

A large salad with dark green lettuces, carrot, cucumber, celery, and
tomato
Olive oil and apple cider vinegar dressing
Quinoa
Nuts and seeds

I've designed the Processed-Free Eating Plan to help you achieve proper alkalinity, but of course it will ultimately be up to you to make the right food choices.

## Determining and Monitoring Your pH

Although your blood pH is always maintained at 7.4, the pH of your other bodily fluids and tissues should be as close to 7.0 as possible. The best way to determine how alkaline or acidic you are is to test what your body secretes—your saliva and urine—with pH test strips (see the resource list in the appendix for a recommended brand). These are similar to the type of pH strips used to test the water in swimming pools. Most pH test strip kits come with instructions about when to take saliva and urine readings, and how to interpret the numbers.

In general, in a healthy, properly balanced individual, urine pH is 6.4 to 6.75, and saliva pH is 7.0 to 7.4. Any variation from this norm indicates an imbalance.

If your pH is not currently in the healthy range, you should test your pH daily until you get there. No matter what your pH reading is, I want to assure you that the Processed-Free Eating Plan will help you to achieve the proper body chemistry.

## Your Body's Main Fat-Burning Organ

According to best-selling author Dr. Sandra Cabot, internationally known as "the Liver Doctor," the liver is what all overweight people dream of—an organ that burns and pumps fat out of their body as fast as possible! If your liver is healthy, your weight loss will be nearly effortless. The practice of

# In Defense of Potatoes

Nearly every diet book and health plan has banished spuds from the menu, claiming their white starch content leads to blood sugar spikes and weight gain. It's time to put an end to that old nutrition myth and save some space on your skinny plate for a favorite comfort food.

I ate a baked potato at least three times a week while I was losing weight, and I still enjoy one every now and then. Potatoes are low in calories; a medium-size baked potato with skin (about 4½ ounces) contains only 115 calories, sans butter, cheese, and sour cream. Potatoes are brimming with many nutrients, including vitamin C; a small amount of protein; and potassium, copper, and manganese. They also contain fiber. But that's only part of why potatoes are a skinny choice.

Plant geneticists at the Agricultural Research Service have identified sixty different kinds of phytochemicals and vitamins in the skins and flesh of one hundred wild and commercially grown potatoes. Analysis of red and Norkotah potatoes revealed that these spuds' phenolic content rivals that of broccoli, spinach, and Brussels sprouts, and includes flavonoids with protective activity against heart disease, respiratory problems, and certain cancers. Among these important health-promoting compounds is a unique tuber storage protein called patatin, which has been shown to stop free radical activity.[6]

Researchers also identified potatoes with high levels of quercetin and compounds called kukoamines, which have blood-pressure-lowering potential, and have only been found in one other plant, the goji berry.[7] It hasn't been determined whether an average portion of potatoes is enough to lower blood pressure in humans, but the evidence of their phytochemical power is enough to prove it's time to do away with their high-carb stigma.

Potatoes are easy to prepare at home and always a good option when eating out. A baked potato is a whole food, whereas other starchy restaurant options, such as white rice, pastas, and breads, are not. There's one caveat if you want to include potatoes in your meals—you have to eat the skins, as that's where most of the nutrients are housed. Potatoes with skins are alkaline forming, whereas without skins they are acid forming. And because potatoes are on the Environmental Working Group's dirty dozen list, you may want

*continues*

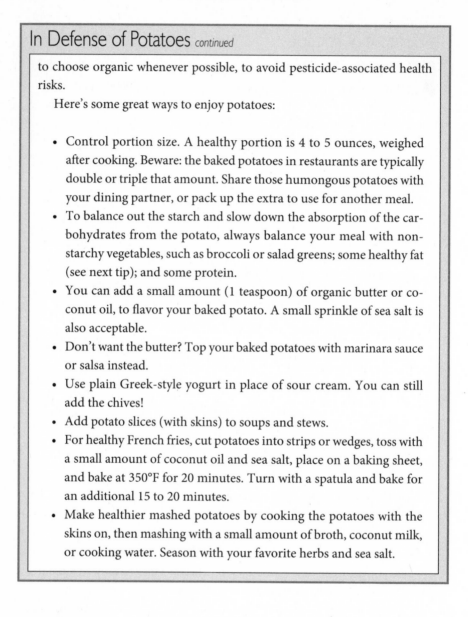

## In Defense of Potatoes continued

to choose organic whenever possible, to avoid pesticide-associated health risks.

Here's some great ways to enjoy potatoes:

- Control portion size. A healthy portion is 4 to 5 ounces, weighed after cooking. Beware: the baked potatoes in restaurants are typically double or triple that amount. Share those humongous potatoes with your dining partner, or pack up the extra to use for another meal.
- To balance out the starch and slow down the absorption of the carbohydrates from the potato, always balance your meal with non-starchy vegetables, such as broccoli or salad greens; some healthy fat (see next tip); and some protein.
- You can add a small amount (1 teaspoon) of organic butter or coconut oil, to flavor your baked potato. A small sprinkle of sea salt is also acceptable.
- Don't want the butter? Top your baked potatoes with marinara sauce or salsa instead.
- Use plain Greek-style yogurt in place of sour cream. You can still add the chives!
- Add potato slices (with skins) to soups and stews.
- For healthy French fries, cut potatoes into strips or wedges, toss with a small amount of coconut oil and sea salt, place on a baking sheet, and bake at 350°F for 20 minutes. Turn with a spatula and bake for an additional 15 to 20 minutes.
- Make healthier mashed potatoes by cooking the potatoes with the skins on, then mashing with a small amount of broth, coconut milk, or cooking water. Season with your favorite herbs and sea salt.

keeping your liver clean is what I call "liver-izing." It simply involves choosing the right foods, spices, and herbs that specifically scrub, flush, and support the liver.

Aside from its role in fat metabolism, the liver is the most important and hard-working organ in the body, performing nearly four hundred different jobs. As it is first and foremost your body's filter, its job is to detoxify the onslaught of toxins that come into your body daily. In the previous chapters, you've learned about some of these toxins, many of which you consume by choice, such as sugars and refined carbohydrates; trans fats; food additives and artificial sweeteners; hormones and antibiotics in your milk, meat, eggs, fish, and poultry; and pesticides and herbicides in your coffee, popcorn, and produce. Other liver toxins you may consume by choice are alcohol, caffeine, and over-the-counter and prescription drugs. Still others sneak into your body without your realizing it, through your personal care products (have you ever read the list of chemical ingredients in your shampoo, lotions, perfumes, deodorant, and sunscreen?); food containers such as BPA-lined cans and plastics; chemicals in the containers of microwaveable products; and the pollution in the air you breathe, including secondhand smoke, car exhaust, and the fumes from paints, carpets, and household cleaners. In other words, everything that you eat, drink, put on your skin, and breathe in is a potential toxin that the liver has to filter. Fortunately, our liver is well designed for this, but we are living in a time where the amount of toxins coming into our body is far greater than ever before in human history.

Whereas a healthy liver will burn and pump fat out of the body easily, a liver that is congested or clogged will do the exact opposite of what it is designed to do—it becomes a fat-storing organ rather than a fat-burning one. Working with people in nutritional counseling over the last decade, I have seen the frustrating effects of this. An increasing number of people are struggling with what should be a simple formula—remove processed foods and exercise, lose weight. When they come to see me, many of them have actually already begun eating processed free and exercising regularly, but they still don't see the results they expect from such valiant efforts. Cleansing and supporting the liver, along with alkalizing, is the key. It works in nearly all cases.

## Breaking Down Toxins

Just as your body has a built-in system for neutralizing acids, it also has a built-in way of dealing with toxins. It can do this by (1) neutralizing them, as antioxidants neutralize free radicals; (2) transforming them, as fat-soluble chemicals are transformed to water-soluble ones; and (3) eliminating them through urine, feces, sweat, mucus, and breath. Working with your lungs, skin, kidneys, and intestines, a healthy liver detoxifies many harmful substances and eliminates them without contaminating the bloodstream.[8]

Many toxins are fat soluble, meaning they have fatlike qualities and cannot dissolve in water or blood. These include pesticides, many drugs, and food additives. These oily substances cannot easily be eliminated from the body through the normal channels. Because of this, the liver has to break them apart and convert them into water-soluble substances.

It does this in two phases that ideally happen quickly, one right after the other: The first phase uses a group of enzymes to break apart the chemical bonds holding fat-soluble toxins together. This chemical reaction, called hydroxylation, changes fat-soluble toxins into more water-soluble substances and temporarily makes them more chemically active. These chemically altered toxins are called intermediates. The second phase, known as conjugation, takes advantage of the temporary chemical availability of the intermediates, by quickly attaching other enzymes to them. These enzymes complete the conversion of the intermediates, producing substances that are nontoxic, water soluble, and easily excreted.

## Breaking Down Fat

Each day, your liver produces about a quart of a yellowish-green liquid called bile. Bile is an emulsifier that helps break down fats and oils into tiny particles so that they are able to mix with water. In your sink, dishwashing soap allows you to mix fats and oils with water and safely flush them down the drain. In your liver, bile breaks down fat globules into smaller particles so that they can be absorbed by the bile and mix with water. This allows fats to be metabolized, to prevent them from being stored in the liver.

The bile is then pumped into the small intestine. If your diet is high in fiber, this unwanted fat will attach to the fiber and will be eliminated from your body through the bowel actions. This is the exact same process that removes excess cholesterol (which is a fat) from your body.

Bile is essential to the liver's ability to burn fat; therefore it is important to make sure your body is producing enough bile, and that the bile it produces is of high quality. Bile comprises water, bile salts, cholesterol, lecithin, bile pigments, and electrolytes (potassium, sodium, and chloride). If the liver is hampered in any way by a lack of any of these bile nutrients, or if the bile becomes thick and congested due to a lack of water, it cannot perform its fat-burning role. Additionally, if the tiny ducts that the liver uses to transport bile to the intestines get clogged with toxins, the liver cannot produce enough bile. If not enough bile is produced, fat cannot be emulsified.

All of these conditions cause the fat-burning process to stop, and you begin to store fat in and around your liver. Because your liver is located near your abdomen, this fat will accumulate around your middle, creating a roll of fat. (Dr. Cabot affectionately refers to this as the "liver roll.") This roll is often the sign of a fatty liver, a condition in which the liver becomes enlarged and swollen with deposits of fatty tissue. Only when you take steps to cleanse and support your liver and bring it back to full function will you be able to lose this fat.

To improve your liver function, you need to liver-ize—by incorporating the following foods into your meals:

Dark green leafy vegetables:  These contain magnesium, one of the key nutrients that your liver needs to manufacture enzymes for toxin breakdown. These vegetables are also highly cleansing to the whole body, as they provide chlorophyll, a phytonutrient that purifies the blood.

Foods rich in sulfur:  These include garlic, onions, eggs, and red peppers. These foods help the liver in the second phase of detoxification through a process called sulfation. Sulfation uses enzymes to attach sulfur compounds onto intermediates and transform them into water-soluble nontoxins. Additionally, eggs contain lecithin, an important nutrient for making quality bile. Garlic and onions also encourage bile secretion.

Foods rich in glutathione:  These include asparagus, avocados, and walnuts. Glutathione is an important conjugating compound that "handcuffs" toxins to other molecules so they can be escorted out of the body.

Foods rich in soluble fiber:  These include pears, oat bran, apples, apple cider vinegar, and legumes. Soluble fiber binds to fats in the intestine and flushes them out of the body.

Cruciferous vegetables:  Foods in the cabbage family, including cabbage, cauliflower, kale, bok choy, broccoli, and Brussels sprouts, also contain sulfur and assist in sulfation.

Artichoke hearts:  These aid in the secretion of bile, and they contain antioxidants known as flavonoids, which protect the liver cells.

Beets:  Beets contains betaine, which thins the bile and helps it flow along the bile ducts more easily.

Brown rice:  This grain acts as a kind of "pipe cleaner." It travels through the intestines, absorbing waste and then flushing it out through the bowel actions.

Oranges, lemons, and limes:  Citrus fruits contain vitamin C, a strong antioxidant that stimulates the production of glutathione.

Turmeric:  This spice is the highest known source of beta-carotene, a powerful antioxidant that helps protect the liver from free radical damage caused by toxins.

Dandelion:  An herb that stimulates the liver to produce more bile, dandelion assists in fat metabolism. This herb can be consumed as a brewed tea, in a dried supplement form, or as a tincture that can be added to water. Dandelion greens can be eaten raw or lightly cooked and can also be juiced.

Milk thistle:  This herb has been used for over two thousand years for its liver-healing properties. More than three hundred studies have now shown that its active ingredient, silymarin, can protect liver cells from the poisonous effects of alcohol and other toxic chemicals. It inhibits free radical formation and boosts glutathione levels in the liver by over 33 percent. Milk thistle is not effective as a brewed tea because the silymarin is not water soluble. It must be extracted using alcohol, therefore it is best consumed in capsules or tincture form. Adding the tincture to a cup of boiling hot water makes a more effective tea.

As you can see, nearly all of these foods are also alkaline forming, which means you can't go wrong with including them in your meals on a regular basis. This is really just about eating your vegetables and staying away from processed foods. That's how I first approached it. I just started replacing the processed foods in my meals with real, whole foods. The more I did this, the better I felt. My aches and pains went away seemingly without explanation and my weight loss was effortless. As time went on, I discovered which key foods can really bump up the alkaline reserve and cleanse the liver, and how to incorporate them into tasty meals and snacks.

Making these significant yet simple shifts is your key to weight loss and optimal health. Eating is supposed to be enjoyable, so I encourage you to focus more on choosing healthy foods, and less on the scientific nuances of alkalinity, pH, and detoxification. Those who have made the choice to eat this way have experienced increased energy, improved metabolism, and weight loss.

## Judy's Story

In 2005, my doctor emphatically stressed, "You should not be eating any sugar! Sugar is very bad for you!" Then he added that my system was very acidic and I needed to get more alkalized. Afterward, I sort of dabbled in not eating sugar, but wasn't really faithful about it.

Then, in 2009, I attended a seminar by Dee McCaffrey and found her stressing the same thing, but elaborating on other foods that make your body acidic, like white rice and pasta that break down into sugar. I knew I was eating lots of them. So I took her challenge and cut out the sugar and the preservatives. As a result I released 27 pounds and found that my gums weren't bleeding any more, that my acne problems had gone away, and that I didn't have head colds anymore! I always had a head cold every winter, but for the last three winters I have not had one. Eating the right foods makes me not worry about acidity any more. Thanks, Dee, for sharing your program with us!

*—Judy Edmond, age 74, retired*

# PART 2
# THE SKINNY

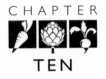
# Putting It All Together
## The Processed-Free Plan for Balanced Eating and Living

*A journey of a thousand miles begins with a single step.*

—LAO-TZU

Everything you have read thus far has given you a clear understanding of the impact your food choices have on your health. You may be a bit overwhelmed and are probably wondering how exactly you're going to make such a huge lifestyle shift. That's where the Processed-Free Plan for Balanced Eating and Living comes in. I've designed the plan to help you transition away from processed foods and begin to incorporate into your life the beautiful, natural, whole foods that your body is designed to eat. In addition to helping you balance your daily meals and snacks, the plan also helps you balance other areas of your life—your quality of fitness, your attitude, the quality of your downtime and sleep, and any emotional barriers that challenge your ability to stick with the process. Each element of the plan is strategically designed with your overall health in mind. Its goal is to continually cleanse and alkalize your body, stabilize your blood sugar levels, and eliminate cravings. Once your body chemistry is clean and balanced, you will have more energy and motivation to exercise, and you will find that you are more willing to make other positive changes in your life.

As you know by now, processed-free eating comprises real foods. It does not include any refined sugars, refined carbohydrates, or harmful oils. Unhealthy foods and poor eating habits may have robbed your body of the ability to support health and/or weight loss by creating chemical imbalances, food allergies, or food addictions. As long as you continue to eat foods that contain refined carbohydrates and too many chemical additives, your body chemistry will remain unbalanced. Therefore, the Processed-Free Eating Plan will help you to focus on the most powerful, cleansing, and alkaline-forming foods, in addition to the right balance of healthy acid-forming foods.

The Processed-Free Eating Plan can be adapted to fit any lifestyle— vegetarian, diabetic, gluten intolerant, or any other food sensitivities. The food guidelines outlined in the plan are just that—guidelines. As I don't believe in a "one size fits all" type of eating plan, each phase and element of the plan can be individualized depending on your preferences and your personal needs. Each person reading this book will be at different levels of awareness, commitment, and enlightenment. Therefore, it's important to remember just one simple principle: *Eat foods in their closest to natural form as possible.* Use your newfound knowledge about how to determine whether a food is natural, and always go with your gut instinct. If you are in doubt, leave it out.

A person who eats processed free generally adopts the following practices:

- Eliminates white sugar, white flour, and other refined foods
- Eliminates artificial sweeteners
- Eliminates trans fats and foods fried in unhealthy oils
- Eats a variety of whole grains
- Minimizes exposure to pesticides
- Minimizes exposure to hormones and antibiotics in animal foods
- Eats full-fat dairy products
- Reads food ingredient lists and avoids as many chemical additives as possible
- Eats an abundance of vegetables and fruits

- Incorporates legumes, nuts, and seeds into daily meals and snacks
- Cooks healthy meals
- Packs healthy meals and snacks
- Makes healthy choices when dining out
- Always eats breakfast and never intentionally skips meals
- Drinks an adequate amount of water
- Minimizes alcoholic beverages
- Stays within healthy portion guidelines, but does not obsess about calories
- Has a healthy relationship with food and approaches it with reverence
- Surrounds him- or herself with a social community supportive of healthy eating and living

This list may seem like a tall order, but those who have been willing to give processed-free living an honest try have found the improvements in their health astounding and remarkable. Our body needs whole foods, as close as possible to the way nature provides them, to function well. Luckily for us, most of nature's foods are readily available, and this plan will show you how to enjoy nature's bounty in a way that is satisfying and delicious!

While most of the recipes in this plan were created with time saving in mind, you should still realize that they are not as quick and convenient as ripping open a bag of chips or shelling out a few bucks for a fast-food value meal. You may have to spend a little more time and money shopping for healthy foods, and a little more time in the kitchen preparing them; however, it will be time well spent now to save yourself from having to spend more time and money later on doctor visits and medications. When you make the effort and adopt the elements of processed-free living, you may begin to rebuild your birthright of good health. Notice the words *elements of.* Processed-free living is not to be approached with an all-or-nothing mind-set, as it is not a diet in the conventional sense of the word.

The word *diet* comes from the Greek word *dieta,* which means "discipline" or "way of living." The Latin root of the word means "a day's journey." I encourage you to approach processed-free living as a steady *process* to be taken *one day at a time.* The key is to make real changes—changes you can live with successfully on a long-term basis—in the way you approach food, fitness, and the challenges and opportunities of living.

The personal stories you've read in these pages illustrate how each person's experience with processed-free living is unique. The willingness to strive for progress, not perfection, brings about results simply by following the guidelines to the best of your ability. Changes are best achieved gradually, as an understanding of food and your own needs deepens. Attempting to change everything all at once may create undue stress and feel overwhelming. Yet, without discipline and commitment, progress will be minimal. You must be committed to sticking with the process, even if results are slow or if you stray from it temporarily.

I have been living processed free for twenty years, and I will tell you that in no way do I claim perfection. Instead, I claim consistency and commitment, and that has made all the difference. The state of your health is all about choices. You can choose to remain the same, wasting your days as I once did struggling with food and weight, or you can choose to make healthy living a true priority. Remember, I was once a morbidly obese junk-food junkie who couldn't see past the next mouthful of M&M's. I know what it's like to be standing in your shoes. The only difference between you and me is that I have more experience with processed-free eating. But my experience was hard won. You have an advantage I didn't twenty years ago: the proven science, advice, wisdom, recipes, and practical tools offered in this plan. These will lay a foundation for transforming your health, and your life, for the long term.

## A Balanced and Cleansing Way of Eating

This chapter details all of the wonderful components of the Processed-Free Eating Plan. These include helpful information about portion sizes, the type of water you'll drink, the beautiful foods you'll enjoy in the right combinations, and the supplements I recommend. As mentioned before, you should incorporate these components into your life as quickly or as gradually as you feel comfortable with. In Chapters 12 and 13, I provide more specifics, including a two-week initial phase to get you acquainted with the alkalizing and liver-izing foods. This Skinny Beginnings phase is designed to kick-start your fat-burning metabolism. It comes with a set of menus and snack ideas and a daily checklist for you to keep track of your food intake. The ongoing Skinny for Life phase continues to alkalize and liver-ize your body, with a wider variety of foods. Skinny for Life is designed to guide you toward long-term health. This information, combined with meaningful fitness, rejuvenating rest, a positive attitude, and a personal commitment to self-care, form the total Processed-Free Plan for Balanced Eating and Living. These final elements will be outlined in detail in Chapter 14.

The Processed-Free Eating Plan emphasizes the following essential components to nourish, cleanse, and support your body.

## Portion Size and Food Quality (not Calories)

As I developed a new relationship with food, my focus was on making sure that I was not eating more food than I needed, and that the food itself was of high quality. In the beginning, I used a kitchen scale to weigh cooked meats, fish, poultry, and baked potatoes, and used measuring cups and measuring spoons for vegetables, whole grains, beans, dairy, and oils. At no time, either during or after my weight loss, did I ever concern myself with the number of calories I was consuming. I would like to encourage you to do the same. You can get rid of your pocket calorie counter and your reliance on online calorie trackers, because you won't need them. I want you to focus on portion sizes instead. Why? Because the traditional method of counting calories does not take into account the nutrient density or the metabolic properties of food. Neither does it account for the alkalizing and liver-izing properties of the food. Which brings us to the seventh Law of Skinny Science: The "calories in, calories out" argument is tragically flawed.

If nutrient density is a new concept for you, here's a quick explanation: An apple containing 100 calories is not the same as a 100-calorie snack pack. The apple alkalizes, cleanses, and nourishes your body with fiber, multiple nutrients, and enzymes. The 100-calorie snack pack contains enriched flour, sugar, hydrogenated oils, TBHQ, and other additives, but has no fiber, few nutrients, and no enzymes; in fact, it robs your body of nutrients, creates acidic body chemistry, leaves you feeling hungry an hour later, and makes you fat! In addition, the number of calories a food contains says nothing of how that food is digested and metabolized by your body. Foods high in fiber have been shown to enhance blood sugar control and assist in the reduction of absorption of between 30 and 180 calories per day. While healthy fats such as avocados, nuts, seeds, omega-3 oils, and coconut oil do have high calorie counts, they actually increase our liver's ability to burn fat more efficiently, thereby increasing our overall metabolism. Some foods, such as celery and lettuce, have what are called negative calories, meaning that we expend more energy (calories) to digest these foods than the foods themselves contain. And legumes contain a type of starch called resistant starch that helps the body burn 20 to 25 percent more fat, when included in the diet on a daily basis.

Even the standard 4-4-9 method (4 calories per gram of protein, 4 calories per gram of carbohydrates, and 9 calories per gram of fat) of calculating calories in foods is an outdated, crude approximation of the actual true caloric values in foods. This general method, called the Atwater General Factor System, was developed at the end of the nineteenth century and applies a single factor for determining calories of protein, fat, and carbohydrates, regardless of the food in which it is found. A more recent and scientifically accurate method, called the Extensive General Factor System, applies more specific factors for calculating the calories provided by proteins, fats, and carbohydrates, *depending on the foods in which they are found.*[1]

The latter system takes into account the differences in the amount of energy provided by the different amino acids in proteins, differing types of sugars and starches, and the differing amounts of energy provided by short-chain, medium-chain, and long-chain fats. The Extensive General Factor System considers other sources of energy from foods, such as the energy from fiber, organic acids (e.g., citric acid found in citrus fruits), and polyols (e.g., xylitol in fruits and vegetables). This results in a huge array of different factors and makes a big difference in how calories are calculated.

The bottom line is, while calorie counting may keep you within a reasonable range, for the most part it is an oversimplified and inaccurate way of achieving optimal health. The whole concept of calorie counting was originally introduced to allow dieters to continue to "have their cake and eat it too," without regard to what that food was doing to their body long term.

Nature supplies food for us in its purest state, and nature has always intended that we eat it in that form. When you improve the quality of the foods you eat and eat them in the proper quantities, there is no need to count calories. In fact, you will find that following the portion guidelines outlined in the Processed-Free Eating Plan will yield a daily calorie level that is within a healthy range.

To help you figure out portions, a detailed list of foods and their portion sizes is provided in Chapters 12 and 13. In general, the following guidelines can be used to help you gauge healthy portion sizes:

- A 1-cup portion is about the size of a baseball.
- A ½-cup portion is about the size of half a baseball.
- A 3-ounce portion of cooked meat, fish, or poultry is about the size of a computer mouse or a deck of cards.
- A small baked potato is about the size of a computer mouse.
- One ounce of cheese looks like three stacked dice or a stick of string cheese.
- One ounce of nuts is a small handful.
- One portion of whole-grain bread is one slice.
- One portion of a whole-grain pancake is the size of a compact disc.

A final note: You don't want your day's worth of food to amount to nothing more than an Excel spreadsheet! Approaching food as a *way of eating for life* helps you put the joy back into eating while supporting health and fitness. This plan emphasizes eating a wide variety of vegetables, fruits, whole grains, legumes, nuts, seeds, oils, and protein foods so you can focus on satisfying meals without undue emphasis on nutritional details that may distract you from the big picture of pleasurable eating.

## Clean Water

Every living and healing process that happens inside your body depends on water. It is vital for absorbing and transporting nutrients, filtering waste from the blood, and cleansing the colon. Water is also what your liver uses to make quality bile so it can metabolize fat into useable energy and flush out toxins. If you don't drink enough water, the bile becomes thick and congested, and your liver's ability to burn fat slows down. When your liver's ability to burn fat slows down, your metabolism slows down right along with it. When your metabolism is low, food has a tendency to turn into fat and you become much more fatigued. It has been medically proven that just a 5 percent drop in body fluids will cause a 25 to 30 percent loss of energy in the average person.[2] When you have no energy, you're not motivated to take care of yourself, and healthy living is difficult to sustain. Drinking an adequate amount of water can make a world of difference in your ability to get and stay skinny and healthy.

Inadequate water intake is dangerous because you typically will not feel thirsty until your cells are already dehydrated. It's kind of like the indicator light on your dashboard that doesn't come on and start flashing until your tank is nearly empty! Thirst does not develop until body fluids are depleted well below levels required for optimal functioning. Unfortunately, chronic dehydration is very subtle and most people don't even realize their body is crying out for water. Symptoms of even mild chronic dehydration include headaches, feeling tired and groggy, constipation, joint pain, back pain, allergies, asthma, high blood pressure, and dry skin. Severe chronic dehydration can lead to more serious problems with blood pressure, circulation, kidney function, immune system function, and digestive disorders.

## How Much Water Do You Need?

Through the normal activities of daily living, the average adult loses about 6 pints (12 cups) of fluid a day in sweat, urine, exhaled air from breathing, and through our bowel movements. We lose approximately 4 to 8 cups of water just from breathing. This water needs to be replaced!

Since we all have a different size body, we all require different amounts of water. To determine how much water your body needs, divide your current weight by two:

> Current weight in pounds ÷ 2 = number of ounces of water you need to drink per day

For example, if you weigh 150 pounds, you need to drink 75 ounces of water per day (2.3 quarts, 2.2 liters, or 9 to 10 cups). You may notice that this amount of water exceeds the typical recommendation of 64 ounces per day for adults. Unless you weigh 128 pounds, 64 ounces of water will not be adequate for proper hydration. If you live in a dry climate, are extremely athletic, or are a person who sweats a lot, you will probably need more than half your body weight in ounces of water. If you are following the Processed-

Free Eating Plan to lose weight, you will need to adjust your water intake according to your reduced weight!

While this is a good method for calculating water requirements, it may be too much water for some people. This is especially true if you are 100 or more pounds overweight. In this case, you may need to use a number that is somewhere between your current weight and your ideal weight, to calculate how much water you need.

A simple test for determining whether you are drinking enough water is to monitor the color of your urine over a period of several days while increasing your water intake. A properly hydrated body will produce nearly colorless or lightly colored urine. If you are somewhat dehydrated, your urine will be yellow. If your urine is dark colored and concentrated, then you are severely dehydrated and should continue increasing water until your urine is nearly colorless. Please be aware that if you are taking any vitamin supplements that contain vitamin $B_2$ (riboflavin), it will turn your urine bright yellow and this test will not be effective. You should stop taking the supplement and wait 24 hours before doing the test. Once you've determined your proper water intake, you can resume taking the supplement.

## Increase Water Gradually

If you are not currently drinking your optimal amount of water per day, you must add water gradually so that your body has a chance to incorporate the water into your cells and keep them properly hydrated. If you try to increase water all at once, you will find yourself in the bathroom frequently, as your body can only absorb so much water at one time, and will need to expel the excess quickly! Therefore, you should add 8 ounces more water per day for one week. The next week, add another 8 ounces of water per day. Do this each week until you reach your optimal amount of water per day.

For example, if you weigh 150 pounds and are currently only drinking 32 ounces of water each day, you need to work your way up to 75 ounces per day. You will need to do it gradually week by week, as follows:

Week 1: Add 8 more ounces of water per day for a total of 40 ounces a day.

Week 2: Add another 8 ounces of water per day for a total of 48
     ounces per day.

Week 3: Add another 8 ounces of water per day for a total of 56
     ounces per day.

Week 4: Add another 8 ounces of water per day for a total of 64
     ounces per day.

Week 5: Add another 13 ounces of water per day for a total of 77
     ounces per day.

When you are always properly hydrated, you will "feel" when you need to replace the water you've lost. You will not feel thirsty, but you will always *want* to drink enough water. When you've had enough, your body will let you know that as well. If you have been chronically dehydrated, it may take your body some time to adjust to being properly hydrated, and you may not experience these intuitive feelings for a while. Therefore, you should drink from a water bottle that lets you know how many ounces you've taken in. For example, I use a 40-ounce refillable stainless-steel water bottle. As I require 55 ounces per day (I weigh 110 pounds), I need to drink one full bottle, plus another 15 ounces of water each day. I do this by drinking a 16-ounce glass of water first thing each morning. Then I fill my 40-ounce bottle and drink from it throughout the day. When my bottle is empty, I know I've fulfilled my water requirement for the day. When I do this, I never feel thirsty, but always want to drink the water.

## Choose Water Wisely

Just as with your food, the quality and source of your water are important to your health. Not all water is created equal. Due to contaminants in tap water, it should be passed through a carbon filter, such as reverse osmosis, Brita, or PUR, before drinking or using for cooking. Reverse osmosis removes chemicals, pesticides, heavy metals, chlorine, fluoride, bacteria, and viruses. This is one of the best methods for filtering water.

In addition to properly filtered tap water, bottled water is another acceptable option. Most bottled water is simply tap water put through conditioning filters, such as those described above, to make it taste better.

Considering that this type of bottled water isn't any better in terms of quality, it is probably more economically feasible (and eco-friendly!) to filter your own tap water and use refillable glass or stainless-steel bottles. Bottled spring water is higher quality than filtered tap water, as long as it does come directly from a natural spring. A certain percentage of bottled water labeled "spring water" is not really from a spring but from a tap. In either case, any bottled water you buy should be bottled in clear, BPA-free plastic or glass containers, not the one-gallon cloudy plastic (PVC) containers, as the latter transfer far too many chemicals into the water.

## What Counts as Water?

Our body is designed to drink clean, clear water that naturally contains various dissolved minerals. Therefore, the best way to hydrate your body is to drink this type of water. This includes spring water, still mineral water, filtered water, structured water, and various other "alkaline" types of water. It is also acceptable to add lemon juice, lime juice, apple cider vinegar, or alkalizing mineral drops to a glass of water in small amounts. These dilute solutions are helpful for hydrating, cleansing, and alkalizing your body and are still clear enough to be considered water. Coconut water can also count as clear water.

Sparkling water, also known as carbonated water, can count as water, but should not be drunk to the exclusion of still water. While it is acceptable to drink sparkling water when you want something fizzy, it should not be an everyday beverage. With the exception of naturally occurring carbonated spring water, most brands of sparkling water are made by dissolving carbon dioxide gas in water. This results in the formation of carbonic acid, which renders the water acidic with a pH between 3 and 4. If you enjoy sparkling water, you should balance it by drinking extra still water.

Beverages that contain water but are not clear, dilute solutions, do not count as water. These include coffee, tea, fruit juices, vegetable juices, and broths. You may consume these beverages, but not to the exclusion of enough clear, natural water. Also, you should be aware that consuming excessive amounts of caffeine can cause your body to excrete more water than normal, due to the diuretic effect of caffeine. Drinking coffee and tea is acceptable, but keep it in moderation, and be careful that you're not dehydrating yourself by doing so. Remember, you can always tell if you're dehydrated by looking at the color of your urine.

*Warning:* Because it has the ability to actively absorb toxic substances from the body and eliminate them, many have claimed that drinking distilled water is advantageous during a detoxification period or when a person is working to heal a serious health challenge. However, it is aggressively acidic, promoting substantial mineral loss throughout the body. The use of distilled water for the purpose of detoxification should only be done for short periods of time, a maximum of two weeks. Overuse of distilled water can be counterproductive to any healing process.

## Warm Lemon Water

One way to begin drinking more water is to drink it first thing in the morning. Because you've been asleep for many hours, and have lost water through your breathing, morning is when you are the most dehydrated. Additionally, your liver does most of its work at night while you are sleeping, and many toxins are released during this time. That's where the warm lemon water comes in.

Drinking warm lemon water in the morning is a health practice that is part of many different health plans and is an easy way to liver-ize. Upon rising, before you consume anything else, drink an 8- to 16-ounce glass of warm water with some freshly squeezed lemon juice added to it. The combination of fresh lemon juice mixed with water benefits the formation of quality bile. The vitamin C in the lemon juice helps produce glutathione, which helps the liver to process toxins and eliminate them.

The warm water also promotes peristalsis, the contraction of muscles in the colon that keeps waste and fat moving along the digestive tract and out of the body for elimination. Also, lemon juice contains the minerals calcium, iron, magnesium, potassium, sodium, and manganese, which makes it highly alkalizing to the body.

*How to prepare:* Add the juice of ½ lemon per 8 ounces of warm water. The warm lemon water counts toward your daily total.

The water should be the temperature of a cup of tea, but not boiling hot. You should be able to drink it down; it should not be so hot that you have to sip it. Wait for twenty minutes after drinking the lemon water before drinking or eating anything else.

You don't want to add the lemon juice to water that is boiling hot, because the vitamin C in the juice is easily destroyed by high temperatures. It is best to use freshly cut lemons, but if you're in a pinch, Santa Cruz Organic sells its bottled 100% Lemon Juice (not from concentrate) that can be used. This bottled lemon juice is better than no lemon juice. But don't make it a habit because bottled lemon juices have been heat pasteurized, which destroys much of the natural vitamin C. Because of this, a synthetic form of vitamin C (ascorbic acid) is added to the juice, which doesn't work as well in the liver.

If you don't have any lemons, you can use limes, but you'll need to use a larger quantity of lime juice, as lemons have twice the vitamin C and alkalizing power of limes. Santa Cruz Organic 100% Lime Juice (not from concentrate) can be used in a pinch if you don't have any limes.

If you don't have any lemons or limes, just drink the warm water. This helps keep you in the habit of drinking water in the morning, and the warm water helps to stimulate peristalsis.

You may add the zest of the lemon to the drink if you want to, but you should chew the zest once you get it into your mouth so that it breaks down in your system for you to get the full benefit. The zest, or peel, of both lemons and limes contain the very powerful phytonutrient limonene. Limonene has been shown to increase the activity of proteins that help eliminate estradiol, a naturally occurring hormone that has been linked with breast cancer. Limonene has also been shown to increase the level of enzymes in the liver that can remove cancer-causing chemicals. As with vitamin C, lemons contain higher concentrations of limonene than do limes.

*Hint:* To save time on squeezing lemons daily, you may freeze a batch by squeezing enough lemon juice to fill an ice cube tray. Each morning you can put your "lemon juice cube" into your warm water, allow it to melt, stir, and drink.

*Note:* If you have acid reflux or other sensitivities that make it painful to drink lemon water, you should still drink just the warm water for its hydrating, flushing, and stimulating qualities. You can support your liver in other ways throughout the day by eating avocados, asparagus, whey protein, and walnuts. Each of these foods can raise levels of glutathione in the liver.

## Vitality Vinegar Tonic

The power of Vitality Vinegar Tonic comes from its main ingredient—raw, unfiltered, organic apple cider vinegar. In combination with proper food choices, Vitality Vinegar Tonic is the most effective food weapon known to help you alkalize. Although acidic on the outside of the body, the minerals in apple cider vinegar (calcium and potassium), when metabolized, leave an alkaline residue in the body.

Raw, unfiltered apple cider vinegar added to water also assists in the reduction of excess weight by improving digestion, adding soluble fiber to stabilize blood sugar levels, blocking absorption of calories, improving metabolism, and creating a feeling of satiety.

The practice of drinking water with apple cider vinegar was developed by health pioneer Paul C. Bragg. Dr. Bragg was a strong advocate of the use of apple cider vinegar, especially with honey, as a healing beverage. While recovering from tuberculosis as a teenager, Dr. Bragg drank this healthful elixir and credited his renewed vigor and strength to it. Dr. Bragg and his daughter, Patricia Bragg, have written several books on the healing powers of apple cider vinegar.

*How to prepare:* Add 1 to 2 teaspoons of raw, unfiltered apple cider vinegar to an 8-ounce glass of water at room temperature. If the tonic is too tart for your taste, ½ teaspoon of raw honey or coconut nectar, or a few drops of stevia may be added. Drink this tonic three times daily, preferably twenty minutes before each meal. If it is too difficult to drink Vitality Vinegar Tonic before each meal, you can drink one in the morning before breakfast, one before retiring at night, and one at another time during the day whenever it is convenient.

Vitality Vinegar Tonic counts toward your daily water total. Here are some ways to make drinking Vitality Vinegar Tonic easy:

- You can prepare a large volume of Vitality Vinegar Tonic by filling a gallon container with water and adding ¾ cup of raw apple cider vinegar. You can then serve your daily quota of the tonic from the larger container. The gallon container will last for five to six days. *Do not refrigerate*; the vinegar will preserve the water and allow you to keep the water at room temperature.

- You can add 1 to 2 teaspoons of apple cider vinegar to your warm lemon water, to combine the two drinks into one morning drink.
- In addition to the company's raw, unfiltered apple cider vinegar, you can purchase Bragg brand bottled, premixed organic apple cider vinegar drinks in natural food markets. They come in several varieties, including Honey, Apple-Cinnamon, Grape-Açai, and Ginger-Spice. While these are convenient ways to alkalize, due to their juice content, these bottled drinks *do not* count toward your daily water total.

*Note:* As with the lemon water, if you have a sensitivity that prevents you from drinking this tonic, you can alkalize in other ways by frequently eating the foods that are highly alkalizing, such as asparagus, parsley, and watermelon.

## Fabulous Fiber Sources

You probably have no clue how much fiber you eat in a day, but if you're like most Americans, it's probably not enough. The Processed-Free Eating Plan will rectify that, as it is high in both soluble and insoluble fiber. Fiber is important for regulating blood sugar levels and normalizing bowel function. It helps lower cholesterol and prevents colon cancer, hemorrhoids, obesity, and many other disorders. Fiber has been found to be helpful in facilitating weight loss because it flushes away fat, promotes satiety, and reduces cravings.

### Soluble Fiber

The *soluble* in *soluble fiber* means that it dissolves in water. Soluble fiber is the type that binds with certain substances, which would normally result in the production of cholesterol, and eliminates them from the body. In this way, soluble fiber helps lower blood cholesterol levels and reduces the risk of heart disease. Soluble fiber also prevents and relieves *both* diarrhea and constipation. Nothing else in the world will do this for you! The soluble fiber in the Processed-Free Eating Plan comes from apple cider vinegar, apples, avocados, bananas, barley, beets, brown rice, carrots, chestnuts, corn, flaxseeds, mangoes, mushrooms, oats, oat bran, papayas, parsnips, potatoes, psyllium husks, quinoa, rutabagas, squash, sweet potatoes, turnips, and yams.

## Insoluble Fiber

Unlike soluble fiber, insoluble fiber, referred to in the past as "roughage," passes through your intestines largely intact. Both types of fiber are found mainly in plant sources such as vegetables, fruits, whole grains, nuts, seeds, and legumes.

Vegetables, beans, and whole grains are some of the best sources of both types of fiber. One cup of cooked carrots has almost the same amount of fiber as three slices of whole wheat bread or two cups of oatmeal. A half-cup of kidney beans contains 7.3 grams of fiber. Many foods such as oats, oat bran, psyllium husks, and flaxseeds are rich in both insoluble and soluble fiber.

Although regulating agencies have made no standard recommendation for daily fiber intake, the National Cancer Institute and the American Dietetic Association suggest between 25 and 35 grams of fiber a day for adults and children, with an approximate ratio of 65 to 75 percent insoluble fiber to 35 to 25 percent soluble fiber. Many clinicians and researchers have come to the conclusion that 35 to 50 grams of fiber daily is optimal.

If you consume the plan's recommended daily servings of vegetables, fruits, nuts, seeds, and whole grains, you will not need to worry about keeping track of the amount or types of fiber.

## Fiber Supplements

If you feel you need additional fiber, a fiber supplement may be helpful. But I'm not talking about Metamucil or Benefiber. The best natural fiber sources are psyllium husks and ground nuts and seeds, such as almonds, sunflower seeds, and flaxseeds, because they are rich in water-soluble fibers. When used as part of a recipe, sprinkled onto foods, or taken with water before meals, these fiber sources bind to the water in the stomach to form a gelatinous mass that makes a person feel full and can help prevent overeating. They will also help block the absorption of calories from carbohydrates, which in turn stabilizes blood sugar levels and facilitates healthy weight loss.

## Health Promoting Fats and Oils

As discussed in Chapter 5, it is absolutely essential to include the right types of fats and oils in your daily meals. Specifically, monounsaturated fats such as avocados and extra-virgin olive oil and medium-chain saturated fats from extra-virgin coconut oil and palm oil can help raise your metabolism and promote weight loss. You will also enjoy a variety of other health-promoting fats and oils including omega-3 oils such as flaxseed oil and fish oil, sesame oil, peanut oil, organic butter, nuts, and seeds. Some of these oils will be discussed in detail in the next chapter.

## High-Quality Protein

The Processed-Free Eating Plan can suit both meat eaters and vegetarians. Therefore I want to make sure that I thoroughly explain how protein works in the plan and in your body, so that you can make sure you're getting enough of this most important nutrient.

Before I speak of protein, I must first speak of amino acids. Amino acids are the basic building blocks that link together in specific numbers and unique combinations to make the proteins our body needs. The human body requires twenty-two amino acids to build the proteins that make up our organs, muscles, hair, nails, skin, ligaments, tendons, and other body structures. Additionally, many of our body's important chemicals—hormones, neurotransmitters, and even our DNA—are at least partially made up of proteins. Altogether, from these twenty-two amino acids, your body builds and uses about *fifty thousand different proteins*, including five thousand specialized proteins called enzymes. The liver uses some of these enzymes to break apart fat-soluble toxins and convert them into water-soluble nontoxic substances.

### Essential and Nonessential Amino Acids

Of the twenty-two amino acids our body uses to make proteins, eight are called essential amino acids. Essential amino acids must be obtained from foods, and more important, they need to be in a specific ratio to one another. The eight essential amino acids are isoleucine, leucine, lysine, methionine, phenylalanine, threonine, tryptophan, and valine.

The other fourteen amino acids are called nonessential amino acids. This does not mean that they are unnecessary; rather, that they do not have to come from foods because our body can make them from other compounds. However, two of the nonessential amino acids, arginine and histidine, are considered essential amino acids for children, because the biological mechanisms that make these amino acids are not fully developed in children's bodies.

## How the Body Makes Proteins

Most people think that when they eat a hamburger or a bowl of beans, that the proteins in those foods are the same ones that their body uses for protein. But our body can't utilize those proteins as they are in animals and plants; when we eat them, our system has to break down those proteins into their individual amino acids and then rebuild them into the type of proteins that we need—human protein. I like to compare this concept to Lego toys. Legos consist of various interlocking plastic bricks that can be assembled and connected in many ways, to construct simple or complex objects. Anything constructed can then be taken apart again, and the pieces can be used to make other objects. As proteins are essentially complex molecules containing amino acids linked together in specific numbers and unique combinations, deconstructing animal and plant proteins into amino acids and reconstructing those amino acids into human proteins is very much the same thing.

We are only able to make the proteins we need when there are sufficient quantities of all the necessary amino acids in the so-called amino acid pool. If we are deficient in even one essential amino acid, we will be unable to make the proteins necessary for the many different functions of protein in our body. We begin to lose muscle, especially heart muscle, which may lead to coronary heart disease. Also, our liver needs amino acids to produce quality bile and the antioxidant glutathione, which prevents free radicals from damaging the liver during detoxification. As a result, it is imperative that our daily intake of food contains enough of each of the essential amino acids.

## Complete Proteins and Incomplete Proteins

Foods are considered to belong to two different groups, depending on the amino acids they provide. *Complete proteins* are foods that contain ample amounts of all eight essential amino acids. *Incomplete proteins,* on the other hand, are foods that lack sufficient amounts of one or more of the eight essential amino acids. Grains, sunflower seeds, peanuts, and vegetables are generally low in lysine, whereas legumes have plenty of lysine but are low in methionine and tryptophan.

Complete proteins are found in the following:

Meat, fish, poultry, eggs, milk, yogurt, and cheeses:  Goat's milk dairy products, whey protein, and goat whey protein are also in this group. Animal proteins supply all eight essential amino acids in the specific ratio to each other that the body needs.

Quinoa (pronounced keen-wah):  This seed, which cooks like a grain, contains an almost perfect balance of all eight essential amino acids.

Amaranth:  Another seed that cooks like a grain, this has respectable amounts of lysine and methionine, two essential amino acids that are not frequently found in grains. A cup of amaranth can supply 60 percent of an adult's daily requirement of protein.

Buckwheat:  This is also a seed that is often eaten as a grain. It is a high-quality source of protein, containing all eight essential amino acids.

Hemp seeds:  This nonhallucinogenic cousin of marijuana appears to be one of nature's perfect foods. No other single plant source contains high amounts of all eight essential amino acids (plus the two essential amino acids necessary for children) in the exact amounts the human body requires. They also contain the ideal ratios of omega-3 and omega-6 essential fatty acids, in addition to being very high in fiber. When it comes to protein sources, hemp outpaces most animal-based sources, pound for pound. According to a study published by Manitoba Harvest, hemp protein powder contains 50 percent protein by weight. Compare that to 35 percent in soybeans, 27 percent in beef, and 26 percent in fish. Tofu contains only 8 percent protein, according to the same study.

Spirulina:  This microscopic green plant found in fresh water ponds contains all eight essential amino acids, though with lower amounts of methionine, cysteine, and lysine than found in meat, eggs, and milk. It is, however, superior to typical plant protein, such as that from legumes.

Soybeans:  contain all eight amino acids; however, as discussed in Chapter 8, only organic fermented forms of soybeans are healthy to consume.

Incomplete proteins are found in a variety of plant foods, including

- Whole grains
- Legumes
- Nuts and seeds
- Dark green leafy vegetables

## Complementary Proteins

Because of the deficiencies of amino acids that exist in some plant foods, you need to combine two or more incomplete protein foods to make *complementary protein*. This dietary strategy allows you to achieve a better amino acid balance than either food would have on its own. For example, when beans and grains are eaten "together," the strengths of one make up for the deficiencies of the other, resulting in a complete protein.

To make complementary protein, use Table 10.1 as a guide. This chart may be helpful to give you ideas on how to put foods together, but you do not need to eat the different complementary protein foods at the same meal. Rather, you can eat them within a few hours of each other or within the same day. Whenever you eat, your body deposits amino acids into a storage bank called an amino-acid pool, where they remain for several hours. Your system then withdraws them whenever you need them. Therefore, it is not necessary to eat complementary protein foods at one sitting to make complete protein. Your body does the necessary assembly automatically from all the foods that you eat over the course of a day. So if you miss getting

## Table 10.1  Complementary Proteins

| Foods with Low Amino Acids | Complementary Foods | Combination Examples |
|---|---|---|
| Legumes: beans, peas, lentils | • Grains<br>• Nuts<br>• Seeds | • Hummus with seed crackers (Mary's Gone Crackers brand)<br>• Naked burrito bowl: brown rice, black beans, salsa, lettuce, avocado, onion<br>• Leafy green salad with kidney beans, sunflower seeds, and almonds |
| Whole grains: wheat, corn, oats, brown rice, barley, rye | • Legumes<br>• Dairy | • Corn tortillas with beans and cheese (basically a taco), or bean and cheese burrito on whole wheat tortilla<br>• Lentil soup with barley |

some amino acids in one meal, you can pick them up at another time during the day.

It has always been my belief that vegetarianism is a health choice, not a health requirement. Whether you eat complete protein sources from animal foods or complementary plant sources, or a combination of both, the most important factor is that the food sources are of high quality. As much as possible, if you eat animal foods, choose from organic sources, as nonorganic sources are by and large the most toxic and tainted foods Americans consume. As of this writing, there are no beans or grains on the Environmental Working Group's 2011 Dirty Dozen List, therefore, if you prefer, you can save some money by buying those conventionally grown (except corn). Although, if you have the resources, organic is always preferred.

I have designed the Processed-Free Eating Plan to meet the protein needs of both omnivores and vegetarians. If you are a meat eater, I highly recommend choosing to eat from the vegetarian guidelines several times a week for at least one of your meals during the day.

## The Best Protein Powders

Protein powder is an excellent supplement that can help build strong healthy muscles and aid in weight loss. It can be added to smoothies; oatmeal or other hot cereals; or mixed with water, juice, or any type of milk. Several types of protein powders are commercially available for you to enjoy, but please keep in mind that some may contain substances that make them inconsistent with the Processed-Free Eating Plan. Check their ingredient lists, especially for artificial sweeteners.

Whey protein concentrate: Whey is the natural liquid by-product of the cheese-making process; therefore it is a dairy product. It has been consumed for thousands of years and revered for its health value. The early ancient Greeks said, "If you drink whey, you live long." Whey is a complete protein because it contains all essential and nonessential amino acids. The best type of whey protein powder is one that contains only "whey protein concentrate." Research indicates that whey protein concentrate has the highest biological value of any other protein source, meaning it is the most easily and fully absorbed type of protein. Whey protein concentrate contains enzymes and other immune supporting nutrients, in addition to CLA (conjugated linoleic acid), the essential fatty acid with strong antioxidant properties found in dairy fat, which also plays a key role in weight loss. Whey protein concentrate is a whole food, and if made from organic raw milk from grass-fed cows, it is an alkalizing food. Whey protein concentrate is also an excellent liver-izing food, as it is high in L-cysteine, an amino acid that helps to synthesize glutathione, a potent liver detoxifer. Because of its fast absorption into the body, whey protein quickly repairs and builds muscle tissue after rigorous exercise.

Beware of whey protein powders consisting of whey protein isolates and/or hydrolyzed whey protein isolates. These have been further processed to remove fat—including the CLA—lactose, carbohydrates, and other nutrients. Unfortunately, the human body was not designed to consume protein in an isolated form devoid of its nutritional cofactors. This leaves these powders deficient in key amino acids and immune supporting nutrients.

*continues*

## The Best Protein Powders *continued*

As I have mentioned before, proteins and fats exist together in nature for a reason.

Recommended brands for whey protein concentrate powders are Action Whey and True Whey, both available from online sources. Whey protein concentrate from goat milk is also an excellent choice.

Hemp protein powder: Hemp protein is another easily digested and absorbed type of protein, which makes it a great alternative for those who choose not to eat dairy products. Like whey protein, hemp is excellent for muscle growth and repair, and is a favorite among vegan athletes. Hemp protein has an advantage over other protein powders in that it is also high in fiber, with 8 grams per serving. Its green color may take some getting used to, but hemp has a great taste. Recommended brands are Nutiva and Manitoba Harvest.

Brown rice protein powder: Brown rice protein powder is a good-quality source of vegetarian protein, although not as high in protein as hemp. It contains fiber, complex carbohydrates, and B vitamins, and it is also easily digested. Studies show that it helps reduce cholesterol and enhances insulin sensitivity. It is important to make the distinction between brown rice protein powder and rice protein powder, the latter of which is made from white rice, a refined food. The recommended brand is NutriBiotic.

## Willow's Story

I was always a slightly overweight child; my weight and health fluctuated throughout high school, college, and veterinary school. I had had numerous attempts at weight loss [starvation diets, temporary banning of a specific food type (meat, cheese, carbs, fats), or excess intense workouts that often resulted in injuries] with minimal success throughout the years. I would lose 10 to 35 pounds and then immediately gain back the weight when I returned to previous habits.

Taco Bell, Mountain Dew, bean burritos, and Cokes were my favorite foods. I would often skip breakfast, sometimes lunch, and then eat most of my calories from late afternoon to bedtime. I would drink one to three large sodas a day and feel the sugar rush and crash throughout the day that would cause food cravings and severe hunger. I was often making nutritional decisions while incredibly hungry and tired. The majority of these decisions led me to fast food, packaged foods, processed foods, and empty calories.

My mom passed away in 2007 from a heart attack brought on by her health. Her death encouraged my entire family to reevaluate our eating habits and lack of regular exercise. I knew that if I kept on my current path I would not even live as long as she had (60 years). In 2008, I was at my heaviest, 260 pounds, and even doing my job as a veterinarian became very difficult. It finally dawned on me that I was twenty-nine but felt at least fifteen years older and I was unable to do any of the physical activities, like hiking and swimming, that I used to enjoy. I was dealing with chronic back pain, acid reflux, what I thought was irritable bowel syndrome, plantar fasciitis, frequent headaches, insomnia, depression, anxiety, and joint pains.

When I first met Dee, I had no idea how to truly eat healthy and how to make changes to my lifestyle that would be permanent and sustainable. The nutrition counseling was geared to my busy lifestyle and encouraged me to plan my meals rather than wait for hunger to drive me to poor choices. The food diary helped keep me honest about what I was eating and evaluate how my diet was affecting my mood, energy level, and intestinal distress. With Dee's help I quickly identified my gluten allergy and was able to eliminate the intestinal problems that had plagued me for nearly my entire life. Within the first four months I had lost 48 pounds. My exercise was initially

*continues*

## Willow's Story continued

just walking, some gentle yoga classes, and elliptical training two to four times a week. After seven months of weight loss, I discovered Bikram Hot Yoga and began to exercise four to six days a week for ninety minutes at 105 degrees. Within the first year of weight loss I had lost 80 pounds and had more energy than ever before. I was now able to add in all those activities that I loved from my childhood, including hiking, camping, biking, trail running, and swimming. I have lost a total of 100 pounds and have kept the weight off for two years!

—*Willow Payton, age 32, veterinarian*

CHAPTER

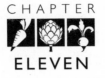

ELEVEN

# Skinny Superfoods

*The doctor of the future will no longer treat the human
frame with drugs but rather he will cure and prevent disease
with nutrition.*

—THOMAS EDISON

This chapter details the health benefits of some of the plan's key foods.
These are the foods that helped me, and the others who you've read about
in this book, get skinny and healthy—the foods you should be incorporating into your meals on a regular, if not daily, basis.

## Vegetables and Fruits

These are the most important foods you should be eating every day. As vegetables and fruits are the most alkalizing foods, and many of them are the
most powerful liver-izers, they are at the top of the list of Skinny Superfoods. These colorful plant foods are perfect packages that deliver health
in remarkable ways and are your best weapon for preventing virtually every
known chronic disease. This fact has been proven many times over by scientific studies on large numbers of people. The evidence in support of the
disease-fighting properties of vegetables and fruits is so strong that it has

221

been endorsed by every major medical organization, including the American Cancer Society.

Vegetables and fruits are so important in the battle against cancer that some experts have said that cancer is a result of a "maladaption" over time to a reduced level of intake of vegetables and fruits. As a study published in the medical journal *Cancer Causes & Control* put it, "Vegetables and fruit contain the anticarcinogenic cocktail to which we are adapted. We abandon it at our peril."[1] Having said that, please remember to be mindful of the most contaminated conventionally grown fruits and vegetables on the Environmental Working Group's Dirty Dozen list mentioned in Chapter 8.

Vegetables and fruits are essential to weight loss. Studies published in *Nutrition Review* and the World Health Organization report *Diet, Nutrition and the Prevention of Chronic Disease* conclude that the more plant foods you eat, the more weight you lose. According to these studies, "energy density" is the key concept to understanding the efficacy of plant foods in regard to weight loss. Most plant foods are high in water and fiber, but comparatively low in energy (calories). Thus they create a feeling of fullness without the hefty load of toxins delivered by many processed foods.

This section gives you an overview of how vegetables and fruits should be incorporated into your meals, highlighting some of the key vegetables and fruits that are essential for obtaining and maintaining a healthy body. As you read about them, you will gain a true appreciation of the perfection of nature's most powerful healers.

## Vegetables

You knew it was coming, our eighth and final Law of Skinny Science: The amount of vegetables you eat is directly proportional to the amount of weight you will lose and the amount of health you will gain. Because vegetables are among the most alkalizing and liver-izing foods, it follows that this would be true. Vegetables are the single most important food to include in your meals if you want to lose weight.

Aside from their weight-loss benefits, vegetables provide the broadest range of nutrients of any food classification and give us the highest amount of Life Force Energy. They are brimming with phytonutrients, vitamins, minerals, complex carbohydrates, protein, and small amounts of essential fatty acids.

In the Processed-Free Eating Plan, the vegetable family has been divided into two categories: nonstarchy and starchy vegetables. The nonstarchy vegetables are further divided into two subcategories: dark green leafy and rainbow (colorful) vegetables. But just how many vegetables are we talking here?

## Nonstarchy, Dark Green Leafy, and Rainbow Vegetables

Each day, you may eat an unlimited amount of nonstarchy vegetables. These include all vegetables *except* potatoes, sweet potatoes, parsnips, pumpkin, winter squash, and yams. To balance your alkalinity and for optimal health and weight loss, *you should consume four or more one-cup servings of nonstarchy vegetables every day.* In this plan, cooked vegetable serving sizes are the same as raw vegetable serving sizes—one cup for each serving.

At least two of those servings should come from dark leafy greens such as beet greens, bok choy, collard greens, dandelion greens, kale, leaf lettuce, mustard greens, and romaine lettuce, spinach, spring mix, Swiss chard, and turnip greens. They are high in fiber and good sources of many vitamins and minerals your body needs to stay skinny, such as vitamin A, vitamin C, and calcium (in fact, you can meet your daily requirement of calcium by eating plenty of dark green leafy vegetables. The darker the leaves of the vegetable, the higher the concentration of chlorophyll and other nutrients it contains.

Because iceberg lettuce is the least "green" of all the leafy vegetables, it does not contain as high amounts of chlorophyll, and has the lowest vitamin and mineral content of all the lettuces, but it is a surprisingly good source of choline (a nutrient that plays a key role in brain health and liver function). If you do include iceberg lettuce in your meals, be sure to also include another dark green leafy vegetable to make up for the nutrients it lacks.

Dark green leafy vegetables are one of our most powerful allies in cleansing the liver, as their high chlorophyll content literally sucks up toxins from the bloodstream. They also have a distinct ability to neutralize chemicals, pesticides, and heavy metals such as lead and mercury. Leafy greens also help increase the creation and flow of bile, the substance that removes waste from the organs and blood.

The other two of your vegetable servings should come from a "rainbow" of other brightly colored vegetables, including red, orange, yellow, green, and purple. It is those biologically active substances in plants, the phytochemicals, which give them their color, flavor, and natural disease-resistant abilities. These include asparagus, beets (all colors), bell peppers (all colors), broccoli, Brussels sprouts, carrots (all colors), cauliflower, cucumbers, eggplant, garlic, leeks, onions (all colors), parsley, radishes, red cabbage, tomatoes, turnips, and yellow squash.

A typical lunch or dinner meal should include at least two full cups of nonstarchy vegetables. Rather than eating two full cups of just one type of vegetable, make sure that you include a variety of them with each meal. For example, instead of eating two cups of just broccoli, try to eat at least three different vegetables, such as a medley of broccoli, carrots, and cauliflower, to make up the two cups to include with your meal. This ensures that you are getting a variety of colors and nutrients.

While it is perfectly healthy to eat your vegetables lightly cooked, the best way to consume nonstarchy vegetables is in their fresh raw form, as the phytonutrients, vitamins, and minerals are in much higher concentrations. Therefore *at least half of your nonstarchy vegetables should be eaten raw,* such as in a salad or slaw. A salad can be any combination of raw vegetables, such as cucumbers, carrots, and onions in a vinaigrette; it does not have to include lettuce.

The tomato is an exception to the raw rule. Its most beneficial cancer-fighting compound, lycopene, is more potent when consumed from cooked tomatoes than from raw ones. Studies show you get up to five times as much lycopene from tomato paste as you do from raw tomatoes, because cooking "liberates" more lycopene from the plant's cells. Therefore, recipes using cooked tomatoes—such as stewed tomatoes, tomato sauce, and tomato paste—provide more anticancer benefits than do the raw tomatoes in your salad.

Dehydrated vegetables, such as the Just Veggies brand, can make a great snack option, but should not be relied upon frequently as an alternative to eating fresh whole veggies.

Here's some quick and easy ways to eat these veggies:

Make a salad: Leafy greens such as spinach, romaine, and arugula taste great when mixed in a salad with different kinds of veggies, such as tomatoes, cucumbers, carrots, celery, and radishes.

Wrap it up: Make a wrap with tuna, chicken, or turkey and add spinach, spring mix, arugula, and other veggies for some extra flavor. Heartier greens such as kale or cabbage can also serve as the wrap itself.

Add to soup: Try mixing some leafy greens with your favorite soup.

Add to tuna salad, chicken, or egg salad: Add chopped carrots, onion, celery, radish, or other crunchy veggies to these classic mayonnaise-based salads. Place a scoop of the salad on top of salad greens.

Add to sandwiches: Add tomato slices, thinly sliced onions, radishes, cucumbers, thinly sliced zucchini, shredded carrots, alfalfa sprouts, lettuce, or spring mix to your favorite sandwich.

Roll them into a meat loaf: Add chopped spinach or other greens into the center of a meat loaf and then bake. Adding spinach is called "meat loaf Florentine."

Sauté or stir-fry: Lightly sauté leafy greens with garlic and onions in coconut oil, or add chopped leafy greens to your stir-fry

Steam: For something new, steam some collard greens, kale, or spinach. Add water to a pot and bring to a simmer. Place a steamer basket with the vegetables into it, cover with a lid, and wait a few minutes until your vegetables are slightly soft.

Juice: If you have your own juicer, freshly juiced vegetables are a great way to get a high amount of raw vegetable nutrients in a refreshing beverage. However, you should not juice your vegetables to the exclusion of eating them whole (unless you are recovering from an illness) because you still need the fiber. You can count one cup of fresh vegetable juice for one of your four cups of vegetables per day. If you want to consume more vegetable juice, you can, but you should still *eat* three cups of whole vegetables each day. Some natural food markets have fresh juice bars, where you can buy a glass of freshly juiced vegetables and fruits for immediately consumption. These are a great option if you don't have your own juicer.

A caveat: Bottled vegetable juices, such as V8, are pasteurized and have fewer nutrients than fresh vegetable juice. They are also high in sodium, and I don't recommend their being used as a vegetable serving on a regular basis. Other bottled juices such as Naked and Odwalla, are fresher than V8 but are still pasteurized, which means the longer they sit in the bottle, the more nutrients they lose. They are typically high in sugar and should not be consumed on a regular basis.

## Starchy Vegetables

Starchy vegetables are also very colorful, mainly deep orange and yellow, owing to their high content of carotenes, which are phytonutrients with strong antioxidant properties. They include sweet potatoes and yams, parsnips, pumpkin, winter squash, and white potatoes (which include those with brown, red, and yellow skins). Other varieties of potatoes that have purple-gray skins and a deep violet flesh also fall into this group.

The serving size for most starchy vegetables, when cooked, is one-half cup, and you will be able to enjoy up to two or three servings per day, depending on your gender and activity level. A 4- to 5-ounce baked potato with skin constitutes one serving.

Acorn squash, butternut squash, pumpkin, and sweet potatoes are some of the richest sources of the antioxidants vitamin C and beta-carotene, which give them their bright orange color. Beta-carotene is converted to vitamin A in the body, and as you may know, vitamin A is good for eye health. High doses of synthetic forms of this vitamin in supplements can cause serious health problems. Food sources of beta-carotene are entirely safe, as the body tightly regulates how much beta-carotene is converted into vitamin A. Winter squash such as acorn and butternut also provide another carotene called beta-cryptoxanthin, which may decrease the risk of developing inflammatory conditions, such as arthritis.

Some of the minerals commonly found in starchy vegetables include potassium, magnesium, and zinc. Potassium and magnesium help lower blood pressure and the risk of heart disease, and they preserve bone health. Magnesium is also important for regulating the body's nerve and muscle tone. Zinc is a mineral that is vital for a strong immune system. It helps keep your skin and hair healthy, and is found in the retina of the eye, where it helps fight macular degeneration.

Because starchy vegetables contain more natural sugars than do non-starchy ones, it is best to eat them in moderation. Starch is a carbohydrate made up of chains of glucose (sugar) molecules. If you eat too much starch, that sugar can be stored as fat if it is not burned for energy. Therefore, if you want to lose weight, you need to limit how much starch you consume. Also, as starchy vegetables raise blood sugar levels more than nonstarchy ones do, you need to be especially careful about limiting their intake if you have diabetes. One notable exception to this is sweet potatoes that, as you will read later, have been shown to help normalize blood sugar levels in diabetics.

## Key Vegetables

Include as many as you can of the following vegetables in your meal plans. You'll find great recipes using these veggies in Chapter 15.

Asparagus: Known for its use in the treatment of arthritis and rheumatism, as well as its cancer-fighting abilities, asparagus also contains high concentrations of the liver-cleansing compound glutathione and an amino acid called asparagine. These compounds quickly alkalize and cleanse the body, which excretes high amounts of toxins and asparagine's distinct odorous residue in the urine. For this reason, it was once thought that asparagus itself was toxic, but we now know that when the urine smells funny, the vegetable is doing its job well! Don't test your urine pH within an hour after eating asparagus, because it so quickly detoxifies, it leaves high acid residues in the urine and may give you a falsely high acid reading.

Raw or cooked asparagus can be added to soups, stir-fries, scrambled eggs, omelets, and casseroles. It can also be tossed into pasta or rice, and makes a great pizza topping. (Even canned asparagus retains its healthy properties, if that form is your only option.)

Beets and beet greens: Beets belong to the same family as chard and spinach. However, unlike those greens, both the root and the leaves of beets can be eaten. The beetroot, commonly just called beets, have long been known for their healing effects on the liver. Beets contain two important compounds that thin the bile in the liver and help it flow more easily. As a result, it protects the liver by breaking down fat deposits in the liver that are often associated with diabetes, high blood pressure, and alcohol consumption. The phytonutrients and high fiber in beets also are powerful cancer-fighting agents and can help protect against heart disease, birth defects, and certain cancers, especially colon cancer.

Although beets are typically red, they also come in white or golden (yellow) varieties. For maximum nutritional benefits, beets are best eaten raw. The next-best option is to cook them briefly. The difference between 15 versus 25 minutes of steaming, or 60 versus 90 minutes of roasting can be significant. It is recommended that you cut beets into small enough pieces that they can completely steam at 15 minutes or less, or roast for under an hour.

Beet greens have a lively taste similar to that of Swiss chard and can be prepared in the same manner as other greens. Like all other dark green leafy vegetables, they are incredibly rich in phytonutrients, calcium, iron, and vitamins A and C. Both the greens and the roots are good sources of magnesium, phosphorus, iron, and vitamin $B_6$.

Here are a few tips for preparing and enjoying beets:

- Wash the beets gently under cool running water. If they were not organically grown, soak them in cold water with a teaspoon of vinegar for a few minutes, then rinse. If you are going to eat them raw, you may remove the outer skin with a vegetable peeler; however, if they're going to be cooked, leave the skins on—this tough outer layer helps keep most of the beets' pigment inside the vegetable. The skins will peel off easily after they've been cooked.
- Beets are typically prepared by steaming. Be sure to cook them lightly to retain their anticancer effects. When boiling beets, leave their root ends on with one inch of stem attached.
- Raw beets can be grated, sliced thinly, or diced for use in salads.
- Beet greens can be used in salads in place of lettuce or can be lightly sautéed with other greens, such as chard or mustard greens.
- Beets can be roasted with other vegetables in the oven or on the grill.

Parsley: This vegetable is one of the highest alkalizing foods (whether raw or dried) and has many valuable health protective properties that are often ignored in its popular role as a plate garnish. In addition to its high chlorophyll and calcium content, parsley contains two classes of unusual components that provide unique health benefits. In animal studies, parsley's volatile oils have been shown to inhibit tumor formation, particularly in the lungs. One of these oils, myristicin, has also been shown to activate glutathione, the powerfully helpful compound involved in liver detoxification. Parsley is a "chemoprotective" food—one that can help neutralize particular types of carcinogens (especially those found in cigarette and charcoal grill smoke). Parsley's volatile oils are also what give this herb its legendary ability to freshen your breath at the end of your meal.[2]

The flavonoids in parsley—especially one called luteolin—are strong antioxidants that protect against free radical damage to the cells. In addition, parsley is an excellent source of two other antioxidant nutrients, vitamins A and C, which are also important for the prevention of many diseases, including lowering the risk of heart disease and stroke, and alleviating rheumatoid arthritis.

Sweet potatoes and yams: Sweet potatoes are not just for Thanksgiving—they can and should be a part of your healthy meals all year long. The sweet potato is not a member of the potato family, and has quite different nutritional qualities than both yams and the common spud. There are nearly four hundred sweet potato varieties in the world; the most common in the Unites States are yellow and orange, whereas the Japanese and Asian varieties of sweet potatoes are purple. Some are shaped like a common potato, while others are shaped like long, skinny tubers. There is often much confusion between sweet potatoes and yams; the larger, moist-fleshed, orange-colored variety that is often called a yam is actually a sweet potato. It was given the name "yam" after it was introduced into the United States in the mid-twentieth century to distinguish it from the white-fleshed sweet potato to which most people were accustomed.

Sweet potatoes contain a high content of vitamin C and beta-carotene, along with unique proteins that work synergistically to increase antioxidants in the body. But perhaps the most interesting nutritional benefit of sweet potatoes is their ability to improve blood sugar levels—even in persons with type 2 diabetes. Unlike many other starchy vegetables, sweet potatoes are classified as an "antidiabetic" food.[3]

It is safe to eat the entire sweet potato, flesh and skin, if they are organically grown. But, if you are eating conventionally grown sweet potatoes, you should peel them before eating, as sometimes the skin is treated with dye or wax. Bake these with the skin on and remove it after cooking.

Sweet potatoes can be boiled, baked, steamed, or stir-fried, but however you cook them, there is one thing you should always have with them (and I'm not talking about mini marshmallows!): always eat sweet potatoes with a small amount of beneficial fat, such as butter, olive oil, coconut oil, or avocado. Multiple studies have shown better absorption of the beta-carotene from sweet potatoes when fat-containing foods are consumed along with them. Additionally, one study has shown that stir-frying in oil is a specific cooking technique for sweet potatoes that can enhance the bioavailability of their beta-carotene. It's interesting to note that the sweet potato stir-fry in this study used a very low stir-frying temperature of 200°F and that only five minutes of stir-frying were required to achieve the beta-carotene bioavailability benefits.[4]

Cruciferous vegetables: Eating cruciferous vegetables not only helps you alkalize and liver-ize, but these are some of the most powerful cancer-fighting foods. This special family of vegetables consists of bok choy, broccoli, Brussels sprouts, cabbages, cauliflower, collards, kale, mustard greens, radishes, rutabagas, and turnips. These vegetables, which belong to the *Brassica* genus, contain multiple nutrients and phytonutrients that are essential in helping you to burn fat, especially the dreaded belly fat associated with a sluggish liver. They also contain natural sulfur compounds called glucosinolates, which enhance the activity enzymes that help the liver convert toxic, fat-soluble compounds into harmless, water-soluble substances that can be safely eliminated from the body through the urine. By including one or more of these vegetables in your meals every day, you will release weight much more easily.

Cruciferous vegetables contain more phytochemicals with impressive and powerful anticancer properties than does any other vegetable family (compounds that have been shown to arrest the growth of both breast and prostate cancer cells, as well as decrease the growth of human papillomavirus—a virus linked to cervical cancer). These vegetables are also high in fiber, making them a serious nutritional weapon against high cholesterol and colon cancer.

To maximize their liver cleansing and anticancer properties, you should consume one-half to one cup per day of these vegetables.

Carrots and pumpkin: Eating these two bright orange foods are an easy and natural way to cleanse the liver. Their most important component, beta-carotene, which the body converts to vitamin A, is a powerful healing antioxidant that improves the overall tissue health within the liver, as well as detoxifies it. Both vegetables have also been shown to protect against heart disease and cancer.

Carrots provide the highest amount of vitamin A of any other vegetable. Two carrots provide roughly four times the recommended daily allowance of vitamin A. In a study of 1,300 elderly Massachusetts residents, those who had at least one serving of carrots and/or squash each day had a 60 percent reduction in their risk of heart attacks compared to those who ate less than one serving per day. Extensive studies suggest that a diet that includes as little as one carrot per day could conceivably cut the rate of lung cancer in half.[5] In addition to cancer and heart disease, a diet rich in beta-carotene also appears to offer protection against developing type 2 diabetes, with pumpkin consumption being the most effective.

Carrots are wonderful either raw or lightly cooked, and make a great addition to muffins, salads, and soups. Although pumpkin is technically classified as a fruit (the botanical definition of a fruit is a plant that contains seeds and has a peel), most people consider it a vegetable, and for the purposes of the Processed-Free Eating Plan, I have categorized it as such. "Pie pumpkins," also called sugar pumpkins, are the type typically used to make pies, soups, muffins, and breads. These varieties are smaller (only about 8 inches in diameter and weighing only a few pounds), sweeter, and less grainy-textured pumpkins than the usual jack-o'-lantern kind. Although pie pumpkin is available year-round as canned pumpkin puree, you can find this vegetable fresh in grocery stores in late September through December in the United States. The pumpkins are easy to cook: cut them in half, scoop out the seeds, and either steam or bake. Fresh and seasonal is always best, but if you have time constraints or if pumpkins are not in season, it is acceptable to eat canned pumpkin puree (just be sure to avoid canned "pie mix" that contains added sugar and flavoring).

Garlic and onions:  Although they are strong on the breath, vegetables from the *Allium* genus are packed with a unique combination of cancer-fighting antioxidants and sulfur compounds that give them their distinct odors— namely allicin, alliin, and others. These, along with vitamin C, vitamin $B_6$, and the antioxidant mineral selenium in garlic, have the ability to activate liver enzymes that flush toxins from the body, hence these are powerful liver-supportive vegetables.

Whole books have been written about garlic's remarkable health supportive properties, especially its role in preventing and healing the effects of heart disease. Garlic has been shown to lower cholesterol, triglycerides, and blood pressure. It also prevents blood vessels from becoming blocked and prevents the formation of blood clots that lead to strokes. Garlic is also known as "Russian penicillin" due to allicin's strong antibacterial and antiviral properties—allicin has been shown to be effective not only against common infections and viruses, but also against such powerful bacterial conditions as tuberculosis and botulism. Studies have also shown that as few as two or more servings of garlic a week can protect against colon cancer. Allicin, along with other substances found in garlic, have been shown not only to protect colon cells from the toxic effects of cancer-causing chemicals but also to stop the growth of cancer cells once they develop.[6]

Onions possess many of the same health properties as garlic, and have been used almost as widely for their medicinal qualities. However, there are some subtle differences that make one more advantageous than the other for certain conditions.

Like garlic, onions have been shown to lower cholesterol, triglycerides, and blood pressure and prevent clot formation. But unlike garlic, onions can significantly lower blood sugar levels in diabetics, with results comparable to the effect of blood sugar lowering prescription drugs such as tolbutamide and phenformin. Onions have also been shown to destroy tumor cells and stop tumor growth.[7] Due to their color, red onions contain 60 percent more cancer-fighting phytonutrients than do yellow or white onions.

For maximum health benefits, you should try to eat both garlic and onions every day, either raw or cooked. Fresh heads of garlic are the best, although prepeeled whole cloves are also acceptable. Minced garlic in a jar has fewer health benefits, but can be used in a pinch. In powdered, flakes, and paste form, garlic loses most of its health-protective benefits.

In terms of cooking, low-heat sautés are the best for both garlic and onions. Boiling onions reduces their cancer-fighting properties by about 30 percent. You'll find that many of my recipes use garlic and onions liberally.

Other *Allium* vegetables include leeks, shallots, scallions/green onions, and chives, which all have some measure of the same health benefits of garlic and onions.

Red bell peppers: When green bell peppers are allowed to ripen on the vine, they become red bell peppers; hence they are much sweeter and contain significantly higher levels of vitamin C, beta-carotene, vitamin K, and B vitamins, than do green bell peppers. Red bell peppers also contain lycopene, the same phytonutrient that gives tomatoes their red color, and that offers protection against cancer and heart disease. As with the other vegetables high in beta-carotene, red bell peppers are strong liver cleansers. They can be used in salads, cut into strips for snacking, sautéed for use in omelets, steamed and stuffed with cooked grains, or roasted with other vegetables.

Avocados: Although technically a fruit (they have a seed and a peel), many people eat avocados as a vegetable. Not only are avocados delicious (they are my absolute favorite) but they contain the vitamins and minerals of green vegetables and the protein of meat, and provide one of the healthiest forms of beneficial fat. In fact, in the Processed-Free Eating Plan, they are categorized as a fat, for their heart-healthy monounsaturated oil.

Avocados contribute nearly 20 vitamins, minerals, and phytonutrients, including vitamin A (the potent antioxidant), B vitamins including folate, lutein (a phytonutrient important for the eyes), magnesium, and 60 percent more potassium than bananas. One medium-size avocado contains a whopping 15 grams of fiber, making it one of the most fiber-rich fruits on the planet. Avocados are also high in a phytochemical that reduces the amount of cholesterol absorbed from foods, so despite its high fat content, the avocado is an excellent cholesterol buster.

According to a study in Brisbane, Australia, eating avocados daily for three weeks improved blood cholesterol levels in middle-aged women better than a low-fat diet did. The daily amount of avocado ranged from ½ avocado for small women to 1½ for large women. The avocado diet reduced total cholesterol by 8 percent, compared with 5 percent for the low-fat diet. Most important, avocados improved the women's good HDL-cholesterol ratio by 15 percent.[8]

The Australian study not only reported that eating either half or a whole avocado per day for a month succeeded in lowering cholesterol levels, but at the same time most people in the study lost weight![9]

Avocados are wonderful in salads, but they can also be mashed into guacamole dip for veggies, and used in place of mayonnaise on sandwiches and in tuna salad or egg salad. Avocados can also be a great addition to smoothies; you'll be amazed at how smooth and creamy they are.

## Fruits

While you may find the idea of increasing your vegetable intake to four or more cups a day somewhat daunting, you probably won't balk at making sure to eat two to three servings of fruit each day. Sweet, succulent, and refreshing, most fruits are high in water, fiber, enzymes, vitamins, minerals, and phytonutrients, making them nature's cleansers. As with vegetables, regular fruit consumption has been shown to prevent many chronic degenerative diseases, including cancer, heart disease, diabetes, cataracts, and strokes.

It is best to eat fruit as fresh, raw, and whole as possible. Dried and dehydrated fruits can also be enjoyed, as long as no added sugar or preservatives, such as sulfur dioxide or sodium metabisulfite, have been added to them.

You may also blend whole fruits, such as those you put in a smoothie, and if you have access to a juicer, you can make your own fresh fruit juices. However, because fruit contains a good amount of natural fruit sugars, such as fructose, you should limit your intake to no more than three servings of whole fresh fruit, or one 8-ounce glass of fresh fruit juice and two servings of whole fresh fruit, per day. As with vegetable juices, pasteurized bottled fruit juices should be avoided due to their loss of nutrients and fiber. This is more important with fruit juices, as the body relies on the fiber contained in fruit to slow down the absorption of its natural sugars.

Whereas there are no acid-forming vegetables, there are a few acid-forming fruits, which does not mean that you should not eat them; it only means that you need to keep them in balance to make sure you are not eating too many acid-forming foods in one day. Blueberries, cranberries, plums, and prunes are acid forming.

## Key Fruits

Apples:  For the thousands of years that humans have been eating apples, it has been well documented that those who eat them regularly experience a certain healthfulness that the non–apple eater never achieves. But it has only been in the last five years that apple research has honed in on the numerous phytonutrients, called polyphenols, found in both the skins and flesh of apples. These special compounds have powerful antioxidant properties that protect against clogging of the arteries and other cardiovascular problems. Apples' strong antioxidant benefits are also related to their ability to lower the risk of asthma and lung cancer. In addition, in study after study, apple consumption is consistently associated with a reduced risk of heart disease, lung cancer, asthma, and type 2 diabetes, compared to other fruits and vegetables.

Additionally, apples are one of the richest sources of potassium. Known as the mineral of youthfulness, potassium is to the soft tissues of the body what calcium is to the bones and harder tissues of the body—it keeps the arteries soft, flexible, and resilient, and fights off bacteria and viruses. Apples also contain pectin, a special type of soluble fiber that lowers cholesterol and blood sugar levels, and improves intestinal health. Eating just one large apple a day has been shown to lower cholesterol by 8 to 11 percent. Eating two apples a day has lowered cholesterol levels by up to 16 percent.[10] New research has shown that it is not just the pectin that lowers cholesterol, but its interaction with the apple phytonutrients that give it a much more powerful cholesterol-lowering effect.

Most of the phytonutrients are found in the skins of apples, so it's best to eat them in their whole raw form to experience their unique benefits. Even if you have a recipe that calls for peeled apples, leave the skins on.

Unfortunately, apples hold the number one position for most contaminated produce item on the Environmental Working Group's 2011 Shopper's Guide to Pesticides in Produce. Therefore, as much as possible, and especially because it is desirable to eat the skins, always eat organic apples. If organic apples are not available, it is still better to eat the apples than to not eat them. Just be sure to thoroughly clean and scrub the skin first.

Dates:  Whenever I get a craving for sweets, I munch on a few dates. Their yummy texture is akin to that of a caramel, which is why dates are world renowned as nature's candy. While you may not have considered eating a few dates for a snack, I'm hoping that once you learn what's packed inside these small, chewy fruits, you'll begin eating them, too. In fact, researchers at the Department of Health and Human Services in London referred to them as an "almost perfect food," based upon dates' nutritional content and numerous health benefits.

Dates contain more than fifteen minerals, with high amounts of alkaline-forming calcium, magnesium, potassium, copper, manganese, and iron; thus they are among the most alkalizing foods. Potassium helps excrete sodium, thus lowering high blood pressure, which can otherwise lead to heart disease. Dates also have a high amount of the antioxidant mineral selenium, which is known to help fight cancer and build the immune system.

Dates are also surprisingly rich in carotenoids, which convert to vitamin A in the body and act as antioxidants. Carotenoids build the immune system and are strong cancer fighters. Studies show that even when exposed to the most potent cancer-causing chemical, benzo(a)pyrene, date extract has the ability to stop the formation of free radicals.[11]

If high levels of minerals and antioxidants weren't enough to garner dates a high position among health-promoting foods, they also contain a special type of soluble fiber that has been shown to slow or delay the absorption of glucose into the bloodstream, thus helping to keep blood sugar levels even. This effect also increases feelings of satiety, and therefore aids in weight loss. The fiber has the ability to absorb and hold water, so it adds bulk and softness to the stools, easing bowel movement and alleviating constipation.

Health benefits aside, dates just taste really good! Medjool dates are my favorite, but other varieties, such as Deglet Noor and Zahidi, are just as tasty and nutritious. You can eat dates by themselves for a snack, as I do, or use them in recipes. Dates are great to add to yogurt, and you can stuff them with nut butters or goat cheese. Adding a date or two to a smoothie is a good way to naturally sweeten it.

Watermelon: Who *doesn't* like watermelon? The subtly crunchy, thirst-quenching fruit is another sweet snack that packs an amazing nutritional profile. As its name implies, watermelon is a good source of pure water, containing approximately 92 percent, which makes it an excellent cleansing food. High in potassium, watermelon is *the* most alkaline-forming fruit, which means you should frequently partake of it when it is in season.

Perhaps the sweet taste of watermelon is nature's way of enticing us to eat it, as it is highly concentrated with some of the most powerful antioxidants in nature, including vitamin C, beta-carotene, and lycopene. Vitamin C and beta-carotene are known to be effective in reducing the risk of heart disease, the airway spasms that occur in asthma, arthritic inflammation, and the risk of colon cancer. In contrast to many other food phytonutrients, whose effects have only been studied in animals, lycopene has been repeatedly studied in humans and found to be powerfully protective against a growing list of cancers, including breast, colon, lung, skin, and prostate cancers.[12] Lycopene also lowers the risk of heart disease, cataracts, and macular degeneration.

Unlike tomatoes, which require heating to release the full power of their lycopene, in watermelon the lycopene is readily available in raw form. In fact, each one-inch wedge of watermelon contains as much lycopene as four medium-size tomatoes, even when the tomatoes are cooked. That's good news for watermelon lovers: you can get all the anticancer benefits of lycopene from your favorite summer food.

Watermelon makes a great, refreshing snack. It is best to eat it between meals, rather than with a meal, as other foods can slow down its digestion and impair absorption of its nutrients.

## Legumes

Legumes, especially beans, have long been called the "poor people's meat"; however, their status has now been elevated to "healthy people's meat." A 2004 study conducted by the U.S. Department of Agriculture found common beans, such as red kidney, pinto, and black beans to be among the plant foods with the highest amounts of disease-fighting antioxidants. In fact, small red kidney beans ranked the highest out of the hundred foods tested, just ahead of blueberries.

Of all the commonly consumed foods eaten worldwide, no other food family has a more health-supportive protein-plus-fiber combination than do legumes (see Table 11.1). They contain both soluble and insoluble fiber, and a one-cup serving of legumes contains anywhere from 11 to 15 grams of total fiber (nearly one-third of your recommended daily fiber intake). When combined with whole grains, legumes form a complete protein providing between 14 and 17 grams of protein (equivalent to the amount in 2 ounces of chicken or fish). The almost magical protein-fiber combination in legumes, coupled with their high antioxidant content, has been shown to be a very powerful food weapon against many of today's common diseases.

Soluble fiber helps lower cholesterol; lowered cholesterol levels decrease the risk of heart disease and heart attacks. However, their soluble fiber is not the only way that legumes protect against heart disease. Their high levels of

## Table 11.1  Fiber and Protein Content in Common Legumes

| Legume (1 cup cooked) | Fiber (grams) | Protein (grams) |
| --- | --- | --- |
| Black beans | 14.96 | 15.24 |
| Black-eyed peas (cowpeas) | 11.1 | 13.22 |
| Garbanzo beans (chickpeas) | 12.46 | 14.53 |
| Green peas* | 8.80 | 9.42 |
| Lentils | 15.64 | 17.86 |
| Lima beans | 13.16 | 14.66 |
| Navy beans | 11.65 | 15.83 |
| Pinto beans | 14.71 | 14.04 |
| Red kidney beans | 11.33 | 15.35 |
| Split peas | 16.27 | 16.35 |
| Tempeh (fermented soybeans)* 4 ounces uncooked | 4.8 | 19.0 |

*These legumes are notable exceptions, with a much lower fiber content than found in other common legumes.

SOURCE: USDA Nutrient Database, www.nal.usda.gov.

phytonutrients, with both antioxidant and anti-inflammatory properties, protect the blood vessels of the arteries from free radical damage. There is also a rich supply of folic acid, vitamin $B_6$, and magnesium in legumes, all important nutrients widely associated with protecting the arteries and the heart. In addition, legumes also improve blood sugar levels (especially in those with diabetes) and reduce the risk of many cancers.

One of the more interesting nutritional qualities legumes have is their high amount of a special type of carbohydrate called resistant starch, so named because it resists the enzymes that normally break down starches during digestion, allowing it to move all the way down to the large intestine without being digested. Once it arrives in the large intestine, probiotics (good bacteria) feed on the starch and produce a compound that has been shown to prevent colon cancer.

Another interesting effect of resistant starch is important for those who want to lose weight. Resistant starch reverses the order in which the body typically burns food for energy. Usually when you eat a meal that contains carbohydrates and fat, the carbohydrates are burned for energy first and the fats get stored for energy later (typically on our butt, hips, and thighs!). But because resistant starch isn't digested until it gets to the colon, the fat gets burned for energy first, before it has a chance to be stored. Because of this digestive anomaly, eating foods that contain the highest amount of resistant starch will help your body resist the accumulation of fat. Research shows that just by eating one meal a day containing resistant starch, a person can burn 20 to 25 percent more fat, and this increase is sustained throughout the day—even if only one meal contains resistant starch. This fat-burning effect is sustained as long as you keep eating foods containing resistant starch on a daily basis.[13]

Research published in the *Journal of Nutrition*, shows that legumes contain a substantially higher percentage of resistant starch than do grains, flours, and grain-based food products. Black beans, for instance, contain the highest amount of total dietary fiber (43 percent), and 63 percent of their total starch content is resistant starch.[14] This makes legumes a miracle food for weight loss.

You will do well to eat one-half cup or more of cooked legumes every day. Although many people have shunned legumes due to their carbohydrate content, few have realized the fat-reducing effect of resistant starch. Whether you eat canned or home cooked legumes, I can't think of a tastier way to improve your health and lose weight. Classic meals such as beans and rice, a bean burrito or taco in a whole wheat or corn tortilla, split pea or lentil soup, bean dips (hummus), hearty mixed-bean chili, and bean salads are great ways to enjoy legumes.

## Raw, Unfiltered Apple Cider Vinegar

In addition to its use in Vitality Vinegar Tonic (see page 208), a dash of raw apple cider vinegar can liven up a plate of steamed vegetables or beans, add zest to a salad, or give just the right amount of flavor to a sauce or dip. It can also be used to make tangy vinaigrettes and salad dressings. But the benefits of consuming apple cider vinegar go beyond its culinary appeal.

Raw apple cider vinegar is made from pressing fresh apples; therefore it is not surprising that this vinegar contains as many health benefits as the apple itself. For this reason, it has been used for generations as a natural remedy for a number of ailments. In particular, raw apple cider vinegar has been known to reduce sinus infections and sore throats, fight allergies, alleviate symptoms of arthritis and gout, prevent and dissolve kidney stones, clear urinary tract infections, and strengthen the immune system.

The best raw apple cider vinegar comes from pressed apples and is matured in wooden barrels. Raw, unfiltered apple cider vinegar is the same cloudy, light-brownish color as unfiltered apple juice. When it's held up to the light, you should see floating particles of a cobweblike substance called the mother, which is naturally formed from the pectin (fiber) and apple residues. The more raw and unfiltered the cider vinegar, the more mother shows in the bottle.

Raw, unfiltered organic apple cider vinegar is different from refined and distilled vinegars found in most grocery stores, which are the refined sugar and flour equivalents of the vinegar world. They have been filtered to remove the mother, as well as pasteurized; therefore, the nutrients have been removed or destroyed. Any vinegar that is clear, without mother, has no nutritional value. Distilled vinegars are better used for cleaning windows and coffeemakers, not for making you healthy.

The effect of apple cider vinegar on blood sugar levels is perhaps the best researched and the most promising of its possible health benefits. This is good news, as blood sugar stabilization is the absolute key to effective weight loss, the prevention and management of diabetes, and long-term weight control. A 2007 study of people with type 2 diabetes found that taking two tablespoons of apple cider vinegar before bed lowered their glucose levels in the morning by 4 to 6 percent.[15]

Other recent studies have shown the positive effects of vinegar consumption on prediabetics and diabetics, and lowered cholesterol and high blood pressure in rats. A significantly lower risk for fatal heart disease was reported among participants in the Nurses' Health Study (one of the largest and longest-running studies of factors affecting women's health) who consumed oil-and-vinegar salad dressings (five or more times per week) compared with those who rarely consumed them. While the study authors suggested that the lowered risk of heart disease could possibly be attributed to the heart-healthy oil, other oil-based salad dressings without vinegar did not show the same risk benefit as the oil and vinegar dressings.[16]

Vinegar has been used for weight loss for thousands of years, yet there have been very few scientific studies to find out why it works. Most research has focused on vinegar's ability to make people feel full for longer periods of time, due to its soluble fiber, thus leading to less eating overall. It certainly does have this effect; however, there are other biochemical forces at work, involving improved utilization of iron. Iron is a key component in substances that carry oxygen to the cells and hold it there. Acids (such as the acetic acid found in apple cider vinegar) help release iron in the food you eat and make it more available to be a building block for oxygen. Oxygen is essential for an efficient, fat-burning metabolism. So, in addition to its fiber, it's apple cider vinegar's ability to increase iron utilization and energy consumption in the body that makes it such a supportive food for weight loss.

Bragg Organic Raw, Unfiltered Apple Cider Vinegar is the superior apple cider vinegar on the market. Other brands are Spectrum and Eden.

# Fats and Oils

As discussed in Chapter 5, *some* fats are good for you.

## Extra-Virgin Coconut Oil (and All Things Coconut)

Of all the health-promoting fats, coconut oil is one of the unique oils on the planet, providing health benefits that surpass even those of other highly regarded oils. After many years of coconut oil's being shunned due to "fat lies," the truth about this oil is now being embraced. Since 2007, a growing body of research is proving scientifically what traditional coconut-eating societies have known for thousands of years: coconut oil is not only a valuable and delicious food, but also a powerful medicine.

So how did coconut oil get such a bad rap? The story is sordid, involving a misinformation campaign by the soy industry and a few others, but it all comes down to the withholding of information about coconut oil studies in the mid-1980s. Prior to that, coconut oil and palm oil (its close cousin) were regarded in high esteem for their many nutritional uses. The darlings of the commercial food supply, these tasty "tropical oils" were used extensively because they are extremely stable, and lend long shelf life to baked goods and many other prepared foods. And, thanks to its sweet, buttery taste, coconut oil was the oil used by movie theaters for popping popcorn.

Coconut oil disappeared from the food supply due to several flawed studies involving rats, rabbits, and a single cow. In each of these separate studies, the animals were fed only coconut oil, which raised their bad cholesterol levels through the roof—which made perfect sense, as no one, not even a cow, can survive with coconut oil as the only source of fat in their diet! The essential fats (omega-3s and omega-6s) had been purposefully removed from these poor animals' diet, and to twist the results even further, the coconut oil that was fed to them was not virgin coconut oil (the type humans have been eating for thousands of years) but hydrogenated coconut oil (laboratory-created trans fats that have only been around since the early 1900s).[17] Hydrogenated coconut oil was used in the studies because it was easier to mix in to the animal's food, ensuring they would lap it all up, thus giving better measurable results of the oil's effect on cholesterol levels. As "science" these studies were completely off the mark, their methods presented to the public somewhat dishonestly (omitting that *hydrogenated* coconut oil was added to and essential oils were missing from the animals' diet). This was the time when the nation was advised to reduce its intake of saturated fats. Because tropical oils contain high amounts of saturated fat, they were lumped with bacon, steaks, and ice cream.

While it's true that coconut oil is a saturated fat, that very fat and its unique molecular structure are what provide many of its health benefits. As mentioned in Chapter 5, fats come in different chain lengths. Coconut oil is mainly comprised of medium-chain fats, which have the unique property of *not* storing easily in your body. They get burned for energy immediately, thereby giving you a burst of energy. This is why the fat in coconut oil has fewer calories than other fats, which give it a special distinction as the only "low-fat" fat. Coconut oil has only 6.8 calories per gram, as opposed to all other fats that typically range from 8.37 to 9.02 calories per gram (that last was for the benefit of any calorie counters who may be reading!).

Also, when you eat medium-chain fats, they help you burn more of your stored fats. This gives coconut oil a unique ability to promote weight loss that no other oil on the planet can claim. Studies show that when a diet contains more coconut oil than long-chain fats, more calories are burned and more weight is lost. Because of its ability to speed up metabolism, coconut oil is my oil of choice for weight loss, and you'll find that it is a key part of the Processed-Free Eating Plan.

Coconut oil has other very special health properties. It has been shown to protect against heart disease, cancer, diabetes, osteoporosis, and a host of other degenerative diseases. It does *not* raise the evil LDL cholesterol, but in fact increases the good HDL. Additionally, the medium-chain fats in coconut oil inhibit platelet stickiness—the kind of stickiness that leads to blood clots, which often trigger heart attacks and strokes. No other oils can inhibit platelet stickiness except for omega-3s.

About half of the medium-chain fats in coconut oil are a special type called lauric acid. In the body, lauric acid is converted into a powerful compound called monolaurin, which is responsible for strengthening the immune system. In addition to warding off colds and flu, monolaurin destroys a wide array of more serious viruses and bacteria, including measles, shingles, herpes, HIV, and the virus *H. pylori,* which has been implicated in the development of stomach ulcers.[18]

As if these virtues weren't enough, the medium-chain fats in coconut oil act as antioxidants, stopping free radicals in their tracks. Because of this, when you put coconut oil on your skin, it acts as a natural sunscreen, protecting against free radical damage from the sun's ultraviolet rays. Additionally, because of its small molecular structure, coconut oil easily absorbs through the skin, giving it a soft, smooth texture. I keep a jar of coconut oil in the bathroom and use it as a face moisturizer and lotion for my whole body. When it is absorbed through the skin, you get the same health benefits as eating the oil. It seems that coconut oil can do everything under the sun, which is why it is called the miracle oil.

Most of my recipes call for coconut oil for sautéing, stir-frying, and baking because of its remarkable stability and resistance to oxidation. As you now know, when oils are heated too high, they become rancid and produce harmful free radicals. Coconut oil is the amazing exception, once again due to its medium-chain structure. It has a very high temperature threshold and is able to take heat up to about 350°F on the stove top and 400°F in the oven, without breaking down the way other fats do.

You might think that using coconut oil will make all of your food taste like coconuts. On the contrary, the coconut flavor you are most familiar with is an artificial flavor that is sweetened with refined sugar. Coconut oil tastes somewhat buttery and is extremely satisfying.

The best way to incorporate coconut into your diet is to use the oil for cooking or adding to foods, but there are many other ways to use it. Because it is a soft solid at room temperature, equal amounts of coconut oil can be used in any recipe calling for butter, margarine, or any other oil. This is highly recommended, as coconut oil is much healthier than margarine, and can be safely eaten in larger quantities than butter. You can mix it into smoothies, oatmeal, and even yogurt, and some people put it in their coffee or tea. Some like to eat it by the spoonful. It works great for greasing pans for baking and is the best oil for popping popcorn. When refrigerated or frozen, the taste of coconut oil changes completely, and it becomes like a candy or white chocolate. Other ways to enjoy the oil from coconut is to use coconut milk, fresh coconut, coconut cream (also called coconut butter), or unsweetened dried coconut.

How much coconut oil should you consume? I recommend 2 tablespoons per day for weight loss; however, each person is individual and some can consume up to 3½ tablespoons per day, provided they reduce the amount of long-chain fats they consume. The more important thing to remember is that coconut oil cannot hurt you; in fact, therapeutic doses for individuals with HIV are as high as 6 tablespoons per day with no weight gain, no rise in bad cholesterol, and no other harmful effects.

Two tablespoons of coconut oil contains 12 grams of lauric acid, plenty to give you its immune-enhancing and metabolism-raising benefits. This amount of lauric acid can also be obtained in 3 tablespoons of coconut cream, a half-cup of canned whole coconut milk, or a half-cup of dried coconut.

The best type of coconut oil to consume is unrefined extra-virgin coconut oil. This is the purest type of coconut oil, pressed from fresh coconut meat, or what is called noncopra. No chemicals or heat are used for pressing. It has a light scent of coconut and a sweet taste.

You don't want to consume refined coconut oil, because it is processed. The oil is extracted from what is called copra, or dried coconut kernel. High heat is used to deodorize the oil, and the oil is typically bleached to remove impurities and prolong shelf life. This type of coconut oil is referred to as RBD, which stands for refined, bleached, and deodorized. While this type of coconut oil has a higher smoke point of about 450°F and has little to no coconut taste, the processing disrupts the balance of medium-chain fats, and so RBD oil does not have the same health benefits as extra-virgin coconut oil does.

You may notice that on the store shelf, coconut oil is a solid white color in the jar, resembling butter when it is cold. That is because coconut oil stays in the solid form at temperatures below 78°F, and most grocery stores maintain lower temperatures. But, like butter, coconut oil will melt when warmed to higher temperatures, so when you get your jar home, it may have melted and turned slightly solid or completely liquid. There is nothing wrong with your oil! It is still healthy to consume. Just as water turns solid when frozen, to liquid at room temperature, and to steam when heated to boiling, coconut oil has different physical phases as well. I don't recommend keeping coconut oil in the refrigerator or freezer, because like butter, it will be very hard and difficult to work with. It's best to store it on your counter or in your cupboard. Unlike other oils, because coconut oil is a saturated fat, it is highly stable and will keep for up to two years without going rancid.

Two new coconut products have been introduced to the marketplace in the past few years—coconut flour and coconut water. Although neither of these contains any oil, each has its own health benefits. Coconut flour is the fiber from the coconut meat after most of the oil has been extracted to make virgin coconut oil. It is a wonderful gluten-free flour that can be used in baking. Coconut water (not to be confused with coconut milk, extracted from coconut meat) is the slightly sweet liquid contained inside the coconut. It is known as a natural sports drink because it contains all of the electrolytes in the exact ratios needed by the human body. It's high in potassium and other minerals, and low in naturally occurring sugars.

You can find coconut oil in natural food markets. My favorite brands of extra-virgin coconut oil are Barlean's, Garden of Life, and Nature's Way. However, as coconut oil can be somewhat pricey in the stores, there is a more economical online source called Tropical Traditions (www.tropicaltraditions .com), which sources the highest-quality coconut oil available anywhere. In addition to coconut oil, the company also sells dried unsweetened coconut, coconut cream, coconut flour, and a large variety of other natural foods. It also sells body lotions and soaps made from coconut and coconut oil.

## Omega-3 Fats: Fish Oil, Flaxseed Oil, and Flaxseeds

As discussed in Chapter 5, most Americans are deficient in omega-3 fats. For this reason, fish oil, flaxseed oil, flaxseeds, and chia seeds are super-skinny foods. Taking fish oil supplements and adding flaxseed oil and flax seeds or chia seeds to your meals will ensure that you are getting the proper amount of omega-3 fats every day.

Omega-3 fats have an amazing ability to provide satiety. You will feel full for a sustained period of time after adding a tablespoon of flaxseed oil at a meal, because the omega-3 fats cause the stomach to retain food for a longer period of time as compared to fat-free or low-fat foods. Flaxseed oil can be blended into yogurt, smoothies, salad dressings, and even maple syrup. Do not use this oil for cooking, and be sure to buy it from only a refrigerated case and to refrigerate it as soon as you get it home from the store. The bottle should have an expiration date of no longer than four months from the date of pressing to ensure freshness and nutritional potency. To extend freshness you may freeze unopened bottles of flaxseed oil prior to use.

Flaxseed oil should not be your only source of omega-3s. Fish oil is really the best source, unless you are a strict vegetarian. I recommend a combination of both fish oil and flaxseed oil. According the USDA, flaxseeds contain twenty-seven identifiable anticancer agents.

Many people like to use flaxseeds instead of their oil. The fat in the seed is well protected by its seed coat and doesn't easily turn rancid. In fact, the seed coat is so tough that if you don't grind the seeds, they will pass right through you unchanged, which means you won't get the benefit of their healthy oils. You can grind the seeds in a coffee grinder, but use them right away, as their oils will tend to go rancid quickly if left exposed to light and air for long periods of time.

## Extra-Virgin Olive Oil

Everyone knows how good olive oil is, so I don't need to espouse its virtues. Aside from coconut oil, olive oil is one of the most digestible of all the fats. It contributes to the prevention of heart disease and cancer, and has been used as a remedy for a wide variety of ailments.

You may use olive oil in your meals for its monounsaturated fat, but don't heat it too much, as you will destroy all of its health-giving qualities. In fact, extra-virgin olive oil is the best because it's "first cold pressed," which means that no heat is used during the pressing. This is important because olive oil has a low heat threshold of 302°F. When heated above this temperature, the oil loses any health benefit it may have had, because it becomes oxidized and turns to free radicals. For this reason, it is recommended that it be used more for salad dressings or very-low-heat sautés. I have included tips for cooking with oils in the sidebar.

## Cooking with Oils

Many oils, such as grape seed oil, are marketed as being good for cooking because they have a high smoke point (meaning they can be used at high temperatures without becoming rancid and producing free radicals). Such oils may be important to modern chefs, but what they fail to understand is that the smoke point of an oil or fat has nothing to do with its health benefits or its safety for cooking at higher temperatures.

Rather than using smoke point as the determining factor for high-heat cooking, be aware of the composition of the oil. As a general rule, if an oil contains 50 percent or more polyunsaturated oil, then it is not good for cooking, *regardless of the smoke point listed on the bottle.* Many oils contain compounds called phenols, which can raise the smoke points, but free radicals can form in the oil at lower temperatures.

*continues*

## Cooking with Oils *continued*

Saturated fats are the best for high-heat cooking—extra-virgin coconut oil, palm oil, butter, ghee, and even lard. If using butter in a skillet, it should never turn brown. If it does, then you have heated it too high and created free radicals. Even saturated fats have a heat threshold. Coconut oil should only go to 350°F on the stove top. If used as part of a baked good, it can go to 400°F in the oven.

For low-heat sautéing, you can use avocado oil, macadamia nut oil, and extra-virgin olive oil. All of these have high percentages of mono-unsaturated fat and low amounts of polyunsaturated fat.

As for other oils, it depends on how much of the oil is composed of poly-unsaturated oil. I always add some saturated fat, either coconut oil or butter, to any monounsaturated fat I cook with, for added protection. The saturated fat can absorb more of the heat, helping to keep the other oil from turning rancid.

The chart on page 249 will give you an idea of the composition of some of the most common oils.

To help you in the kitchen, here are some my rules for cooking with oils:

- *Never* allow the oil to touch a hot pan.
- *Preheat* your empty pan over medium heat.
- *Have your vegetables and/or meat ready* (as if for stir-frying), so the pan doesn't heat excessively while you are busy with prep.
- *Put some water or broth into the pan first,* enough to cover the bottom, to cool the pan down to 212°F. The liquid creates a barrier between the hot pan and the oil; that way, the oil never gets as hot as the pan.
- Toss in your vegetables and/or meat.
- Drizzle a bit of your favorite oil *after* you've added the other ingredients, and stir it around so it's always moving and doesn't have a chance to burn. This minimizes the damage to the oil and preserves the flavor.

As a rule of thumb, you should never see smoke coming off your oil. If you do, that means you are burning it and creating free radicals. You can smell the difference between smoking oil and steam coming off your food. And finally, you should never see any black or brown residue in your pan after you've cooked with oil. If you do, that means you burned your oil and created free radicals.

*continues*

# Cooking with Oils *continued*

## Table 11.2 Composition of Common Oils

| Type | % Polyunsaturated | | | % Monounsaturated | % Saturated |
|------|------|------|------|------|------|
| | Total | % Omega-3 | % Omega-6 | | |
| Almond | 17 | 0 | 17 | 78 | 5 |
| Avocado | 10 | 0 | 10 | 70 | 20 |
| Beef tallow | 4 | 1 | 3 | 43 | 46 |
| Brazil nut | 24 | 0 | 24 | 48 | 24 |
| Butter (cow) | 3 | 1 | 2 | 29 | 56 |
| Canola (rapeseed) | 37 | 7 | 30 | 54 | 7 |
| Cashew | 6 | 0 | 6 | 70 | 18 |
| Chia | 70 | 30 | 40 | 0 | 0 |
| Cocoa butter | 3 | 0 | 3 | 32 | 63 |
| Coconut | 3 | 0 | 3 | 6 | 91 |
| Corn | 59 | 0 | 59 | 24 | 17 |
| Cottonseed | 50 | 0 | 50 | 21 | 25 |
| Evening primrose | 81 | 0 | 81 | 11 | 8 |
| Filbert | 16 | 0 | 16 | 54 | 5 |
| Flaxseed | 72 | 58 | 14 | 19 | 9 |
| Grape seed | 73 | 0 | 73 | 15 | 12 |
| Hemp | 80 | 20 | 60 | 12 | 8 |
| Lard (pork fat) | 10 | 0 | 10 | 44 | 42 |
| Macadamia | 10 | 0 | 10 | 71 | 12 |
| Olive | 8 | 0 | 8 | 76 | 16 |
| Palm | 10 | 0 | 10 | 40 | 50 |
| Palm kernel | 2 | 0 | 2 | 15 | 79 |
| Peanut | 29 | 0 | 29 | 47 | 18 |
| Pecan | 20 | 0 | 20 | 63 | 7 |
| Pistachio | 19 | 0 | 19 | 65 | 9 |
| Pumpkin | 57 | 0–15 | 42–57 | 34 | 9 |
| Rice bran | 36 | 1 | 35 | 48 | 17 |
| Safflower | 75 | 0 | 75 | 13 | 12 |
| Salmon oil | 40 | 34 | 6 | 20 | 29 |
| Sesame | 45 | 0 | 45 | 42 | 13 |
| Soybean | 57 | 7 | 50 | 26 | 15 |
| Sunflower | 65 | 0 | 65 | 23 | 12 |
| Walnut | 56 | 5 | 51 | 28 | 16 |
| Wheat germ | 55 | 5 | 50 | 25 | 18 |

SOURCE: USDA Nutrient Database, www.nal.usda.gov/fnic/foodcomp/search/.

## *Organic Butter*

Some believe that butter is bad for us. But that would be a surprise to many people around the globe who have used butter for its life-sustaining properties for millennia. Butter can especially protect against heart disease (yes, that's right, I'm busting the "fat lies" wide open!). It contains vitamin A, which is needed for the health of the thyroid and adrenal gland, both of which play a role in the proper functioning of the heart. Butter is America's best and most easily absorbed source of this vitamin, which, along with vitamin E and the mineral selenium, also contained in butter, are strong antioxidants that protect us against free radical damage.[19]

Additionally, butter is a good source of iodine, a nutrient many people are deficient in. Iodine protects the thyroid gland, thereby helping to regulate metabolism. Butter has many other health benefits, from improving the immune system and preventing cancer, to assisting the body in the absorption of calcium and building strong bones. All the nutrients in butter make it an essential food, capable of supplying many of our daily nutrient needs.[20]

It is best to get butter from cows that have been fed their natural diet—grass—and that the butter is organic. This type of butter is much higher in health-supportive nutrients. My recipes call for only organic butter, not margarine.

## Almonds

The list of health benefits derived from eating almonds is long and impressive—they lower cholesterol and reduce the risk of heart disease, stabilize blood sugar levels, protect against diabetes, promote weight loss, and prevent gallstones. Almonds are one of only a few alkaline-forming nuts, owing to their high content of calcium, magnesium, and potassium. They are also high in fiber and protein—a quarter-cup contains 4.07 grams of fiber and 7.62 grams of protein—more protein than is provided by the typical egg, which contains 5.54 grams. And eating almonds with their skins provides you with twenty antioxidant flavonoids, which team up with the vitamin E found in their meat to more than double these nuts' antioxidant power than when eaten skinned.

A study published in the *International Journal of Obesity and Related Metabolic Disorders* followed sixty-five overweight and obese adults who ate almonds as part of a diet consisting of 39 percent fat, as opposed to another group on a low-fat (18 percent) diet that omitted almonds. Both groups ate the same amount of protein and total calories. After six months, those eating almonds experienced a 62 percent greater reduction in their weight and body mass index, 50 percent greater reduction in waist circumference, and 56 percent greater reduction in body fat, compared to those on the low-fat, no-almond diet! Among those subjects who had type 1 diabetes, diabetes medication reductions were sustained or further reduced in 96 percent of those on the almond diet, versus in 50 percent of those on the no-almond diet.[21]

It is very important to eat almonds and any other nuts *in their raw form*. Heating and roasting nuts destroys their health-promoting natural oils, the same as heating vegetable oil has a detrimental effect on health.

Almonds make great snacks, and can also be added to yogurt, oatmeal, salads, and smoothies. Almond butter and almond milk are two more great ways to enjoy the nutrients from almonds.

## Wild-Caught Salmon

Salmon is an incredibly healthful fish full of essential omega-3 fatty acids, but you need to make sure that you are eating wild-caught salmon instead of farm-raised salmon. Wild salmon roam freely in the ocean and eat little crustaceans called krill, a big part of their natural diet. Krill contain the powerful antioxidant carotenoid.

A farm-raised salmon lives a very different life from its wild cousin: fed grains, an unnatural diet for fish, and antibiotics to prevent diseases that can result from living in its close quarters. Farmed salmon have more antibiotics administered by weight than does any other form of livestock. The natural color of farmed salmon is an unappetizing gray, so they're fed colorings to turn them pink. On the packaging of all farm-raised salmon you will see the statement, "Farm raised, color added." What's more, according to the Environmental Working Group, farmed salmon contained high levels of contaminants called PCBs (polychlorinated biphenyls) when the organization tested farmed salmon purchased in U.S. grocery stores.

Most farmed salmon is called Atlantic salmon, whereas wild salmon is called Alaskan, sockeye, or chum. As a general rule, you should strive to eat only wild-caught fish of any kind, as opposed to farm raised.

While fresh is best, most canned salmon is wild. Just make sure the can says "wild" on it. High-quality canned salmon—king (chinook), sockeye, or coho is fine. I prefer skinless and boneless myself; but the bones, which are quite soft, and the skin are good sources of calcium and other nutrients. Canned salmon is high-quality "fast food" that can easily be used to top a salad, for a sandwich filling, or to make salmon patties and salmon loaf.

## Organic Eggs

Banish the boring egg-white-only omelets, and start eating whole eggs! Organic eggs contain nearly all known nutrients except for vitamin C and are a nearly perfect form of protein. They are good sources of the fat-soluble vitamins A and D, plus they contain essential fatty acids. While many people have been afraid to eat eggs due to their high cholesterol levels, studies suggest that eggs contain several nutrients that promote heart health and actually lower the risk of heart disease.

The best thing about eggs is their ability to assist in weight loss. Eggs are rich in lecithin and sulfur compounds, which help to cleanse and detoxify the liver. In one study of 160 overweight and obese people, the group that ate two eggs for breakfast for eight weeks, as part of a low-fat diet, lost twice as much weight as the other group that ate a bagel breakfast, and also the egg eaters had an 83 percent greater decrease in waist circumference. The egg-eating group had no significant difference in the levels of total, HDL, and LDL cholesterol.[22] As with other animal products, you should eat organic eggs.

## Plain, Organic Whole-Milk Yogurt

Yogurt is a fermented dairy product made by adding bacterial cultures to milk. These "live and active" cultures carry on the conversion of the milk's lactose sugar into lactic acid. This clever process gives yogurt its unique tart and sour flavor and puddinglike texture. The texture is the reason the Turks gave it the name *yoghurmak*, meaning "to thicken." The lactic acid bacteria that are traditionally used to make yogurt—*Lactobacillus bulgarius, Lactobacillus acidophilus, Bifidobacterium lactis,* and *Streptcoccus thermophilus*—are also responsible for many of yogurt's health benefits.

Yogurt containing live and active cultures has been demonstrated to improve intestinal health by suppressing harmful bacteria in the intestine. Yogurt also lowers cholesterol. In a study of older adults, intake of about 1 cup of yogurt with live cultures per day for one year prevented an increase in blood total and low-density lipoprotein (LDL) cholesterol levels.[23]

Several other studies have suggested that the consumption of high levels of cultured milk products, such as yogurt and buttermilk, may reduce the risk of colon cancer. They also play a critical role in the detoxification of many cancer-causing substances, including hormones, meat carcinogens, and environmental toxins.[24]

When buying yogurt, the more natural the product is, the more beneficial it will be to your health. Plain organic yogurt is best, as it will have the lowest amount of naturally occurring sugars (from lactose) and the highest amount of live and active cultures. Greek yogurt or European-style yogurts are some of my favorites.

Beware of yogurts containing artificial colors, flavorings, or sweeteners such as aspartame or sucralose (Splenda), modified food starch, gelatin, and added sugars such as high-fructose corn syrup. Vanilla and other flavored yogurts, and yogurts with fruit already mixed in are usually inferior yogurts in terms of nutritional value and levels of live and active cultures. The same goes for frozen yogurts—they are really just glorified ice cream.

# Grains and Grain Products

## Quinoa

Pronounced "KEEN-wah," this unique grainlike food has only recently become part of the North American cuisine, but has been cultivated and enjoyed in South America for more than five thousand years. A dietary staple among early South American civilizations, it was known to give strength and stamina, and was called "the gold of the Aztecs." While it is often referred to and eaten as a grain, quinoa is technically the seed of a plant. When cooked, it resembles a cross between couscous and brown rice. It is small, light, and fluffy, yet slightly crunchy, with a delicate and subtly nutty flavor.

Quinoa is one of only a few alkaline-forming grains, owing to its high content of magnesium, the mineral that relaxes blood vessels. Since low levels of magnesium are associated with increased rates of high blood pressure and heart disease, this tiny grain can offer yet another way to protect against strokes and heart attacks. Other nutrients contained in quinoa are folate, manganese, iron, copper, and phosphorous.

As quinoa is technically a seed, it does not contain gluten, the highly allergenic protein found in several other grains. This makes quinoa a fantastic food for those who are gluten intolerant. It is a good source of fiber (quinoa has 5 grams per cup vs. 3.5 grams in one cup of brown rice) and a protein powerhouse, containing all of the essential amino acids needed to make a complete protein. This makes quinoa an excellent food for vegetarians.

Like legumes, quinoa is a resistant-starch food, meaning it raises metabolism and burns more fat. Quinoa also has a good amount of fiber and phytochemicals, which have been shown to fight a variety of chronic diseases, including cancer, heart disease, and diabetes. Quinoa contains saponins on the outer coat, which gives it a bitter taste if not rinsed before cooking. See the Basic Quinoa recipe in Chapter 15 for cooking instructions.

While the most popular varieties of quinoa are transparent yellow and red, other varieties are orange, pink, purple, or black. Quinoa makes a great side dish alternative to rice or pasta, and can also be eaten as a warm breakfast porridge. Like other grains, quinoa can be ground into flour and made into pasta.

## Oat Bran

The most virtuous and versatile component of the oat resides in its outer layer—the bran. Since 1963, study after study has proven that oat bran significantly lowers cholesterol. Individuals with high cholesterol consuming just 3 grams of soluble oat fiber per day (an amount found in one cup of oatmeal or one-half cup of oat bran) typically lowers total cholesterol by 8 to 23 percent. This is highly significant since each 1 percent drop in cholesterol translates to a 2 percent decrease in the risk of developing heart disease.[25]

Unique to oats, and in particular oat bran, are special antioxidant compounds that help prevent free radicals from damaging cholesterol, providing another powerful mechanism for oat bran to reduce the risk of heart disease.

Because oat bran is high in fiber, it promotes weight loss by reducing cravings, stabilizing blood sugar levels, and by providing a prolonged feeling of fullness along with a steady boost of energy. Also, because it is mainly fiber, one cup of oat bran has less calories and carbohydrates than a cup of oatmeal or any other grain. It is considered an excellent food for diabetics because the fiber causes dietary sugars to be absorbed more gradually and increases tissue sensitivity to insulin. In fact, studies show that people with type 1 diabetes who incorporate oat bran into their balanced diet reduce their insulin requirements.

The fiber in oat bran helps regulate bowel function and can alleviate constipation—a health problem that many people suffer from which can lead to a number of bowel diseases, including colon cancer. The soluble fiber in oat bran activates white blood cells, which in effect strengthens the immune system and may prevent some cancers.

Most natural food stores carry raw oat bran in the bulk food section, which is the most economical way to purchase it. Packaged oat bran tends to be higher priced. Quaker Oats sells it in a 1-pound box that you will find in the hot cereal section of most grocery chains. Bob's Red Mill also sells it in a 1-pound clear plastic package.

Oat bran can be eaten raw or cooked. You can sprinkle raw oat bran into yogurt, add it to smoothies, and use it in place of bread crumbs in recipes. Oat bran can be cooked and eaten just like oatmeal, and you can use it in baked goods. It is the main ingredient in Dee's Naturals Flourless Oat Bran Muffins, sold in select natural food markets.

## Sprouted Whole-Grain Bread

There are two ways to make whole-grain bread: (1) harvest the whole grains, dry them, grind them into flour, make dough, form into loaves, then bake at 350°F for 30 to 40 minutes; or (2) harvest the whole grains, sprout them, blend them into a thick puree, form into loaves, then bake at 250°F for 2½ hours. The second is a more digestible bread with more available enzymes and nutrients.

Sprouting grains is a process similar to fermentation, where grains are soaked in water for several days until a sprout begins to form. Once the sprouting starts, natural enzymes break down the starch into simpler molecules that are easier to digest. Sprouting increases many of the grains' key nutrients, including B vitamins, vitamin C, folate, fiber, and essential amino acids often lacking in dried grains, such as lysine. Because the grains are not ground into flour, such breads are often referred to as "flourless." Although sprouted grains do still contain gluten, the sprouting process changes the gluten to a more digestible or tolerable state. Many people with mild gluten sensitivities are able to tolerate sprouted grain products. Also, the serotonin "high" described in Chapter 4, which is associated with dried grains that have been ground into flour, does not happen when you eat sprouted grains. Therefore, this type of bread is a better choice for curbing sugar and flour cravings.

As the popularity of eating sprouted grains has been increasing, there have been a number of studies documenting a wide range of health benefits for different sprouted grains. Here are just a few:

- Sprouted brown rice fights diabetes.
- Sprouted buckwheat protects against fatty liver disease.
- Cardiovascular risk is reduced by sprouted brown rice.
- Sprouted brown rice decreases depression and fatigue in nursing mothers.
- Decreased blood pressure is linked to sprouted barley.[26]

Once the puree is made from the sprouted grains, it can be used to make bread, tortillas, English muffins, burger buns, hot-dog buns, pita bread, breakfast cereals, and other "flourless" products. These breads are ideal for weight loss because they are filling, regulate blood sugar levels, and do not cause cravings. Believe me, you will not want to overeat on this bread!

Just so you know, companies making sprouted grain products currently use two different approaches once the grains are sprouted. Due to the differences between these two approaches, the ingredient lists for sprouted grain products will list either "sprouted whole wheat, sprouted whole rye, sprouted whole barley, etc." or "sprouted whole wheat flour, sprouted whole rye flour, etc." Some companies use a combination of both types in one product.

You will find sprouted grain breads in natural food markets and many mainstream grocery stores. They are highly perishable due to their lack of chemical preservatives and are usually kept in the freezer or refrigerated section of the store. You need to keep them refrigerated or frozen also once you get them home. Several nationally available brands of flourless bread include Food for Life, which makes Ezekiel 4:9–type breads, and Alvarado Street Bakery. Some grocers, such as Trader Joe's, sell sprouted grain breads under their private label.

Whole wheat berries and other whole grains can be purchased from the bulk section of natural food markets, and you can sprout them yourself to make your own flourless bread. You can also buy or make your own sprouted grain flour. See the appendix (page 403) for more information.

You can use sprouted bread in the same way you use other whole-grain breads. I use it for sandwiches, toast, and making my own "flourless" bread crumbs.

## Chocolate

For the past decade, researchers all over the world have been discovering the myriad compounds locked inside the seeds of the tropical fruit known as cacao (pronounced "ka-KOW"), from which all forms of chocolate are derived. As a result, chocolate's bad rap as a fattening guilty pleasure has been given a complete 180. Cacao is loaded with flavonoids, has at least twice as many antioxidants as any other fruit or vegetable, and has taken the crown from the reigning superstars green tea and red wine for its role in preventing heart disease. It truly is the granddaddy of all superfoods. In February 2011, new research published in *Chemistry Central Journal* demonstrated that dark chocolate and cocoa powder have more antioxidant activity and contain more flavonoids than do any of the new super fruits—açai berries, blueberries, cranberries, and pomegranates.[27]

Cacao is a hard-shelled tropical tree fruit. Each pod, which somewhat resembles a papaya in shape, contains thirty to forty seeds. These seeds, which are very bitter, need to be fermented to activate enzymes that develop and release the compounds that give chocolate its characteristic flavor and aroma. (Interestingly, this is very similar to the fermentation required to activate enzymes that release the isoflavones in soybeans.) Raw cacao nibs are fermented seeds that have been dried but not roasted, or roasted at temperatures below 118°F. Natural cocoa powder and natural dark chocolate emerge from their minimal processing (pressing and low-heat friction) still loaded with the nibs' antioxidant flavonoids. One particularly active flavonoid, called epicatechin, greatly reduces the risk of a heart attack or stroke by inhibiting the oxidation of cholesterol, thus preventing the formation of the bad cholesterol (LDL). Epicatechin also raises levels of HDL (the good cholesterol), and performs the same blood-thinning activity as taking a baby aspirin. Research performed at the University of California–Davis, found that epicatechin in dark chocolate thins the blood and prevents the blood platelet clumping that leads to atherosclerosis and strokes. Study participants consumed 1.6 ounces of dark chocolate every day for two weeks. At the end of the study, blood tests showed that high levels of epicatechin were coursing through their arteries.[28]

An immense amount of other research has also demonstrated that chocolate's flavonoids can reduce blood pressure, enhance brain function, lift depression, improve blood sugar levels, ease chronic fatigue syndrome, suppress coughs, and more. Chocolate also contains magnesium, a crucial mineral for heart health. It seems that chocolate, like its tropical cousin the coconut, can do no wrong!

Like coconut oil, cocoa butter is a saturated fat, a long-chained kind called stearic acid that, in the body, acts like a monounsaturated fat—the same type of fat in olive oil and avocados. The stearic acid in cocoa butter has similar heart protective properties as the epicatechin found in cocoa powder—it protects cholesterol in the body from becoming oxidized by free radicals, makes blood platelets less sticky, and protects against blood clots and atherosclerosis. Cocoa butter is solid at room temperature and melts slightly below body temperature, at 89° to 93°F. Like coconut oil, its remarkable stability and resistance to oxidation gives it an exceptionally long shelf life. Under normal storage conditions, cocoa butter will keep for years without going rancid.

The best chocolate of all is raw cacao nibs, which can be purchased in natural food markets and from online sources. They have a natural ratio of

47 percent cocoa solids to 53 percent cocoa butter, unmatched by any form of manufactured chocolate. Raw cacao is the number one antioxidant food in the world—thirty times higher than red wine and twenty times higher than green tea. It provides good amounts of magnesium, chromium, and iron, which are the top three mineral deficiencies in the United States. It is also extraordinarily high in vitamin C and is one of the best sources of natural fiber. And cacao contains two potent phytochemicals—theobromine and phenylethylamine. Theobromine has a molecular structure similar to caffeine's, but unlike caffeine, does not affect the central nervous system. Its stimulatory effects are mild, about ten times weaker than caffeine. Because it dilates blood vessels, theobromine can lower blood pressure and also relax bronchi muscles in the lungs. For this reason is has been used medicinally as a cough medicine. Phenylethylamine is the compound that makes us feel like we're in love. It stimulates the feel-good brain chemicals serotonin and endorphins, which is why we all *love* chocolate.

The next best source of antioxidants is natural cocoa powder, which for antioxidants still ranks higher than any other plant food.

Dark chocolate contains higher amounts of cocoa powder and smaller amounts of cocoa butter than do raw cacao nibs, plus sugar and vanilla, and sometimes soy lecithin as an emulsifier. Very high-quality milk chocolate has much less cocoa powder and even smaller amounts of cocoa butter, with higher amounts of sugar and milk, plus the soy lecithin. Lower-quality chocolate does not contain any cocoa butter; partially hydrogenated oils (trans fats) are used instead.

So how much chocolate can you have? I hate to disappoint, but most studies suggest only small amounts are needed to obtain its benefits. Beyond these amounts the beneficial effect tends to disappear, according to research. Therefore, the type of chocolate and how much you eat are critical. Just as critical is to make sure that you don't consume the chocolate with milk, as milk prevents the absorption of polyphenols. Also, read labels carefully to avoid alkali-treated (Dutch-process) cocoa or chocolate, which has little to no health benefits.

The best effect is obtained by consuming about a tablespoon or two a day of either raw cacao powder or unsweetened cocoa powder. About one-quarter ounce of raw cacao nibs is your next best source. Or, a little farther down the list, eat about 6.7 grams (one-quarter ounce, or one small square) per day of extremely dark chocolate—the type used in most studies. Although you were probably wishing for more, once you start eating processed free, you will find that these small amounts of chocolate are very satisfying, and you won't feel the need to overindulge.

Choose the purest dark chocolate you can find—the more raw and unprocessed, the higher the flavonoid content. The best dark chocolate has at least 80 percent cacao content and not more than 5 or 6 grams of sugar per serving. (The typical serving size for dark chocolate bars is half a bar, so for a quarter-ounce square, the sugar content should be less than 1 gram per square.) Organic dark chocolate is preferred, because it will typically contain a higher quality of sugar, and if you can find a dark chocolate bar without soy lecithin or dairy (cocoa butter, derived from cacao, is fine), that would be the best.

For daily chocolate benefits, I recommend mixing unsweetened cocoa powder into smoothies that do not contain cow milk (nut milks and rice milk are fine). Drinking your chocolate will minimize any unhealthy attachments or food addictions to its being in the form of candy. On occasions when you want a small indulgence, you can make the chocolate truffle recipe Allowable Sin, in Chapter 15, or purchase a high-quality dark chocolate bar and eat it in small daily increments. If you make Allowable Sin to the exact truffle size specified, you can eat two pieces, which will give you the beneficial 6.7 grams of dark chocolate.

## Kombucha, Yerba Maté, and Rooibos Teas

### Kombucha

If you haven't yet discovered a unique fizzy beverage in your natural food market, I'd like to introduce you to its virtues. Pronounced "kom-BOO-cha," it is a sparkling fermented tea made from green or black tea, sugar, and a healthy fungus. I know it sounds terrible, and you're probably wondering why I would approve of something made from sugar, but this tea has alkalizing abilities similar to those of apple cider vinegar, plus it's loaded with probiotics, B vitamins, and free-radical-stopping polyphenols. The sugar is used to start the fermentation process, and gets completely converted to acetic acid and carbon dioxide (hence the fizziness), so there is no sugar left in the tea once the fermentation is complete.

Kombucha tea reputedly has been used in Asia and Russia for centuries as a healing beverage. It is a potent detoxifier and an efficient enhancer of metabolism. It can also help curb food cravings, because it balances alkalinity.

If you can get used to its tartness, kombucha makes a great replacement for sodas; however, you should not drink more than 16 ounces of it in one day. While the original flavor of kombucha is almost identical to the taste of the vinegar drink, many companies that brew kombucha have come up with wonderful fruit and botanical flavors that make the beverage absolutely delightful. I've grown accustomed to the original flavor, but I also like the cranberry and other fruity varieties. Of the several brands on the market, my favorite is Synergy. The going price for this fizzy health elixir is about three bucks a bottle, so you probably won't be making drinking it a habit; however, you can make it yourself at home by ordering a kombucha starter kit from online sources.

## Yerba Maté

Yerba maté (pronounced "yer-bah mah-tay"), also called maté, is a small shrub indigenous to the rainforests of South America. It is said to have the "strength of coffee, the health benefits of tea, and the euphoria of chocolate," owing to its combination of three xanthines: caffeine, theophylline, and theobromine, well-known stimulants found in tea, coffee, and chocolate. Yerba maté was first cultivated and consumed over 1,500 years ago by the Guarini peoples of Paraguay, who used it as a rejuvenative medicinal tea. Today, it is the national drink of several South American countries. The steeped leaves produce a bitter herbal tea whose taste is similar to that of green tea. The xanthine combination in yerba maté is different from that in other plants containing caffeine; it has a relaxing effect on the body, especially the muscles, rather than a stimulating effect on the nervous system.

Those who drink yerba maté tea claim that it provides tremendous invigoration and focus. Yerba maté leaves contain twenty-four vitamins and minerals, fifteen amino acids, and eleven antioxidant polyphenols. In 1964, the Pasteur Institute and the Paris Scientific Society concluded, "It is difficult to find a plant anywhere in the world equal to maté in nutritional value" and that it contains "practically all of the vitamins necessary to sustain life."[29] Yerba maté tea can be prepared in a variety of ways—in a coffeepot, French press, tea infuser, and even espresso maker. Enjoy maté as a hot brew or iced.

## Rooibos

Rooibos (pronounced "roy-boss," a.k.a. "red bush") is a unique tea from a bush that grows only in a small region of South Africa. It is considered more of an herbal drink than a true "tea" because it does not derive from the same plant as do most other teas. Its small green leaves become red when oxidized and produce a beverage with a rich red color and a slightly sweet and nutty taste. Rooibos, called the new "wonder tea," is naturally caffeine free, and has become increasingly popular around the world. Its health benefits rival those of green and white teas. Its high levels of antioxidants have been shown to protect against cancer and inflammation, and its high mineral content—namely, calcium, copper, iron, fluoride, magnesium, manganese, potassium, and zinc—aids in boosting the immune system and promoting strong bones and teeth. Rooibos tea has been widely studied for its therapeutic role in heart health, lowering blood pressure, fighting HIV, managing diabetes, regenerating damaged liver cells, and alleviating respiratory ailments. While studies are still preliminary, rooibos tea is emerging as another one of nature's powerful healers.

## Organic Popcorn

It was a glorious day in August 2009 when a new study out of the University of Scranton, in Pennsylvania, announced that my favorite snack food can actually help prevent cancer. Research revealed that popcorn contains surprisingly large levels of polyphenols, the antioxidant compounds that help reduce the risk of heart disease, cancer, and other diseases. Scientists examined a variety of whole-grain breakfast cereals and snack foods and found that popcorn had the highest amount of antioxidants of all the snack foods studied.

Previous researchers always thought fiber was the active ingredient responsible for whole grains' ability to reduce the risk of cancer and heart disease. But polyphenols are emerging as potentially more important. Whole-grain products are proving to have comparable antioxidants per gram to fruits and vegetables.

In laboratories, popcorn is air-popped to determine its antioxidant content, so I'm guessing that movie theater popcorn is probably not a healthy choice, due to the bad oils that are used and the potential pesticide residues on nonorganic popcorn. If it's organic and air-popped, or even better, if it's popped in coconut oil, popcorn gets a high ranking in my plan. But of course, I was biased all along! Check out my recipe for the World's Best Popcorn in Chapter 15.

## High-Quality Natural Vitamin and Mineral Supplements

Consuming enough of the right foods is certainly the foundation for overall wellness, but even the best foods in today's world may not provide you with all of the nutrients that are essential for optimal health. Additionally, you may be missing out on some nutrients because you eat a limited variety of foods. Most people buy the same vegetables and fruits, the same bread, the same cereal, the same meats, and so on, every time they shop for groceries. When was the last time you tried a new vegetable in your salad? Are you familiar with every item in your grocer's produce section, or do you skip by many items because you don't know what they are or you don't know how to eat them? Perhaps you just don't like some foods, which is understandable (I didn't like Brussels sprouts for the longest time).

For any or all of these reasons, you may be unintentionally depriving your body of the vitamins, minerals, and phytonutrients that it needs to function at its best. Vitamin and mineral supplements can help to fill in the gaps that may be lacking in your food choices. However, you need to make sure that the supplements you take are high quality.

Vitamin and mineral supplements can be divided into two groups: synthetic and natural. Most over-the-counter multivitamin and/or mineral supplements are synthetic—meaning they are made in a laboratory from isolated chemicals that mirror their counterparts found in nature but are not from real food. They're kind of like those "natural flavorings" and the aspirin I synthesized in my college chemistry lab. On the other hand, natural multivitamin and/or mineral supplements (also called whole food supplements) are derived from real food sources, specifically vegetables, fruits, herbs, sprouts, and seaweeds.

Although the chemical differences between a vitamin or mineral found in food and one created in a laboratory are slight, synthetic supplements contain the isolated vitamins and minerals only, whereas natural supplements provide all of the other nutrients in foods not yet discovered, such as antioxidants and phytochemicals that help the vitamins and minerals do their jobs. Natural vitamins and minerals also retain the necessary enzymes that are specific to the foods they are derived from, which assist the body in utilizing these supplements properly.

Another difference is that synthetic vitamins and minerals always contain a bunch of "other" ingredients, such as artificial colorings; preservatives and stabilizers, such as maltodextrin; stearates and dioxides; sugars, cornstarch, or modified food starch; and even hydrogenated palm oil. They also often contain added lactose, which can cause digestive problems in those sensitive to it.

Natural whole food supplements are made by condensing or compressing real whole foods and then evaporating off the water at a very low temperature. The low temperature is crucial so as not to destroy the enzymes and cofactors contained in the foods. The enzymes are very important synergists required for digesting and assimilating vitamins and minerals. The remaining dried "powders" are then placed in capsules or combined with vegetable cellulose to form solid tablets.

To know whether your vitamin and mineral supplement comes from whole foods, you have to carefully read the "Supplement Facts" labels. Read down to scan the "ingredient list" on the bottom of the label. If you see such chemical terminology as *thiamine mononitrate* (vitamin B$_1$), *pyridoxine hydrochloride* (vitamin B$_6$), and *dl-alpha tocopheryl acetate* (vitamin E), this means that the vitamins and minerals are synthetically made. If you see the names of real foods and herbs, such as apple, carrots, celery, parsley, asparagus, sprouts, grapes, garlic, and ginger, the vitamins and minerals come from natural sources.

To help facilitate and ensure vitamin and mineral efficiency, you should always take your multivitamins with food. Vitamins A, D, E, and K are only soluble in fat; that is, when oil or fat is present in the meal. All other vitamins are water soluble, meaning they can be dissolved by any food containing water. Because multivitamins are very concentrated, they need a full or nearly full stomach to get adequate absorption into the body through the digestive process. To obtain its greatest benefit, take your nutritional supplements in the middle of or at the end of a meal, *not* at the beginning of a meal and not with just a snack.

Just as you need to eat more than once a day to get vitamins from your food, you should take your supplements in divided doses—one with the morning meal and one with the evening meal. It is important to do the latter because your body needs the extra nutrients for regeneration at night.

Aside from a natural multivitamin-mineral supplement, I also recommend green superfood drink powders and probiotics. These will help balance your alkalinity, detoxify your liver, ensure a strong immune system, and if needed, aid in weight loss.

*Green superfood drink powders* refers to products containing highly concentrated carefully dehydrated green plants and vegetables. They can provide the nutritional benefits of the green plants and vegetables that are often lacking in the typical American diet. Green drink powders contain many different alkalizing foods, and the regular consumption of these greens can assist you in achieving and maintaining an alkaline body chemistry. For this reason, I like to refer to green powders as *alkalizing green superfood.*

Green drinks typically contain grasses, such as barley grass and wheat grass, sprouts, and green vegetables (e.g., spinach and broccoli), and the superfood algae chlorella and spirulina, which infuse your body with easily absorbed vitamins, minerals, phytochemicals, and amino acids. Many green drink powders also contain fruits and other vegetables, such as carrots and beets, along with ground stevia leaves for added sweetness. All of these foods are also powerful liver-izers.

You can "drink your greens" by mixing them with water, juice, any type of milk, or adding them to a smoothie. You can also "eat your greens" by mixing them into yogurt or oatmeal. You can supplement with green powders up to three times per day.

Probiotics, otherwise known as "friendly flora" or "good bacteria," are a crucial part of your immune system. Their main job is to keep bad bacteria and yeast from growing in your intestinal tract. They also help to make vitamin K in your body. Vitamin K prevents hardening of the arteries and also plays a crucial role in anchoring calcium into the bones.

Ideally you should have about 100 trillion of these good bacteria lining your intestinal tract. However, if at any time in your life you have ever taken a round of antibiotics, you probably have far less than this amount. Antibiotics can't distinguish between good and bad bacteria in your body; therefore, they not only kill off infectious bacteria in your tissues and blood but also the good bacteria in your digestive tract. If you do not replace the good bacteria by eating a high-quality diet that provides probiotics and "prebiotics"—fibrous food for the good bacteria so they can grow and multiply—you will end up with a bacterial imbalance in your intestines called dysbiosis. Dysbiosis is an overgrowth of bad bacteria and yeast, and has been linked with such disorders as yeast infections (both vaginal and intestinal), irritable bowel syndrome, colitis, and rheumatoid arthritis. Intense sugar cravings, weight gain, and bloating are also signs of dysbiosis. The standard American diet—high in sugar, processed foods, and toxic food additives, while low in prebiotic-type foods—is another main contributor to dysbiosis.

To maintain a high level of probiotics in your intestine, the most important factor is eating processed free, making sure to include the types of foods that have been discussed in this chapter. Second to that, especially if you are not eating a daily serving of a fermented type of food containing probiotics such as plain organic yogurt, kefir, kimchee, or kombucha tea, you should take a high-quality probiotic supplement. Such supplements should contain at least 15 billion colony-forming-units (CFU) of probiotics and eight to ten strains of probiotics, including *L. bulgarius, L. acidophilus, L. bifidus,* and *S. thermophilus.* The best probiotics are shipped and stored refrigerated, to ensure that they do not die off, although a few types of probiotics do not require refrigeration.

Finally, supplements are supposed to be just that—supplements. They are not intended to replace what you would get from eating the actual food. You cannot take vitamins or alkalizing green drinks in place of eating fruits and vegetables. *No vitamin pill or supplement can make up for a diet that is lacking in variety and nutrients.* The Processed-Free Eating Plan ensures that you get a variety of food as well as the proper amount of nutrients from whole food supplements. Please see the list of recommended foods and supplements in the appendix (page 403).

## Terri's Story

I am a mother of six who has gained and lost 315 pounds over the last twelve years due to all of my pregnancies. I have always been determined to lose my pregnancy weight, but it was never easy and required a lot of work. I have struggled with hypoglycemia most of my life and have had a lifelong battle with consuming too much sugar. Once I read Dee's book and realized what white sugar does to my body, I have eliminated sugar, white flour, canola oil, and as much nonorganic processed food from my diet as possible. The change has enabled me to conquer my sugar cravings, stabilize my energy levels, and to feel so much healthier than I ever have. The changes suggested in Dee's book have made me a more stable, less emotional mom and has helped reduce the sugar levels in my children, helping them to be happier, healthier, and more obedient. This is the first year in over six years that we have not had a major illness travel through our family during cold and flu season and I attribute it to our new processed-free eating habits! Dee's plan has changed our lives and my prayer is that others will pick up your book and let their lives be revolutionized!

*—Terri Hunter, age 40, homemaker*

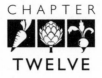
# Skinny Beginnings

## *The Initial Two-Week Cleansing and Alkalizing Phase*

*We can't expect to have a sharp mind and luminous spirit if
our body is polluted.*

—ANONYMOUS

Skinny Beginnings, the initial two-week phase of my processed-free plan,
is designed to kick-start your metabolism, reduce cravings, and gently release toxins that can inhibit weight loss. In this phase you will begin increasing water intake and choosing foods that are both high alkalizers and
liver-izers. You will see in the food lists that many whole grains and dairy
products are limited, but vegetables are plentiful and you will be able to
enjoy a variety of healthful snacks. Let me assure you that even though
some foods are omitted during this phase, you will not feel hungry between
your meals. That's because you will be incorporating a balance of health-
promoting oils into your meals, which, along with high-fiber foods, will
help you feel satisfied for longer periods of time. This phase also includes
some optional alkalizing and liver-izing supplements that are not intended

to replace any of your food portions, but are helpful in ensuring that your alkalinity will be balanced and your liver cleansing will be thorough.

Here are some basic steps to get you going:

Begin to hydrate your body.  A week or two before you embark on Skinny Beginnings, I recommend that you prepare your body. Start drinking more water, by first incorporating the warm lemon water in the morning. Then add more pure water between meals. This will begin to hydrate you and get you into the habit of drinking more water.

Wean yourself off coffee and sodas.  If you're a heavy coffee drinker (more than two cups of coffee per day), or if you drink more than three cups of caffeinated tea per day, I recommend weaning off it gradually rather than cold turkey. Eliminate one cup every other day until you are down to just one or no cup per day. Hopefully, the morning lemon water will begin to take the place of morning coffee or tea. You may also replace coffee or non-caffeine-free tea with herbal tea or an herbal coffee substitute, such as Teeccino.

The same goes for sodas, especially diet sodas, because they create acidic body chemistry and slow your metabolism. Wean yourself gradually down to zero sodas.

You will have better results if you do not consume any caffeine during this phase. Caffeine is a nonnutritive substance that has been found to elicit cravings. Just two cups of coffee will make your body secrete 80 percent more adrenaline than normal. Adrenaline increases insulin secretion, which in turn lowers blood sugar levels and triggers feelings of hunger, which you may identify as cravings. Second, caffeine is a liver stressor, which will inhibit your body's ability to effectively burn fat.

If you just can't fathom life without coffee (or tea), then at least make sure it's organic.

Breakfast is a must.  If you are not already doing so, make sure to eat breakfast every day within one hour of waking up, even if it is just a piece of fruit. This gets your metabolism started and will help burn more energy overall throughout the day.

Start replacing processed foods with higher-quality whole foods. **Replace** margarine with extra-virgin coconut oil or organic butter, and phase out canola and vegetable oils. Read every food ingredient list and avoid anything with partially hydrogenated or hydrogenated oils. These are trans fats, and even though they have a bad rap, you'd be surprised at how prevalent they still are in the food supply. Unless you dine in New York City, where they have been banned, fast-food joints and restaurants use trans fats liberally. Beware!

Begin stocking your pantry and fridge with healthier options. **Discard sugars** and artificial sweeteners and invest in a bottle of liquid stevia extract, raw honey, or coconut nectar. Switch from white rice to brown rice or quinoa, and taper off from processed flour products. And most important, stock up on colorful veggies and fruits, and try some new ones for a change. Get in the habit of eating raw veggies or a salad every day.

Yep, organic is still key. Because this is a cleansing phase, the more organic foods you eat, the better. However, do not let issues of affordability or availability of organic foods deter you. The most important thing is to eat the recommended food selections and follow the plan to the best of your ability. If you can't get grass-fed beef, wild-caught fish, and organic yogurt, don't despair. Remember, you do not have to follow this plan perfectly. You will still get results, so just do your best. My recommendations are designed to maximize your results and get your body back to where it functions best, but you can achieve it piecemeal if you need to.

Reduce grains and dairy. You are more likely to see quick and significant weight loss during this phase, due to the reduction of most grains and breads and the addition of beneficial oils. Milk and dairy products, with the exception of plain whole-milk yogurt, are also removed during this phase, as they have a tendency to clog your system. You will gradually add them back during the Skinny for Life phase.

Rest. It is also important that you get more rest and sleep than normal during this time. It may be a good idea to start this phase on the weekend, rather

## Withdrawal Symptoms Are Normal

White sugar, artificial sweeteners, caffeine, and food additives can create addictions that you may not even be aware of until you stop eating them. So, while most people make the transition to processed-free eating quite easily, others may experience temporary withdrawal symptoms that can range from mild to briefly uncomfortable. Headaches and fatigue are normal in the first few days, as are cravings for sugar and carbohydrates, irritability, and even changes in your bowel habits. Some people may feel as though they are coming down with the flu. If you experience any of these symptoms, don't worry, I have some suggestions to help ease you through it.

Remember the phrase, "You are what you eat." If you've been eating low-quality foods, the tissues in your body are also low quality. When you start eating whole natural foods, your body begins to *regenerate*. It makes new, higher-quality tissues and gets rid of the old low-quality tissues. As this is happening, you may feel worse before you feel better, and you may say to yourself, "This new way of eating is making me sick! I should stop and go back to my old way of eating so I can feel better." Don't! These symptoms, while they may temporarily feel bad, are actually a good sign that the cleansing is *working*! Old toxins that have been stored in your fat tissues over the years are being released into your bloodstream so they can be flushed out. While they are circulating around, they register in your brain as pain and you feel yucky! But please don't fail to give your body a chance to adjust and complete its first phase of cleansing. Just be patient and take care of yourself.

To help relieve headaches from caffeine and sugar withdrawal, I recommend a natural herbal remedy called feverfew. Feverfew is like a natural ibuprofen, specific for afflictions and pain related to changes in the amount of blood flow in the brain. If the headaches are severe, I recommend a product called Headache Take Care by New Chapter. Both products can be found at natural food markets.

To tame those sugar cravings, one of the best things to help you is bee pollen. Bee pollen contains many key nutrients to help your brain and your blood sugar levels; most notably, it contains B vitamins and amino acids. A key amino acid needed to help with sugar cravings is the brain-feeding nutrient L-glutamine. It converts to glutamic acid, which is the only source of

*continues*

## Withdrawal Symptoms Are Normal *continued*

glucose besides sugar that the brain can use for energy. Bee pollen has worked wonders for many of my clients with sugar withdrawal. It also allows you to think more clearly and feel more positive and focused, and improves the quality of your sleep. You can purchase bee pollen granules at natural food markets. I recommend taking 1 teaspoon of bee pollen, placed under the tongue, and allowing it to dissolve. This way the nutrients absorb subcutaneously into your bloodstream. You can work your way up to more bee pollen throughout the day. Note: if you are allergic to bee stings, you will also be allergic to bee pollen and cannot safely consume it. A supplemental form of L-glutamine (500 mg three times a day) can be taken instead.

Also, as I mentioned in Chapter 4, raw honey naturally suppresses the desire for other sweets and helps quell sugar cravings. Take 1 teaspoon of raw honey in your lemon water or with a cup of herbal tea.

than during the week, so that you will have the opportunity to take it easy for the first two days. Withdrawal symptoms typically pass after five days, as your body begins to normalize to a new level of health. When you give your body what it needs to constantly create healthy new tissue, you will feel even better than before you started.

Abstain from alcohol (at least, at first).  During Skinny Beginnings, I recommend that you abstain from alcohol, as it is a liver stressor and an acid-forming substance. However, as part of the ongoing Skinny for Life processed-free lifestyle, it is acceptable to enjoy a glass of wine or a beer every now and then. Mixed drinks and sugary cocktails such as margaritas and daiquiris should be much more limited, as they have a higher sugar and alcohol content. Organic, sulfite-free wine is the best choice.

Although I do recognize that there have been studies pointing to the health benefits of drinking small amounts of red wine for heart health, there are some downsides, and you can get equal amounts of cardiovascular benefits from other heart-healthy foods and from exercise. When you drink alcohol, it gets processed in the liver the same as fructose, and disrupts that organ's fat-burning efficiency. Additionally, if you consume too much alcohol at once, whatever doesn't get burned for energy will be stored as fat, just like the fructose from sugar.

Be aware, that as a by-product of grain fermentation, alcohol does not merely contain sugar, it is in and of itself a *type* of sugar and will cause sugar cravings. Therefore, if sugar is a problem for you, I urge you to abstain from alcohol while you're withdrawing from sugar. Everyone should always be mindful of possible sugar cravings that can occur within one to several days after consuming alcohol.

Avoid processed soy. Products made from soy in its *unfermented* state should be avoided. These include edamame, most tofu, and most soy milks. Small amounts of unfermented tofu (about an ounce) are acceptable, but should not be eaten daily. If you can find tofu made from sprouted soybeans, or fermented tofu, that would be the best choice. Processed foods made from soy milk or unfermented tofu should also be avoided. These include soy yogurt, soy cheese, soy milk, and soy ice cream, among others. Highly processed soy foods such as Tofurky, soy burgers, soy hot dogs, soy crumbles, soy protein powder, frozen dinners, most protein bars, and anything containing soybean oil, isolated soy proteins, soy protein concentrate, hydrolyzed soy protein, texturized soy protein (TVP), and any other soy proteins.

Limit or eliminate pork and shellfish. Pigs are the scavengers and garbage collectors of their environment. They happily eat dead carcasses and even their own feces (and anyone else's they happen upon), not bothered in the least by the grossness of it. You may say, "But other animals such as chickens, cows, deer, and buffalo, also search through feces and eat unnatural items. What makes them different?" The difference is in their digestive physiology.

Chickens, cows, deer, buffalo, and other animals have a multichambered stomach that effectively cleanses whatever is being digested. Pigs do not have the ability to "wash and rinse" what they ingest because whatever they eat goes straight into a single, simple stomach, where it is rudimentarily digested in a short period of time. Any viruses and worms that pigs eat do not get filtered out of their body. Like humans, pigs store toxins in their fatty tissues. When you eat pork, their toxins are transferred to you. Ann Louise Gittleman, the "First Lady of Nutrition" in the United States, and author of

*Guess What Came to Dinner?* (2001), says, "If you've ever looked at pork under a microscope, you would understand why it's not recommended. The *Trichinella spiralis* organism, which causes trichinosis, is rampant in American pigs. The encysted larvae can hatch in your intestines and migrate to your muscles, where they mimic at least fifty other illnesses characterized by a persistent flu-like feeling and severe muscle aches and pains. Need I say more?"[1]

The reason I don't recommend shellfish is very similar. Shellfish are bottom feeders and feed on parasites and dead skin, many times from dead animals. They do not have appropriate digestive and filter systems to purify toxins and parasites from their body. Most shrimp, for example, come from places where there are little to no restrictions on contaminants such as PCBs and dioxins. Shellfish also are among the most well-known allergens and you can react at any time to them, even after having consumed such seafood for years (most likely due to your repeated exposure to different toxins in the shellfish).

Although the decision will ultimately be up to you whether you give up these foods for good, at least give them up during this initial two-week cleansing phase. Going forward, if you do decide to occasionally indulge in some ham or crisp bacon, make sure it comes from an organic source and is uncured without added nitrates, nitrites, or chemical preservatives.

Note: If you have more than 25 pounds to lose, you may want to stay on the Skinny Beginnings phase for three or four weeks. However, if you begin to get bored with the food choices, and want to incorporate a wider variety, you should move on to the Skinny for Life phase after the initial two weeks.

## Suggested Daily Portions

The food charts on the following pages outline the variety of foods that you will be selecting from. The more meals you build around these foods, the skinnier you will be! It is best to follow the portion guidelines as closely as possible, but they may need to be adjusted to fit your own individual needs by adding either more protein, whole grains, or starchy vegetables sooner rather than later. Just make sure to focus on liver-izing foods as you do so. If you don't like avocados, you can substitute one portion of another health-promoting fat or oil in its place. If you are gluten intolerant, you will have to stick to the gluten-free options, of which there are plenty for you to choose from. Each day, in addition to the other foods on the list, you have the option of having one cup of either unsweetened almond milk or unsweetened rice milk.

The supplements are optional but are highly recommended for maximum results, especially the milk thistle and dandelion root extracts. As these extracts are to be mixed into water and drunk, that water can count toward your total for the day.

I offer both omnivore and lacto-ovo (dairy and eggs) vegetarian meal plans to suit your needs. If you are a meat eater, I recommend that you take at least one day a week to try the vegetarian guidelines. If you are a vegan, you can omit the dairy and eggs and substitute a serving of quinoa, legumes, or a high-quality vegan protein powder.

## Table 12.1  Skinny Beginnings Daily Regimen

| Omnivore (Meat Eater) | Vegetarian (Lacto-Ovo) |
|---|---|
| **Nonstarchy Vegetables**<br>Dark leafy greens: unlimited, minimum 2 portions<br>Rainbow vegetables: unlimited, minimum 2 portions | **Nonstarchy Vegetables**<br>Dark leafy greens: unlimited, minimum 2 portions<br>Rainbow vegetables: unlimited, minimum 2 portions |
| **Legumes and Starchy Vegetables**<br>1 legume portion or 1 starchy vegetable portion | **Legumes and Starchy Vegetables**<br>1 legume portion and 1 starchy vegetable portion, *OR*<br>2 legume portions |
| **Whole Grains**<br>1 portion | **Whole Grains**<br>1 portion |
| **Fruits**<br>2 portions (lemon and lime juice are in addition to these portions) | **Fruits**<br>2 portions (lemon and lime juice are in addition to these portions) |
| **High-Quality Proteins**<br>3 portions from meat, fish, poultry, yogurt, whey, or eggs<br>(For a dairy alternative, you may choose hemp protein powder instead of whey or yogurt.) | **High-Quality Proteins**<br>2 portions from yogurt, whey, eggs, quinoa, or tempeh<br>(For a dairy alternative, you may choose hemp protein powder instead of whey or yogurt.) |

*continues*

## Table 12.1  Skinny Beginnings Daily Regimen *continued*

| Omnivore (Meat Eater) | Vegetarian (Lacto-Ovo) |
| --- | --- |
| **Health-Promoting Fats and Oils** | **Health-Promoting Fats and Oils** |
| Coconut oil/coconut products: 2 portions | Coconut oil/coconut products: 2 portions |
| Omega-3 oils: 2 portions | Omega-3 oils: 2 portions |
| Other fats/oils: ½ to 1 whole avocado plus 1 other fat portion | Other fats/oils: ½ to 1 whole avocado plus 1 other fat portion |
| Nuts/seeds: 1 portion | Nuts/seeds: 1 portion |

**Optional Extras**

1 cup nondairy milk (almond, rice, or coconut)

1 tablespoon ground flaxseeds (in addition to your nut/seed portion for the day)

1 tablespoon unsweetened cocoa powder

**Natural Supplements**

Whole food multivitamin/mineral: Take as directed on package, one dose in the morning, one dose in the evening.

Alkalizing green powder: 1 to 3 servings per day

Milk thistle tincture: 28 drops of tincture added to water, drink 3 times per day

Dandelion root tincture: 3 cups of brewed tea, *or* 28 drops of tincture added to water, drink 3 times per day

(Tinctures may be mixed into the same glass of water and drunk together. This water counts toward your total water for the day!)

**Warm Lemon Water**

One 8-ounce glass, drink upon arising

**Vitality Vinegar Tonic**

Three 8-ounce glasses, preferably one glass 20 minutes before each meal

**Pure Water**

(Body weight in pounds ÷ 2) = ounces of pure water per day

**Meaningful Fitness**

30 minutes minimum, 6 days/week

## Skinny Beginnings Food List

Choose from the following food categories to make balanced meals. All vegetables, fruits, and most whole grains listed are alkaline forming.

### *Dark Green Leafy Vegetables*_____

PORTION SIZE: 1 cup raw, cooked, or raw juiced

| | |
|---|---|
| Arugula | Green loose-leaf lettuce |
| Beet greens | Kale |
| Bok choy | Mustard greens |
| Butterhead lettuce | Radicchio |
| Cabbage, green and red | Red loose-leaf lettuce |
| Chard, all types | Romaine lettuce |
| Chinese cabbage (napa cabbage) | Spinach |
| Collard greens | Spring mix |
| Dandelion greens | Turnip greens |
| Endive | Watercress |
| Escarole | Kelp and seaweeds |
| Frisée | |

### *Rainbow Vegetables*_____

PORTION SIZE: 1 cup (unless otherwise noted) raw, cooked, or raw juiced

| | |
|---|---|
| Artichokes | Carrots |
| Alfalfa sprouts | Cauliflower |
| Asparagus | Celery |
| Bamboo shoots | Chives |
| Bean sprouts | Cucumbers |
| Beets | Daikon |
| Bell peppers (all colors) | Eggplant |
| Broccoli | Jicama |
| Brussels sprouts | Kohlrabi |

Leeks

Mexican gray squash

Mushrooms

Okra

Onions, all types

Parsley

Radishes

Rutabagas

Rhubarb

Sauerkraut

Scallions and green onions

Shallots

String beans, green and yellow

Snap peas

Snow peas

Sorrel

Sprouts, all types

Tomatoes

Turnips

Water chestnuts

Yellow summer squash

Zucchini

## Legumes

PORTION SIZE: Each of the following equals 1 portion (cooked).

| | |
|---|---|
| Beans, all types | ½ cup |
| Lentils, all types | ½ cup |
| Split peas | ½ cup |
| Bean burgers | 1 burger |

## Starchy Vegetables

PORTION SIZE: Each of the following equals 1 portion (cooked).

| | |
|---|---|
| Winter squash | ½ cup |
| Parsnip | ½ cup |
| Pumpkin | ½ cup |
| Spaghetti squash | ½ cup |
| Sweet potato or yam | ½ cup measured if boiled, mashed, or fried; 4 ounces by weight if baked |

## Whole Grains _____

PORTION SIZE: Each of the following equals 1 portion (cooked).

Amaranth . . . . . . . . . . . . . . . . . . . . . . . . . . . . . . . . . ½ cup
Brown rice . . . . . . . . . . . . . . . . . . . . . . . . . . . . . . . . ½ cup
Buckwheat . . . . . . . . . . . . . . . . . . . . . . . . . . . . . . . . ½ cup
Millet . . . . . . . . . . . . . . . . . . . . . . . . . . . . . . . . . . . . ½ cup
Quinoa . . . . . . . . . . . . . . . . . . . . . . . . . . . . . . . . . . . ½ cup
Red rice . . . . . . . . . . . . . . . . . . . . . . . . . . . . . . . . . . ½ cup
Wild rice. . . . . . . . . . . . . . . . . . . . . . . . . . . . . . . . . . . ½ cup
Sunshine Burger or other veggie burger . . . . . . . . I burger

### Whole-Grain Crackers

PORTION SIZE: Each of the following equals 1 portion.

San-Jay Tamari Brown Rice Crackers. . . . . . . 6 crackers
Brown rice cakes (any unsalted). . . . . . . . . . . 2 rice cakes
Mary's Gone Crackers . . . . . . . . . . . . . . . . . Check package for portion size

### Bran and Whole-Grain Cereals

PORTION SIZE: Each of the following equals 1 portion.

Oat bran. . . . . . . . . . . . . . . . . . . . . . . . . . . ¼ cup uncooked, ½ cup cooked
Bob's Red Mill gluten-free hot cereal . . . . . . . ¼ cup uncooked, ½ cup cooked
Crispy brown rice cereal . . . . . . . . . . . . . . . . I cup, cooked
Puffed brown rice cereal . . . . . . . . . . . . . . . I cup, cooked
Puffed millet cereal. . . . . . . . . . . . . . . . . . . . I cup, cooked

## Fruits _____

PORTION SIZE: Each of the following equals 1 portion.

Apple . . . . . . . . . . . . . . . . . . . . . . . . . . . . . . . . . . . I large
Applesauce, unsweetened . . . . . . . . . . . . . . . . . . . I cup

Apricot, fresh . . . . . . . . . . . . . . . . . . . . . . . . . . . 4 medium

Banana . . . . . . . . . . . . . . . . . . . . . . . . . . . . . . . . . I medium

Berries

    Blackberries . . . . . . . . . . . . . . . . . . . . . . . . . . I cup

    Raspberries. . . . . . . . . . . . . . . . . . . . . . . . . . . I cup

    Strawberries. . . . . . . . . . . . . . . . . . . . . . . . . . I cup

Cherries . . . . . . . . . . . . . . . . . . . . . . . . . . . . . . . 20 large

Dates . . . . . . . . . . . . . . . . . . . . . . . . . . . . . . . . . . 3 whole

Fig, fresh or dried. . . . . . . . . . . . . . . . . . . . . . . . 2 whole

Grapefruit. . . . . . . . . . . . . . . . . . . . . . . . . . . . . . . ½ large

Grapes, all types. . . . . . . . . . . . . . . . . . . . . . . . . I cup

Kiwifruit . . . . . . . . . . . . . . . . . . . . . . . . . . . . . . . 2 small

Lemon . . . . . . . . . . . . . . . . . . . . . . . . . . . . . . . . . 2 whole

Lime . . . . . . . . . . . . . . . . . . . . . . . . . . . . . . . . . . 2 whole

Melon

    Cantaloupe. . . . . . . . . . . . . . . . . . . . . . . . . . . ½ small

    Honeydew . . . . . . . . . . . . . . . . . . . . . . . . . . . . ¼ medium

    Watermelon . . . . . . . . . . . . . . . . . . . . . . . . . . 2 cups cubed

Nectarine . . . . . . . . . . . . . . . . . . . . . . . . . . . . . . 2 small

Orange . . . . . . . . . . . . . . . . . . . . . . . . . . . . . . . . I large

Papaya . . . . . . . . . . . . . . . . . . . . . . . . . . . . . . . . I cup

Peach . . . . . . . . . . . . . . . . . . . . . . . . . . . . . . . . . I medium

Pear . . . . . . . . . . . . . . . . . . . . . . . . . . . . . . . . . . I medium

Persimmon. . . . . . . . . . . . . . . . . . . . . . . . . . . . . 2 medium

Pineapple . . . . . . . . . . . . . . . . . . . . . . . . . . . . . . I cup cubed

Tangelo. . . . . . . . . . . . . . . . . . . . . . . . . . . . . . . . I large

Tangerine . . . . . . . . . . . . . . . . . . . . . . . . . . . . . . 2 medium

Frozen fruit, natural unsweetened. . . . . . . . . . . . . I cup

## High-Quality Protein

PORTION SIZE: For meats, poultry, and fish, the portion size is 3 to 4 ounces for women, 4 to 5 ounces for men, weighed after cooking. For other proteins, the portion size varies depending on the type of protein; refer to the following list for portion sizes.

## Fish (wild caught is best)

Cod

Grouper

Haddock

Halibut

Herring

Mahimahi

Mackerel

Orange roughy

Sardines, canned in water or olive
  oil only

Salmon, fresh

Salmon, canned, in water

Sea bass

Snapper

Sole

Tilapia

Trout

Whitefish

Tuna, fresh

Tuna, canned in water only

## Poultry

Chicken

Chicken, canned (no additives)

Cornish game hen

Duck

Turkey

Chicken or turkey bacon (no
  nitrates or nitrites)

Chicken or turkey sausage
  (no pork casings, nitrates,
  or nitrites)

Chicken or turkey deli meats
  and hot dogs (no synthetic
  additives, nitrates, or nitrites)

## Meat (all lean types)

Beef

Buffalo

Lamb

Liver (must be organic)

Veal

Venison

Beef deli meats and hot dogs
  (no synthetic additives, pork
  casings, nitrates, or nitrites)

## Other Protein Foods

Eggs . . . . . . . . . . . . . . . . . . . . . . . . . . . . . . . . . . . . . 2 eggs

Dairy

  Whole-milk organic plain yogurt . . . . . . . . . . . . I cup

Whole-milk organic plain yogurt, Greek style . . . 1 cup

Whole-milk goat yogurt . . . . . . . . . . . . . . . . . . 1 cup

Fermented soy foods

Tempeh . . . . . . . . . . . . . . . . . . . . . . . . . . . . . 4 ounces after cooking

Tofu . . . . . . . . . . . . . . . . . . . . . . . . . . . . . . . . 4 ounces after cooking

## Protein Powders

Whey protein powder concentrate (unsweetened or naturally sweetened brands only): 1 scoop (about 8–10 grams protein)

Goat whey protein powder concentrate (unsweetened or naturally sweetened brands only): 1 scoop (about 13 grams protein)

Hemp protein powder (unsweetened or naturally sweetened brands only): 4 tablespoons (about 15 grams protein)

Brown rice protein powder (unsweetened or naturally sweetened brands only): 2 tablespoons (about 15 grams protein)

## Health-Promoting Fats and Oils

### Extra-Virgin Coconut Oil and Coconut Products

PORTION SIZE: The portion size varies depending on the type of coconut product. Refer to the following list for portion sizes.

NOTE: Coconut oil is best used for cooking; however, it can also be added to smoothies, soups, and oatmeal and other hot cereals, and used as a spread in place of butter.

Extra-virgin coconut oil . . . . . . . . . . . . . . . . . . . . . 1 tablespoon

Coconut milk, fresh or canned, unsweetened . . . . . 1/3 cup

Fresh coconut meat . . . . . . . . . . . . . . . . . . . . . . . 2 ounces

Coconut cream, unsweetened . . . . . . . . . . . . . . . . 1 tablespoon

Dried coconut, unsweetened . . . . . . . . . . . . . . . . . 2 tablespoons

## Omega-3

PORTION SIZE: The portion size varies depending on the type of oil. Refer to the following list for portion sizes.

NOTE: Always take omega-3 oils with a meal. *Do not take more than two portions at the same meal.* You must divide the portions equally and take them at different times throughout the day. These oils are extremely sensitive to heat and light, therefore *they should never be heated or used for cooking.* Keep them in dark bottles in the refrigerator.

| | |
|---|---|
| High-lignan flaxseed oil | I tablespoon |
| Hemp seed oil | I tablespoon |
| Fish oil | I teaspoon |
| Cod liver oil | I teaspoon |

## Other Health-Promoting Fats and Oils

PORTION SIZE: The portion size varies depending on the type of fat/oil. Refer to the following list for portion sizes.

| | |
|---|---|
| Avocado | ½ avocado |
| Butter, organic | I teaspoon |
| Extra-virgin olive oil | I tablespoon |
| Mayonnaise, safflower or Wilderness Family | I tablespoon |
| Olive oil–based salad dressings | 2 tablespoons |
| Peanut oil, expeller pressed, unrefined | I teaspoon |
| Sesame oil, expeller pressed, unrefined | I teaspoon |
| Sweet Skinny Apple Cider Vinaigrette (see Chapter 15) | 2 tablespoons |

## Seeds

PORTION SIZE: Each of the following equals 1 portion.

| | |
|---|---|
| Flaxseeds | I tablespoon |

Hemp seeds . . . . . . . . . . . . . . . . . . . . . . . . . . . . I tablespoon

Pumpkin seeds (pepitas). . . . . . . . . . . . . . . . I tablespoon

Sesame seeds (includes tahini) . . . . . . . . . . . I tablespoon

Sunflower seeds . . . . . . . . . . . . . . . . . . . . . . . I tablespoon

## Nuts

PORTION SIZE: Each of the following equals 1 portion.

Almonds, raw . . . . . . . . . . . . . . . . . . . . . . . . . . I ounce, 20 to 24 almonds

Pine nuts, raw. . . . . . . . . . . . . . . . . . . . . . . . . I ounce, 150 to 157 pine nuts

Walnuts, raw . . . . . . . . . . . . . . . . . . . . . . . . . I ounce, about 14 walnut halves

## *Alkalizing and Liver-izing Herbs and Spices*

PORTION SIZE: There are no specific serving sizes for herbs and spices. Use them liberally in your cooking or added to foods. The herbs and spices listed are thermogenic, meaning they create heat in the body, raise metabolism, and burn fat. You may use other spices as well, but these also alkalize and liver-ize.

| | |
|---|---|
| Allspice | Cumin |
| Anise | Curry powder |
| Bay leaves | Dill |
| Cardamom | Fennel |
| Cayenne | Garlic |
| Cilantro/Coriander | Ginger |
| Cinnamon | Mustard, dried |
| Cloves | Turmeric |

## Beverages

PORTION SIZE: Unlimited quantities, except for cocoa and coffee. Teas may be sweetened with stevia or a small amount of raw honey or coconut nectar.

All naturally decaffeinated herbal teas

Unsweetened cocoa: 1 tablespoon daily, mixed in to smoothie or nondairy milk

Coffee: 1 cup daily, black or sweetened with a natural sweetener. No cow's milk or cream. Nondairy milks are okay. Make the coffee organic!

Dandelion tea
Green tea
Kombucha tea
Milk thistle tea
Red rooibos tea
White tea
Yerba maté

### Alternatives to Dairy Milk

PORTION SIZE: Each of the following equals 1 portion.

Almond milk, unsweetened . . . . . . . . . . . . . 1 cup
Hemp milk, unsweetened . . . . . . . . . . . . . . 1 cup
Rice milk, unsweetened . . . . . . . . . . . . . . . 1 cup

## Sweeteners

PORTION SIZE: Enjoy unlimited quantities of stevia; for other listed sweeteners, consume no greater than a total of 1 tablespoon per day (combined).

Stevia
Coconut nectar . . . . . . . . . . . . . . . . . . . . . 2 teaspoons
Raw honey . . . . . . . . . . . . . . . . . . . . . . . . 1 teaspoon
Pure maple syrup . . . . . . . . . . . . . . . . . . . 1 tablespoon

## Condiments and Seasonings _____

PORTION SIZE: Enjoy these condiments and seasonings added to foods and recipes.

Apple cider vinegar, raw, unfiltered
Bragg oil-free vinaigrettes
Brown rice vinegar
Herbamare seasoning salt
Herbs, fresh or dried, all types
Ketchup (no added sugar)
Miso
Mustard (no added sugar)
Pure extracts, e.g., vanilla,
   almond, mint

Salsa, fresh or jarred
Sea salt or Himalayan salt
   (use sparingly)
Spices (no added stabilizers; read
   labels carefully)
Tomato sauce and paste, canned
   (no additives)
Wheat-free tamari sauce
   (reduced sodium)

# Skinny Beginnings Daily Checklist, Omnivore

| | |
|---|---|
| **Dark Leafy Green Vegetables:** *minimum of 2 cups daily* ❑ ½ cup ❑ ½ cup ❑ ½ cup ❑ ½ cup ❑ ½ cup ❑ ½ cup | **Rainbow Vegetables:** *minimum of 2 cups daily* ❑ ½ cup ❑ ½ cup ❑ ½ cup ❑ ½ cup ❑ ½ cup ❑ ½ cup |
| **Legumes and Starchy Vegetables** ❑ I portion ❑ I portion | **Whole Grains** ❑ I portion |
| **Fruits** ❑ I portion ❑ I portion | **High-Quality Protein** ❑ I portion ❑ I portion ❑ I portion |
| **Coconut Oil/Coconut Products** ❑ I portion ❑ I portion | **Omega-3 Oil** ❑ I portion ❑ I portion |
| **Avocado, Other Fats and Oils, and Nuts/Seeds** ❑ I portion ❑ I portion ❑ I portion | **Morning Lemon Water** ❑ 8 oz. |

*continues*

## Skinny Beginnings Daily Checklist *continued*

| Vitality Vinegar Tonic | Pure Water |
|---|---|
| ☐ 8 oz. ☐ 8 oz. ☐ 8 oz. | ☐ 8 oz. ☐ 8 oz. ☐ 8 oz. ☐ 8 oz.<br>☐ 8 oz. ☐ 8 oz. ☐ 8 oz. ☐ 8 oz.<br>☐ 8 oz. ☐ 8 oz. ☐ 8 oz. ☐ 8 oz.<br>☐ 8 oz. ☐ 8 oz. ☐ 8 oz. ☐ 8 oz. |
| **High-Quality Multiple Vitamin**<br>☐ I dose, morning ☐ I dose, evening | **Alkalizing Green Powder**<br>☐ I portion ☐ I portion ☐ I portion |
| **Milk Thistle Supplement**<br>☐ I dose ☐ I dose ☐ I dose | **Dandelion Supplement**<br>☐ I dose ☐ I dose ☐ I dose |

## Skinny Beginnings Meal Plan

Here is a set of sample menus to help you plan your meals. They incorporate all of the components of the daily plan, but keep in mind that these menus are not set in stone; they are intended to help you understand how to create balanced meals. In general, a balanced meal should contain protein, fiber, healthy fats, and colorful phytonutrients. You can mix and match the meals and snacks; just make sure that you get all of your components every day. The ultimate goal is to understand how to select and balance foods, whether preparing your own meals or eating away from home.

A kitchen scale and a set of measuring cups and spoons are essential kitchen tools. As you are getting used to the meals and the portion sizes, I highly recommend measuring your foods at first so that you can see what they look like on your plate or in your bowl. This will give you an idea of what a half-cup of rice, three or four ounces of chicken, and two cups of vegetables look like. Also, you'll be able to see how they look in relation to one another on the plate. In general, for lunch and dinner, half the plate should be covered with vegetables; one-fourth should have starchy foods such as grains, legumes, or starchy vegetables; and one-fourth should be protein. For vegetarians, two-thirds of the plate should be vegetables; one-third should be a mixture of beans, grains, nuts, seeds, or fermented soy foods. This visual will help you "eyeball" a reasonable serving when you are in a restaurant.

Breakfast is the most important meal of the day and should not be skipped. My experience has shown that most people feel safe eating the same breakfast nearly every day, and that is fine. However, I suggest selecting a few breakfasts that work the best for you and rotating them every few days. Eggs should be eaten at least three times a week, so to save prep time, I recommend boiling some eggs to have them on hand to grab quickly. Also, you can make up a quiche or two on the weekend, divide it into four equal portions and wrap them to store in the fridge or freezer to eat later in the week. The more advance planning you do, the easier it is to eat healthy.

Most lunches and dinners are interchangeable, as you will see that both of these meals always contain lots of vegetables, protein, and health-promoting fats. Most lunch and dinner menus include meat, poultry, or fish, but you can also eat eggs for lunch or dinner. If you're a vegetarian, the staples for lunch and dinner are quinoa, other whole grains, and legumes.

Each menu consists of three meals and two snacks. You can move one of the snacks to the evening after dinner if you need to. It is important not to exceed the portion sizes, as they are designed for balancing your blood sugar levels and releasing weight. If you are too hungry between meals, eat an additional ounce of protein, a teaspoon or two more of fats, a piece of fruit, or any amount of nonstarchy vegetables. *Do not eat more legumes or whole grains, as they may affect the rate of your weight loss.*

Finally, you'll find recipes for the asterisked (*) items in Chapter 15.

## Menu 1

| Breakfast | Snack |
| --- | --- |
| Berry Blast Smoothie* | 1 medium-size orange |
| **Omnivore Lunch** | **Vegetarian Lunch** |
| Mixed greens plus a mixture of chopped assorted rainbow veggies; 1 portion salmon or other fish; 1/4 avocado; 1 portion baked sweet potato; 4 sprigs fresh parsley; 2 tablespoons Sweet Skinny Apple Cider Vinaigrette* | Mixed greens plus a mixture of chopped assorted rainbow veggies; 1 1/2 cups lentil soup; 1/4 avocado; 4 sprigs fresh parsley; 2 tablespoons Sweet Skinny Apple Cider Vinaigrette* |

*continues*

## *Menu 1* continued

| Snack | |
| --- | --- |
| 1 ounce almonds | |
| **Omnivore Dinner** | **Vegetarian Dinner** |
| 2 cups Farmers' Market Coconut Curry\*; 1 portion grass-fed ground beef patty; ¼ avocado; ½ cup brown rice | 2 cups Farmers' Market Coconut Curry\*; ¼ avocado; 1 cup Minty Quinoa\* |

## *Menu 2*

| Breakfast | Snack |
| --- | --- |
| Pumpkin Smoothie\* | 1 apple |
| **Omnivore Lunch** | **Vegetarian Lunch** |
| 1 portion chicken; ½ cup Lemon-Dill Rice\*; ½ avocado, onions, salsa; 1 cup salad greens; 4 sprigs fresh parsley; 1 cup Cucumber Tomato Salad with Honey Mustard Vinaigrette\* | ½ cup black beans; ½ cup Lemon-Dill Rice\*; ½ avocado, onions, salsa; 1 cup salad greens; 4 sprigs fresh parsley; 1 cup Cucumber Tomato Salad with Honey-Mustard Vinaigrette\* |
| Snack | |
| 14 walnut halves | |
| **Omnivore Dinner** | **Vegetarian Dinner** |
| 1 portion Turkey Meatloaf\*; 1 portion Sautéed Greens with Garlic and Cannellini Beans\*; 1 cup steamed broccoli | 1 portion Sautéed Greens with Garlic and Cannellini Beans\*; 1 portion quinoa; 1 cup steamed broccoli |

## Menu 3

| | |
|---|---|
| **Breakfast** | **Snack** |
| Proatbran: I portion cooked oat bran, | Pear |
| prepared with water; I portion | |
| coconut oil mixed into cooked oat | |
| bran; I portion protein powder mixed | |
| into cooked oat bran | |
| or I cup of whole-milk yogurt, | |
| ½ ounce chopped walnuts (about | |
| 7 walnut halves), | |
| splash of almond milk (optional) | |
| **Omnivore Lunch** | **Vegetarian Lunch** |
| I portion Wild Alaskan Salmon Stuffed | I portion Wild Alaskan Salmon Stuffed |
| Tomatoes* over 2 cups mixed salad | Tomatoes* (replace salmon with |
| greens; ½ avocado; 4 sprigs fresh | Minty Quinoa*); mixed salad greens; |
| parsley; I portion Mary's Gone | ½ avocado; 4 sprigs fresh parsley; |
| Crackers | I portion Mary's Gone Crackers |
| **Snack** | |
| 2 cups watermelon | |
| **Omnivore Dinner** | **Vegetarian Dinner** |
| I portion Dijon-Garlic Chicken*; I cup | I cup 4-Bean Chili*; 2 cups mixed |
| Sesame-Sautéed Brussels Sprouts*; | greens with cucumbers and carrots; |
| I cup steamed carrots; 4 sprigs fresh | 4 sprigs fresh parsley; I portion |
| parsley; I portion baked sweet potato | Creamy Honey Mustard Dressing* |

## Menu 4

| Breakfast | Snack |
|---|---|
| Over-Easy Egg Florentine* | I portion strawberries |

| Omnivore Lunch | Vegetarian Lunch |
|---|---|
| Dee's Everyday Rainbow Salad* | Dee's Everyday Rainbow Salad* |

| Snack | |
|---|---|
| I cup Sugar-Free Strawberry Frozen Yogurt* | |

| Omnivore Dinner | Vegetarian Dinner |
|---|---|
| Beef stir-fry: I portion lean beef with greens, broccoli, carrots, onions, and snow peas sautéed in coconut oil with garlic and ginger and a dash of wheat-free tamari; raw cucumber slices | I cup Split Pea Soup*; I cup Skillet-Steamed Lemon and Butter Asparagus*; cucumbers and tomatoes with vinaigrette |

## Menu 5

| Breakfast | Snack |
|---|---|
| Skinny Yogurt Supreme* | I peach |

| Omnivore Lunch | Vegetarian Lunch |
|---|---|
| Spinach salad: 2 cups spinach with I hard-boiled egg, ½ portion chicken, shredded carrots, cucumber, cherry tomatoes, sliced red onion; ½ avocado; 2 tablespoons Sweet Skinny Apple Cider Vinaigrette*; I portion hummus | Spinach salad: 2 cups spinach with 2 hard boiled eggs, shredded carrots, cucumber, cherry tomatoes, sliced red onion; ½ avocado; 2 tablespoons Sweet Skinny Apple Cider Vinaigrette*; I portion hummus |

| Snack | |
|---|---|
| ¾ ounce almonds | |

*continues*

**Menu 5** *continued*

| Omnivore Dinner | Vegetarian Dinner |
|---|---|
| I portion baked halibut: brush fish with I tablespoon of toasted sesame oil; bake at 350°F for 20 minutes; I portion baked sweet potato, mashed with splash of coconut milk and pinch of cinnamon; 2 cups mixed steamed broccoli, cauliflower, carrots | I portion baked tempeh; I portion baked sweet potato, mashed with splash of coconut milk and pinch of cinnamon; 2 cups mixed steamed broccoli, cauliflower, carrots |

Mix and match these menus for two weeks to kick-start your healthy, skinny life.

## Join a Processed-Free Support Group!

Do you desire to be part of a supportive community of like-minded healthful eaters? If so, you can join or start a Processed-Free Support Group!

It is unfortunate that we live in a world that doesn't always support healthy eating, so we have to support ourselves! The Processed-Free Support Groups allow us to come together to support, affirm, and uphold our choice, and our right, to live processed free.

The first Processed-Free Support Group was formed in January 2010. Since then, other groups have formed all over the United States. The Processed-Free Support Group is a safe place to express victories and challenges; ask questions; exchange ideas, recipes, and information; and experience the magic of working together to achieve a common goal.

No weigh-ins, no calorie counting. The intention of this group is to create a space for change; to educate and enlighten ourselves on the value of proper nutrition; and to support one another in our transition to happy, healthy living.

To find a group, or to start a group in your area, log on to www.processed freeamerica.org.

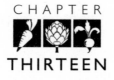

CHAPTER

THIRTEEN

# Skinny for Life
## *Ongoing Phase for Optimal Health*

You've been alkalizing and liver-izing for two whole weeks—congratulations! Now it's time to transition to the Skinny for Life phase. This is your "way of eating for life" guideline—it will help keep your body chemistry balanced and will not put stress on your liver. The elements of the Skinny Beginnings phase are still in place, such as the Morning Lemon Water, Vitality Vinegar Tonic, and supplements. You may continue with the milk thistle and dandelion root tinctures for six more weeks, for a total of eight weeks. The vitamins and the alkalizing green powder are meant to be ongoing for life as frequently or as infrequently as you like.

The first change you will notice in the Skinny for Life phase is that you have more portions of whole grains, starchy vegetables, legumes, and dairy products, in addition to a wider variety of foods in those categories to select from. In this phase, I have given ranges of portion sizes for some foods because, as each person's body is different, some may be able to handle more food than may others. You should increase your portions gradually, and evaluate how your body is responding. If you start to put on weight, you may need to cut back down to the lower end of the range.

It is also important to point out that your level of exercise will also determine how well your body tolerates the extra food. If you have developed a good routine and are exercising five to six days per week, you should have no problem at all. However, if you are still sedentary or only exercising a few days per week, your weight loss may slow down.

I want you to be able to transition into this phase without feeling overwhelmed. The most important thing to remember is that you are eating processed free! And you are focusing on eating delicious foods. You will find the meal plans in this phase have more variety, and you can begin to partake in a few allowable indulgences, such as Allowable Sin, granola, and popcorn. Leave the cookies, banana bread, and other sweet treats as occasional extras.

### Table 13.1  Skinny for Life

| Omnivore (Meat Eater) | Vegetarian (Lacto-Ovo) |
|---|---|
| **Nonstarchy Vegetables** <br> Dark leafy greens: unlimited, minimum 2 portions <br> Rainbow vegetables: unlimited, minimum 2 portions | **Nonstarchy Vegetables** <br> Dark leafy greens: unlimited, minimum 2 portions <br> Rainbow vegetables: unlimited, minimum 2 portions |
| **Legumes and Starchy Vegetables** <br> 1 to 2 starchy vegetable portions *OR* <br> 1 to 2 legume portions | **Legumes and Starchy Vegetables** <br> 1 legume portion and 1 starchy vegetable portion *OR* <br> 1 to 2 legume portions |
| **Whole Grains** <br> 1 to 2 portions | **Whole Grains** <br> 1 to 2 portions |
| **Fruits** <br> 2 to 3 portions (lemon juice and lime juice are in addition to these portions) | **Fruits** <br> 2 to 3 portions (lemon juice and lime juice are in addition to these portions) |
| **High-Quality Proteins** <br> 2 portions from meat, fish, poultry, or eggs <br> 1 to 2 portions from dairy <br> (For a dairy alternative, you may choose hemp protein powder instead of whey or yogurt, or an egg or half of a meat protein portion.) | **High-Quality Proteins** <br> 1 to 2 portions from dairy (optional) <br> 1 portion from eggs (optional) <br> (For a dairy alternative, you may choose vegetarian protein powder, tempeh, or quinoa instead of dairy or eggs.) |
| **Health-Promoting Fats and Oils** <br> Coconut oil/coconut products: 2 portions <br> Omega-3 oils: 2 portions <br> Other fats/oils: ½ to 1 whole avocado plus 1 other fat portion <br> Nuts/seeds: 1 portion | **Health-Promoting Fats and Oils** <br> Coconut oil/coconut products: 2 portions <br> Omega-3 oils: 2 portions <br> Other fats/oils: ½ to 1 whole avocado plus 1 other fat portion <br> Nuts/seeds: 1 portion |

*continues*

## Table 13.1  Skinny for Life *continued*

### Optional Extras
1 cup nondairy milk (almond, rice, or coconut) in place of dairy
1 tablespoon ground flaxseeds (in addition to your nut/seed portion for the day)
2 tablespoons unsweetened cocoa powder, or 1 ounce dark chocolate

### Natural Supplements
Whole food multivitamin/mineral: Take as directed on package, one dose in the morning, one dose in the evening.
Alkalizing green powder: 1 to 3 servings per day
Milk thistle tincture: 28 drops of tincture added to water, drink 3 times per day
Dandelion root tincture: 3 cups of brewed tea, or 28 drops of tincture added to water, drink 3 times per day
(Tinctures can be mixed into the same glass of water and drunk together. This water counts toward your total water for the day!)

### Warm Lemon Water
One 8-ounce glass: drink upon arising

### Vitality Vinegar Tonic
Three 8-ounce glasses: preferably one glass 20 minutes before each meal

### Pure Water
(Body weight in pounds ÷ 2) = ounces of pure water per day

### Meaningful Fitness
30 minutes minimum, 6 days per week

# Skinny for Life Food List

Choose from the following food categories to make balanced meals. All vegetables and most of the fruits listed are alkaline forming. You may eat all the foods on this list, but keep these liver-izing choices as your main focus.

## *Dark Green Leafy Vegetables*

PORTION SIZE: 1 cup raw, cooked, or raw juiced

Arugula

Beet greens

Bok choy

Butterhead lettuce

Cabbage, green and red

Chard, all types

Chinese cabbage (napa cabbage)

Collard greens

Dandelion greens

Endive

Escarole

Frisée

Green loose-leaf lettuce

Kale

Mustard greens

Radicchio

Red loose-leaf lettuce

Romaine lettuce

Spinach

Spring mix

Turnip greens

Watercress

Kelp and seaweeds

## *Rainbow Vegetables*

PORTION SIZE: 1 cup raw, cooked, or raw juiced

Artichokes

Alfalfa sprouts

Asparagus

Bamboo shoots

Bean sprouts

Beets

Bell peppers (all colors)

Broccoli

Brussels sprouts

Carrots

Cauliflower

Celery

Chives

Cucumbers

Daikon

Eggplant

Jicama

Kohlrabi

Leeks

Mexican gray squash

Mushrooms

Okra

Onions, all types

Parsley

Radishes

Rutabagas

Rhubarb

Sauerkraut

Scallions and green onions

Shallots

String beans, green and yellow

Snap peas

Snow peas

Sorrel

Sprouts, all types

Tomatoes

Turnips

Water chestnuts

Yellow summer squash

Zucchini

## Legumes

PORTION SIZE: Each of the following equals 1 portion (cooked).

Beans, all types . . . . . . . . . . . . . . . . . . . . . . . . . ½ cup

Lentils . . . . . . . . . . . . . . . . . . . . . . . . . . . . . . . . ½ cup

Split peas . . . . . . . . . . . . . . . . . . . . . . . . . . . . . ½ cup

Bean burgers . . . . . . . . . . . . . . . . . . . . . . . . . . I burger

## Starchy Vegetables

PORTION SIZE: Each of the following equals 1 portion (cooked).

Winter squash . . . . . . . . . . . . . . . . . . . . . . . . . ½ cup

Parsnips . . . . . . . . . . . . . . . . . . . . . . . . . . . . . . ½ cup

Pumpkin . . . . . . . . . . . . . . . . . . . . . . . . . . . . . . ½ cup

Spaghetti squash . . . . . . . . . . . . . . . . . . . . . . . . ½ cup

Potatoes . . . . . . . . . . . . . . . . . . . . . . . . . . . . . . ½ cup measured if boiled,
mashed, or fried; 4 ounces
by weight if baked

Sweet potatoes and yams . . . . . . . . . . . . . . . . ½ cup measured if boiled,
mashed, or fried; 4 ounces
by weight if baked

## Whole Grains _____

PORTION SIZE: Each of the following equals 1 portion (cooked).

| | |
|---|---|
| Amaranth | ½ cup |
| Barley | ½ cup |
| Brown rice | ½ cup |
| Buckwheat | ½ cup |
| Bulgur | ½ cup |
| Corn kernels | ½ cup |
| Corn on the cob | ½ cob |
| Cornmeal, whole grain with germ | 2 tablespoons, dried |
| Kamut | ½ cup |
| Millet | ½ cup |
| Oats | ½ cup |
| Polenta, cooked | ½ cup |
| Quinoa | ½ cup |
| Red rice | ½ cup |
| Rye | ½ cup |
| Spelt | ½ cup |
| Wild rice | ½ cup |
| Whole wheat | ½ cup |
| Sunshine Burger or other veggie burger | 1 burger |

### Whole-Grain Breads

PORTION SIZE: Each of the following equals 1 portion.

| | |
|---|---|
| Sprouted-grain bread | 1 slice |
| Sprouted-grain English muffin | ½ muffin |
| Sprouted-grain bagel | ½ bagel |
| Sprouted-grain burger bun | ½ bun |
| Sprouted-grain hot dog bun | ½ bun |
| Sprouted-grain tortilla | 1 tortilla |
| Corn tortilla (6-inch) | 2 tortillas |
| Baked blue corn tortilla chips | 1 ounce, about 18 chips |

Dee's Naturals Flourless Oat Bran Muffin . . . . . . 1 muffin

Whole-grain pancakes . . . . . . . . . . . . . . . . . . . . 2 (4-inch) pancakes

100% whole spelt bread . . . . . . . . . . . . . . . . . . 1 slice

100% whole wheat bread . . . . . . . . . . . . . . . . . 1 slice

Dee's Naturals Whole-Grain Tortilla . . . . . . . . . 1 tortilla

Gluten-free breads. . . . . . . . . . . . . . . . . . . . . . . 1 slice

## Whole-Grain Pastas

PORTION SIZE: Each of the following equals 1 portion (cooked).

Ezekiel sprouted-grain pasta . . . . . . . . . . . . . . ½ cup

Brown rice pasta . . . . . . . . . . . . . . . . . . . . . . . ½ cup

Corn pasta . . . . . . . . . . . . . . . . . . . . . . . . . . . . ½ cup

Quinoa pasta . . . . . . . . . . . . . . . . . . . . . . . . . . ½ cup

Whole spelt pasta. . . . . . . . . . . . . . . . . . . . . . . ½ cup

Whole wheat pasta. . . . . . . . . . . . . . . . . . . . . . ½ cup

## Whole-Grain Crackers

PORTION SIZE: Each of the following equals 1 portion (cooked).

Ak-mak 100% whole wheat crackers . . . . . . . . 5 sections

San-Jay tamari brown rice crackers . . . . . . . . . . 6 crackers

Brown rice cakes, unsalted . . . . . . . . . . . . . . . . 2 rice cakes

Mary's Gone Crackers . . . . . . . . . . . . . . . . . . . Check package
for portion size

RYVITA 100% rye crackers . . . . . . . . . . . . . . . . 2 crackers

## Whole-Grain Cereals, Bran, Germ

PORTION SIZE: Each of the following equals 1 portion.

Ezekiel sprouted-grain cereal . . . . . . . . . . . . . . ½ cup

Granola (low sugar content) . . . . . . . . . . . . . . . ½ cup

Kasha . . . . . . . . . . . . . . . . . . . . . . . . . . . ¼ cup uncooked, about ½ cup cooked

Oat bran . . . . . . . . . . . . . . . . . . . . . . . . . . ¼ cup uncooked, about ½ cup cooked

Oatmeal . . . . . . . . . . . . . . . . . . . . . . . . . . ¼ cup uncooked, about ½ cup cooked

Bob's Red Mill gluten-free hot cereal . . . . . . . ¼ cup uncooked, about ½ cup cooked

Crispy brown rice cereal . . . . . . . . . . . . . . . I cup

Puffed millet cereal . . . . . . . . . . . . . . . . . . . I cup

Puffed cereal, unsweetened . . . . . . . . . . . . . I cup

Shredded wheat cereal . . . . . . . . . . . . . . . . I cup

Uncle Sam's cereal . . . . . . . . . . . . . . . . . . . ¾ cup

Wheat bran . . . . . . . . . . . . . . . . . . . . . . . . . ¼ cup uncooked

Wheat germ . . . . . . . . . . . . . . . . . . . . . . . . ¼ cup

Whole-grain hot cereals, unsweetened . . . . . ¼ cup uncooked, about ½ cup cooked

Other whole-grain unsweetened cereal . . . . . ¾ cup, or check package for serving size

## Fruits

PORTION SIZE: Each of the following equals 1 portion.

Apple . . . . . . . . . . . . . . . . . . . . . . . . . . . . . I large

Applesauce, unsweetened . . . . . . . . . . . . . . I cup

Apricots, fresh . . . . . . . . . . . . . . . . . . . . . . 4 medium

Apricots, dried . . . . . . . . . . . . . . . . . . . . . . 8 halves

Banana . . . . . . . . . . . . . . . . . . . . . . . . . . . . I medium

Berries

    Blackberries . . . . . . . . . . . . . . . . . . . . . . . I cup

    Blueberries . . . . . . . . . . . . . . . . . . . . . . . . I cup

    Cranberries . . . . . . . . . . . . . . . . . . . . . . . I cup

    Raspberries . . . . . . . . . . . . . . . . . . . . . . . I cup

    Strawberries . . . . . . . . . . . . . . . . . . . . . . . I cup

Cherries . . . . . . . . . . . . . . . . . . . . . . . . . . 20 large

Dates . . . . . . . . . . . . . . . . . . . . . . . . . . . 3 whole

Figs, fresh or dried . . . . . . . . . . . . . . . . . . . 2 whole

Grapefruit. . . . . . . . . . . . . . . . . . . . . . . . . ½ large

Grapes, all types . . . . . . . . . . . . . . . . . . . . . I cup

Kiwifruit . . . . . . . . . . . . . . . . . . . . . . . . . . 2 small

Mango. . . . . . . . . . . . . . . . . . . . . . . . . . . . I small

Melon

    Cantaloupe. . . . . . . . . . . . . . . . . . . . . . . ½ small

    Honeydew . . . . . . . . . . . . . . . . . . . . . . . ¼ medium

    Watermelon . . . . . . . . . . . . . . . . . . . . . . 2 cups cubed

Lemon . . . . . . . . . . . . . . . . . . . . . . . . . . . 2 whole

Lime . . . . . . . . . . . . . . . . . . . . . . . . . . . . 2 whole

Nectarines . . . . . . . . . . . . . . . . . . . . . . . . 2 small

Orange . . . . . . . . . . . . . . . . . . . . . . . . . . . I large

Papaya. . . . . . . . . . . . . . . . . . . . . . . . . . . . I cup

Peach . . . . . . . . . . . . . . . . . . . . . . . . . . . . I medium

Pear . . . . . . . . . . . . . . . . . . . . . . . . . . . . I medium

Persimmons . . . . . . . . . . . . . . . . . . . . . . . 2 medium

Pineapple . . . . . . . . . . . . . . . . . . . . . . . . . I cup cubed

Plums . . . . . . . . . . . . . . . . . . . . . . . . . . . . 4 medium

Prunes. . . . . . . . . . . . . . . . . . . . . . . . . . . . 4 medium

Prune juice . . . . . . . . . . . . . . . . . . . . . . . . ½ cup

Raisins. . . . . . . . . . . . . . . . . . . . . . . . . . . . 4 tablespoons

Tangelo. . . . . . . . . . . . . . . . . . . . . . . . . . . I large

Tangerines . . . . . . . . . . . . . . . . . . . . . . . . 2 medium

Frozen fruit, natural unsweetened . . . . . . . . . I cup

Dried fruit, unsweetened (no sulfites) . . . . . . ¼ cup

Fruit juice, fresh . . . . . . . . . . . . . . . . . . . . . I cup (8 ounces)

100% fruit jams and preserves. . . . . . . . . . . I tablespoon

## High-Quality Protein

PORTION SIZE: For meats, poultry, and fish, portion size is 3 to 4 ounces for women, 4 to 5 ounces for men, weighed after cooking. For other proteins, the portion size varies depending on the type of protein. Refer to the following list for portion sizes.

### Fish (wild caught is best)

Cod
Grouper
Haddock
Halibut
Herring
Mahimahi
Mackerel
Orange roughy
Sardines, canned in water or
    olive oil only

Salmon, fresh
Salmon, canned, in water
Sea bass
Snapper
Sole
Tilapia
Trout
Whitefish
Tuna, fresh
Tuna, canned in water only

### Poultry

Chicken
Chicken, canned (no additives)
Cornish game hen
Duck
Turkey
Chicken or turkey bacon
    (no nitrates or nitrites)

Chicken or turkey sausage
    (no pork casings, nitrates,
    or nitrites)
Chicken or turkey deli meats and
    hot dogs (no synthetic additives,
    nitrates, or nitrites)

### Meat (all lean types)

Beef
Buffalo
Lamb
Liver (must be organic)
Veal

Venison
Beef deli meats and hot dogs
    (no synthetic additives, pork
    casings, nitrates, or nitrites)

## Other Proteins

Eggs . . . . . . . . . . . . . . . . . . . . . . . . . . . . . . . . . . . . . . . 2 eggs

Dairy

    Milk . . . . . . . . . . . . . . . . . . . . . . . . . . . . . . . . . . . . I cup

    Whole-milk organic plain yogurt . . . . . . . . . . . . . I cup

    Whole-milk organic plain yogurt, . . . . . . . . . . . I cup
        Greek style

    Whole-milk goat yogurt . . . . . . . . . . . . . . . . . . . I cup

    Kefir . . . . . . . . . . . . . . . . . . . . . . . . . . . . . . . . . . . . I cup

    Cottage cheese . . . . . . . . . . . . . . . . . . . . . . . . . . ½ cup

    Ricotta cheese . . . . . . . . . . . . . . . . . . . . . . . . . . . ½ cup

    Goat cheese, soft . . . . . . . . . . . . . . . . . . . . . . . . . I ounce

    All other soft cheeses . . . . . . . . . . . . . . . . . . . . . I ounce
        (blue cheese, feta, etc.)

    Hard cheeses . . . . . . . . . . . . . . . . . . . . . . . . . . . . I ounce
        (Cheddar, Jack, mozzarella, etc.)

Fermented soy foods

    Tempeh . . . . . . . . . . . . . . . . . . . . . . . . . . . . . . . . 4 ounces after cooking

    Tofu . . . . . . . . . . . . . . . . . . . . . . . . . . . . . . . . . . . . 4 ounces after cooking

## Protein Powders

Whey protein powder concentrate (unsweetened or naturally sweetened
    brands only): I scoop (about 8–10 grams protein)

Goat whey protein powder concentrate (unsweetened or naturally sweetened
    brands only): I scoop (about 13 grams protein)

Hemp protein powder (unsweetened or naturally sweetened brands only:
    4 tablespoons (about 15 grams protein)

Brown rice protein powder (unsweetened or naturally sweetened brands only:
    2 tablespoons (about 15 grams protein)

## Health-Promoting Fats and Oils _____

### Extra-Virgin Coconut Oil and Coconut Products

PORTION SIZE: The portion size varies depending on the type of coconut product. Refer to the following list for portion sizes.

NOTE: Coconut oil is best used for cooking; however, it can also be added to smoothies, soups, and oatmeal and other hot cereals, and used as a spread in place of butter.

Extra-virgin coconut oil . . . . . . . . . . . . . . . . . . . . . . 1 tablespoon
Coconut milk, fresh or canned, unsweetened . . . . $\frac{1}{3}$ cup
Fresh coconut meat . . . . . . . . . . . . . . . . . . . . . . . . 2 ounces
Coconut cream, unsweetened . . . . . . . . . . . . . . . . 1 tablespoon
Dried coconut, unsweetened . . . . . . . . . . . . . . . . . 2 tablespoons

### Omega-3

PORTION SIZE: The portion size varies depending on the type of oil. Refer to the following list for portion sizes.

NOTE: Always take omega-3 oils with a meal. *Do not take more than two portions at the same meal.* You must divide the portions equally and take them at different times throughout the day. These oils are extremely sensitive to heat and light, therefore *they should never be heated or used for cooking.* Keep them in dark bottles in the refrigerator.

Cod liver oil . . . . . . . . . . . . . . . . . . . . . . . . . . . . . . 1 teaspoon
Fish oil . . . . . . . . . . . . . . . . . . . . . . . . . . . . . . . . . . 1 teaspoon
Hemp seed oil . . . . . . . . . . . . . . . . . . . . . . . . . . . . 1 tablespoon
High-lignan flaxseed oil . . . . . . . . . . . . . . . . . . . . . 1 tablespoon

## Other Health-Promoting Fats and Oils

PORTION SIZE: Consume up to 2 portions daily. The portion size varies depending on the type of fat/oil. Refer to the following list for portion sizes.

Avocado ................................. ½ avocado
Butter, organic ........................... 1 teaspoon
Extra-virgin olive oil ...................... 1 tablespoon
Mayonnaise, safflower or Wilderness Family ..... 1 teaspoon
Olive oil–based salad dressings ............... 2 tablespoons
Peanut oil, expeller pressed, unrefined ......... 1 teaspoon
Sesame oil, expeller pressed, unrefined ........ 1 teaspoon
Sweet Skinny Apple Cider Vinaigrette .......... 2 tablespoons
  (see Chapter 15)

## Seeds

PORTION SIZE: Each of the following equals 1 portion.

Flaxseeds ................................. 1 tablespoon
Hemp seeds ............................... 1 tablespoon
Pumpkin seeds (pepitas) ..................... 1 tablespoon
Sesame seeds .............................. 1 tablespoon
Sunflower seeds ............................ 1 tablespoon

## Nuts

PORTION SIZE: Each of the following equals 1 portion.

Almonds.................................. 1 ounce, 20 to 24 almonds
Brazil nuts ............................... 1 ounce, about 5 nuts
Cashews ................................. 1 ounce, about 18 nuts
Hazelnuts ................................ 1 ounce, about 20 nuts
Macadamias .............................. 1 ounce, about 10 nuts
Nut and seed butters, includes sesame tahini ..... 1 tablespoon
Peanuts, dry roasted, unsalted ............... 1 ounce, about 28 nuts

Pecans ............................ I ounce, about 19 pecan halves
Pine nuts ........................... I ounce, 150 to 157 nuts
Pistachios ........................... I ounce, about 47 nuts
Walnuts ........................... I ounce, about 14 walnut halves

## Alkalizing and Liver-izing Herbs and Spices

PORTION SIZE: There are no specific portions sizes for herbs and spices. Use them liberally in your cooking or added to foods. These herbs and spices are thermogenic, meaning they create heat in the body, raise metabolism, and burn fat.

| | |
|---|---|
| Allspice | Curry powder |
| Anise | Dill |
| Bay leaves | Fennel |
| Cardamom | Garlic |
| Cayenne | Ginger |
| Cilantro/Coriander | Mustard, dried |
| Cinnamon | Turmeric |
| Cloves | |

## Beverages

PORTION SIZE: Unlimited quantities, except for cocoa and coffee. Teas may be sweetened with stevia or a small amount of raw honey or coconut nectar.

| | |
|---|---|
| All naturally decaffeinated herbal teas | Dandelion root tea |
| | Green tea |
| Unsweetened cocoa powder: I to 2 tablespoons daily | Kombucha tea |
| | Red rooibos tea |
| Coffee: I cup daily, black or sweetened with a natural sweetener. No cow's milk or cream. Nondairy milks are okay. Make the coffee organic! | White tea |
| | Yerba maté |

Alternatives to Dairy Milk

PORTION SIZE: Each of the following equals 1 portion.

Almond milk, unsweetened . . . . . . . . . . . . . . . . . . I cup
Hemp milk, unsweetened . . . . . . . . . . . . . . . . . . . I cup
Rice milk, unsweetened . . . . . . . . . . . . . . . . . . . . I cup

## Sweeteners

PORTION SIZE: Enjoy unlimited quantities of stevia; for other listed sweet-eners, consume no greater than a total of 1 tablespoon per day (combined).

Stevia
Coconut nectar . . . . . . . . . . . . . . . . . . . . . . . . . . 2 teaspoons
Raw honey  . . . . . . . . . . . . . . . . . . . . . . . . . . . . I teaspoon
Pure maple syrup  . . . . . . . . . . . . . . . . . . . . . . . . I tablespoon

## Condiments and Seasonings

PORTION SIZE: Enjoy these condiments and seasonings added to foods and recipes:

Apple cider vinegar, raw, unfiltered
Bragg oil-free vinaigrettes
Brown rice vinegar
Herbamare seasoning salt
Herbs, fresh or dried, all types
Mustard
Pure extracts, e.g., vanilla, almond,
    mint
Salsa, fresh or jarred
Sea salt or Himalayan salt
    (use sparingly, not more than
    I teaspoon per day)

Soy sauce, reduced sodium
Spices (no added stabilizers; read
    labels carefully)
Tomato sauce and paste, canned
    (no additives)
Wheat-free tamari sauce
    (reduced sodium)
Miso

# Skinny for Life Daily Checklist

| | |
|---|---|
| **Dark Leafy Green Vegetables:**<br>*minimum of 2 cups daily*<br>☐ ½ cup ☐ ½ cup ☐ ½ cup<br>☐ ½ cup ☐ ½ cup ☐ ½ cup | **Rainbow Vegetables:**<br>*minimum of 2 cups daily*<br>☐ ½ cup ☐ ½ cup ☐ ½ cup<br>☐ ½ cup ☐ ½ cup ☐ ½ cup |
| **Legumes and Starchy Vegetables**<br>☐ I portion ☐ I portion | **Whole Grains**<br>☐ I portion ☐ I portion |
| **Fruits**<br>☐ I portion ☐ I portion ☐ I portion | **High-Quality Protein**<br>☐ I portion ☐ I portion<br>☐ I portion ☐ I portion |
| **Coconut Oil/Coconut Products**<br>☐ I portion ☐ I portion | **Omega-3 Oil**<br>☐ I portion ☐ I portion |
| **Avocado, Other Fats and Oils,**<br>**Nuts/Seeds**<br>☐ I portion ☐ I portion<br>☐ I portion ☐ I portion | **Morning Lemon Water**<br>☐ 8 oz. |
| **Vitality Vinegar Tonic**<br>☐ 8 oz. ☐ 8 oz. ☐ 8 oz. | **Pure Water**<br>☐ 8 oz. ☐ 8 oz. ☐ 8 oz. ☐ 8 oz.<br>☐ 8 oz. ☐ 8 oz. ☐ 8 oz. ☐ 8 oz.<br>☐ 8 oz. ☐ 8 oz. ☐ 8 oz. ☐ 8 oz.<br>☐ 8 oz. ☐ 8 oz. ☐ 8 oz. ☐ 8 oz. |
| **High-Quality Multiple Vitamin**<br>☐ I dose, morning ☐ I dose, evening | **Alkalizing Green Powder**<br>☐ I portion ☐ I portion ☐ I portion |
| **Milk Thistle Supplement**<br>☐ I dose ☐ I dose ☐ I dose | **Dandelion Supplement**<br>☐ I dose ☐ I dose ☐ I dose |

# Pay Attention to Your Digestion

Good nutrition is not just a question of *what* we eat, but how efficiently the food is digested and utilized by our body. Most people don't think much about digestion unless it isn't working well. The function of digestion is to break down foods into basic components for the cells to use for energy. The uninterrupted flow of these nutrients into our system is critical to our long-term health. When we eat poorly or our digestion becomes blocked and sluggish, we compromise the ability of all our cells to work efficiently and healthfully. A poorly functioning digestive system can manifest in many ways, from an upset stomach to chronic constipation, acid reflux, irritable bowel disorders, liver disease, and cancers.

In 1911, Dr. William Howard Hay introduced a theory called "food combining," which in its most boiled-down form states that starchy foods neutralize protein foods in the stomach, slowing down digestion of both. Long-term poor digestion leads to poor health and weight gain. He recommended eating certain foods separately and other foods together, to optimize digestion. Since Dr. Hay's theory was first introduced, many more after him have devised elaborate eating systems based on food-combining rules. While I don't adhere strictly to these rules, there a few that I want you to know about because you may benefit from them yourself. One of my clients is a ten-year-old boy who had chronic stomachaches and would eat few foods because he was always in such severe pain. By eating starchy foods at different times than protein foods, he experienced great relief. I have witness the improved health of many of my other clients who have adopted these rules. Weight loss comes easier, with little to no bloating, gas, constipation, or diarrhea.

## Poor Food Combinations

The following combinations can slow down digestion:

Vegetables with fruits: The complex carbohydrates in vegetables require different enzymes for digestion than do the sugars in fruits. If fruits and vegetables are eaten together, there is competition in the stomach for digestive

*continues*

## Pay Attention to Your Digestion *continued*

enzymes. Usually the vegetables win, and the fruit goes partially undigested, leading to fermentation in the small intestine.

Meat with fruit:  Sugars and animal proteins don't combine well.

Liquids with meals:  Water is good for many things, but too much of it dilutes digestive enzymes and has a numbing effect on the cells that secrete stomach acid. No more than a few ounces of liquid, especially cold liquids, should be taken with meals. It is recommended you wait at least 30 minutes after eating before drinking large amounts of liquids.

More than one type of animal protein food at a meal:  This means no steak and lobster dinners, or chicken and fish combinations. When more than one type of animal protein is eaten, digestion is impaired and toxicity may result.

Eggs are the exception to the protein rule:  They are considered neutral and can be combined with other animal proteins. They go particularly well with dairy products (e.g., in frittatas) and add to the protein value of bean dishes. Eggs can be combined with sprouted-grain products.

Animal proteins with gluten grains:  Dairy, meats, fish, and poultry do not combine well with gluten grains (e.g., wheat, rye, oats, and barley). This means bread and meat do not combine well together, nor do wheat pastas with meat. However, animal proteins do combine well with sprouted grains, nongluten grains, baked potatoes, sweet potatoes, corn, or peas as long as you also include leafy greens in the meal.

### Healthy Food Combinations

The following combinations digest well together:

> In general, vegetables combine well with proteins and should always be eaten together.

*continues*

## Pay Attention to Your Digestion *continued*

> Starches combine well with vegetables and should always be eaten together.
>
> Yogurt and whey protein combine well with fruit, except the acidic citrus fruits.
>
> Citrus fruits don't combine well with cow's milk.
>
> As mentioned before, these rules are not hard and fast. You are encouraged to listen to your body. You may find that you feel fine with some combinations and not others.

## Skinny for Life Meal Plans

Here are some sample menus for both omnivores and vegetarians. I have designed them to use the lower ranges on some of the portions for fruits, whole grains, legumes and starchy vegetables, so please feel free to adjust them to suit your needs. In the Skinny for Life Meal Plans, you can be more flexible with the portions. Some days you might eat more, some days you might eat less. Remember, the most important thing is to eat processed free.

In these meal plans I have allowed for a few "treat" days, where I included some healthy treats into the snacks. Please understand that these are to be exceptions, rather than the rule. I recommend healthy treats only occasionally, such as once every month or less. Treats such as dried fruits, popcorn, or those that are sweetened with stevia can be more frequent, as long as you don't go overboard. For chocolate treats, please be satisfied with the small amount that will give you health benefits, and don't become obsessed about the chocolate. If you want to get the daily benefit of chocolate, it is best to blend it into a smoothie.

If weight loss and long-term maintenance are your goals, you will be wise to moderate your treats—be honest with yourself about how much you are thinking about them and how frequently you are eating them. It took me years to get to the point where I was able to handle chocolate in a healthy manner. If anything on this plan becomes a problem for you, you should leave it out. There are plenty of healthy options to suit everyone's needs.

You'll find recipes for the asterisked (*) items in Chapter 15.

## Menu 1

| **Breakfast**<br>Chocolate PB&B Smoothie* | **Snack**<br>1 Flourless Oat Bran Pumpkin Muffin* |
| --- | --- |
| **Omnivore Lunch**<br>2 cups green salad with carrot, cucumber, celery, 1 oz. goat cheese, and Sweet Skinny Apple Cider Vinaigrette*; ½ tablespoon pine nuts sprinkled on salad;<br>½ avocado; 1 portion chicken | **Vegetarian Lunch**<br>2 cups green salad with carrot, cucumber, celery, 1 oz. goat cheese, and Sweet Skinny Apple Cider Vinaigrette*; ½ tablespoon pine nuts sprinkled on salad; ½ avocado;<br>1½ cup Carrot-Ginger Soup*; 1 slice sprouted-grain bread |
| **Snack**<br>1 orange, 3 Medjool dates | |
| **Omnivore Dinner**<br>1 cup 15-Minute Steamed Beets* with 1 cup Sautéed Beet Greens with Goat Cheese*; 1 portion Turkey Meatloaf*; 1 portion wild rice | **Vegetarian Dinner**<br>Asian Cold Noodle Salad*; 1 portion tempeh |

## Menu 2

| **Breakfast**<br>Breakfast Waldorf Salad* | **Snack**<br>1 Flourless Oat Bran Pumpkin Muffin* |
| --- | --- |
| **Omnivore Lunch**<br>Salmon salad: 1 portion canned salmon; 3 cups salad greens, ½ cup chickpeas, chopped celery, cucumber, red cabbage; Balsamic Ginger Vinaigrette* | **Vegetarian Lunch**<br>Smoky Black Bean and Avocado Pitas*; 3 cups salad greens, chopped celery, cucumber, red cabbage; Balsamic Ginger Vinaigrette* |

*continues*

## Menu 2 *continued*

| **Snack** |
| --- |
| 14 walnut halves |

| **Omnivore Dinner** | **Vegetarian Dinner** |
| --- | --- |
| 1 cup Quick-Braised Red Cabbage*; 1 cup steamed broccoli; 1 portion Extremely Easy Oven-Baked Salmon*; 1 portion baked potato with 1 portion butter | 1 cup Quick-Braised Red Cabbage*; 1 cup steamed broccoli; ½ cup kidney beans; 1 portion baked potato with 1 portion cheese |

## Menu 3

| **Breakfast** | **Snack** |
| --- | --- |
| Breakfast Baked Apple*; 1 cup yogurt | ½ portion almonds |

| **Omnivore Lunch** | **Vegetarian Lunch** |
| --- | --- |
| 1 portion Creamy Beef and Carrot Topped Baked Potatoes*; 2 cups mixed green salad with chopped beets and cucumbers; 2 tablespoons Sweet Skinny Apple Cider Vinaigrette* | Bean soft tacos: 2 corn tortillas, ½ cup pinto beans, diced red bell peppers, diced onions, ½ avocado, 1 ounce cheese, 2 tablespoons salsa, 1 cup shredded lettuce |

| **Snack** |
| --- |
| 2 Allowable Sin* |

| **Omnivore Dinner** | **Vegetarian Dinner** |
| --- | --- |
| Grass-Fed Beef and Vegetable Stew for the Slow Cooker*; 2 cups mixed green salad with chopped carrots, radish, zucchini, yellow squash; 2 tablespoons Sweet Skinny Apple Cider Vinaigrette* | Creamy Spaghetti Squash with Asparagus and Rosemary*; 2 cups mixed green salad with chopped carrots, radish, zucchini, yellow squash; 2 tablespoons Sweet Skinny Apple Cider Vinaigrette* |

## Menu 4

| Breakfast | Snack |
|---|---|
| Sprouted French Toast à la Mode* | 1 cup strawberries |

| Omnivore Lunch | Vegetarian Lunch |
|---|---|
| 1 portion Too Easy Chicken and Rice Soup*; 2 cups mixed green salad with chopped celery, carrot, cucumber, tomato; 2 tablespoons Sweet Skinny Apple Cider Vinaigrette* | Quinoa Tabbouleh*; 2 cups mixed green salad with chopped celery, carrot, cucumber, tomato; 1 table-spoon pine nuts; 2 tablespoons Sweet Skinny Apple Cider Vinaigrette* |

| Snack | |
|---|---|
| Chocolate Sweet Potato Brownie* | |

| Omnivore Dinner | Vegetarian Dinner |
|---|---|
| Wild Alaska Salmon Croquettes*; Sesame Sautéed Brussels Sprouts*; Tamari Roasted Sweet Potato Fries* | Cheddar Sweet Potato Wrap*; 2 cups mixed baby greens with 1 cup mixed chopped rainbow veggie; 2 tablespoons Sweet Skinny Apple Cider Vinaigrette* |

## Menu 5

| Breakfast | Snack |
|---|---|
| Skinny Yogurt Supreme* | 1 peach |

| Omnivore Lunch | Vegetarian Lunch |
|---|---|
| Spinach salad: 2 cups spinach with 1 hard-boiled egg, ½ portion chicken, shredded carrots, cucumber, cherry tomatoes, sliced red onion; ½ avocado, 2 tablespoons Sweet Skinny Apple Cider Vinaigrette*; 1 portion hummus | Avocado Black Bean Veggie Wrap*; Spinach salad: 2 cups spinach with shredded carrots, cucumber, cherry tomatoes, sliced red onion; ½ avocado, 2 tablespoons Sweet Skinny Apple Cider Vinaigrette* |

*continues*

**Menu 5** continued

| Snack |
|---|
| The World's Best Popcorn* |

| Omnivore Dinner | Vegetarian Dinner |
|---|---|
| Skinny Sweet-and-Sour Meatballs*; ½ cup brown rice; 2 cups steamed broccoli, carrots, cauliflower | Homemade Sunshine Burger*; Tamari Roasted Sweet Potato Fries*; 2 cups steamed broccoli, carrots, cauliflower |

You can mix and match these menus to your heart's—and stomach's—content!

## Shopping Tips

To make your kick-start and lifelong eating plans simpler, here are some additional tips and information to help you create the healthiest, skinniest—and most delicious—meals possible.

- Make a trip to the natural food store and explore its bounty. There, you'll discover many frozen vegetable medleys and varieties of frozen fish that would be easy for you to prepare.
- Look in the freezer section of a natural food store for a box that contains three pouches of precooked organic brown rice. What could be simpler? Stock up! Note: It is not recommended to microwave the rice. You can put the pouches in a steamer and heat them that way.
- Buy already roasted chickens at a natural food store and use them for dinners or to add to salads.
- Hummus is a garbanzo bean dip that can be purchased at any grocery store, or you can make it yourself. Hummus contains no saturated fat, no cholesterol, and no sugars and is high in protein and fiber. Aside from being good for you, it also tastes great. Hummus is a perfect food for processed-free living. Make sure to select a brand that is sold fresh in the refrigerated case and made without preservatives.

*continues*

## Shopping Tips continued

- Several companies make healthy jarred marinara sauce without sugar or other additives. This is good for topping baked potatoes, cooked vegetables, or pastas. Read ingredient lists carefully.
- It is best to make your own salad dressings, as most commercially prepared dressings are loaded with undesirable oils or additives.
- If you must buy a salad dressing, a good brand is Bragg, which offers several varieties of vinaigrettes containing apple cider vinegar, which is extremely helpful for weight loss, lowering cholesterol, and overall good health.
- Most commercial canned soups are loaded with sodium and harmful chemical preservatives. Go to a natural food market and look for such brands as Health Valley or Amy's. Better yet, make your own large pot of soup and freeze the rest to enjoy later.
- Some good whole-grain crackers are ak-mak, Back to Nature brand Harvest Whole Wheats, RYVITA, and Wasa. Also, Mary's Gone Crackers and San-Jay tamari brown rice crackers are gluten free. You may also purchase crackers made from flaxseeds. Do not eat any other types of crackers.
- Healthy frozen entrées are hard to find, but natural food markets carry some acceptable frozen items. Amy's Organics is a line of organic vegetarian frozen entrées, with several gluten-free varieties. Organic Bistro is another acceptable frozen entrée that contains organic vegetables, grains, meats, and poultry. Sunshine Burgers are my favorite organic vegetarian patties, made from organic brown rice, nuts, and seeds. All of these frozen items are organic and free of preservatives. They come in one- or two-serving sizes, so it's easy to control portions.

# Raising Processed-Free Children

As a nutrition educator, I am often asked, "How do I get my children to eat fruits and vegetables?" I have even had concerned mothers bring their young ones into my office so that I could "help" them see the value of eating broccoli. Every parent faces this challenge. It's tough—but not insurmountable. As you begin your processed-free journey, you'll probably run into some mutiny when you start bringing "healthy" foods into the house. But just like yourself, ease your kids into it gently and gradually. Start with one or two foods, and work up from there.

Start with what they like, and buy a healthier version of it. For instance, if your kids like microwave popcorn, start making it yourself on the stove top, and get them involved in making it. If they're old enough to shake the pot while it's popping, that's great; otherwise, just let them watch you do it. Once the popcorn is done, you can season it with a variety of toppings, such as Parmesan cheese or taco seasoning.

Make the food visually appealing. While I worked as a personal chef, I managed to get a three-year-old and two seven-year-olds eating salmon patties every week. Aside from the tasty recipe, the secret was how I presented them. I served their parents larger patties the size of burgers; the kids didn't like the larger patties one bit. One day, I offered my young clients the same salmon patties in small slider shapes that I called "Sponge Bob Krabby Patties." They loved them!

Along with presentation, kids enjoy a multisensory experience. When I teach kids about how grapes grow and what vitamins give strawberries their color, they get to touch, smell, and create something with the colorful components of their lessons. When this happens, they *always* want to eat it. So, the notion that "kids won't eat healthy foods" isn't always necessarily so, but it does truly depend on how the foods are presented to them. It has been well observed and documented that when a child is involved in the selection and preparation of the food, or even better in the growing of some of it, they are more likely to eat it.

*continues*

## Raising Processed-Free Children continued

Don't try to "hide" vegetables in foods. That gives children the impression that the vegetable is undesirable. Let your kids know exactly what's in their meals. Keep in mind that it can take them up to ten times of eating a new food before they decide that they like it. Don't give up trying to get them to try new foods!

Be a good example and role model for eating healthy foods yourself. Teach your children as much as you can about the foods you are eating. Take ingredient lists, for example. Cue the kids especially to watch out for sugar as one of the first few ingredients. An easy exercise to get your kids thinking about what's in their food is to compare breakfast cereal box ingredients with the ingredients listed on a container of oatmeal or other whole-grain cereal. Your child can immediately see the differences.

I've experimented with some great recipes to help get kids to try healthier foods. In Chapter 15 you'll find a macaroni and cheese recipe that replaces some of the cheese with butternut squash. The bright orange color is intact— with the addition of a vegetable in the meal. There is also a recipe for home-made chocolate syrup, which you can make together with your children and then make chocolate milk with it. While you're making it, you can explain how natural cocoa contains nutrients that help keep them healthy so they don't get sick from colds and flu.

Wrapping foods up in whole wheat tortillas is a great way to get them to try a new food. I've included an easy recipe for pinwheels, which rolls up baby spinach leaves and red bell pepper strips into a tortilla with healthy cream cheese.

Many blogs and websites offer a wealth of videos and recipes to help you get your kids on board. The following are excellent resources:

> http://weelicious.com: Hundreds of healthy recipes and videos that often involve the kids in the kitchen.
>
> http://kellythekitchenkop.com: A true processed-free approach to using traditional foods.
>
> http://smartparentprogram.blogspot.com: A great site for tips and techniques to teach your children to love healthy food.

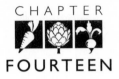

CHAPTER

FOURTEEN

# A Lifetime of Gentle, Balanced Living

*The process of changing a lifestyle is more important than reaching a goal or measuring a performance.*

—THEODORE ISAAC RUBIN

In Chapter 1 I shared with you that true change must happen on a soul level. I've spent a great many pages so far discussing our society's lack of priority on food choices, but you now have a strong nutritional foundation for changing that. If you want to stop eating processed foods, lose weight, and be skinny and healthy for the rest of your life, you have to take the time to care for yourself on other levels beyond diet. This type of balance will not be accomplished overnight; rather, it will be a steady, lifetime process. Specifically, four areas of our life need constant attention and nurturing, yet few of us take the time to make them a priority. These key elements—a positive attitude, meaningful fitness, rejuvenating rest, and journaling—contribute to the total Processed-Free Plan for Balanced Eating and Living. As you begin to make each of these a working part of your life, you will find that healthful eating is enjoyable and manageable. Cultivating a strong

321

foundation for good balanced health requires that you spend time on yourself every day—a gift you give to yourself that gives back to you in return!

## Positive Mental Attitude

The key to physical healing is having a positive mental attitude and a strong belief that you will be successful in achieving your health goals.

A positive mental attitude results from a life dedicated to self-improvement. With a personal commitment to living processed free to the best of your ability today, you don't have to be overly concerned about yesterday or tomorrow. As I have mentioned several times before, it is not recommended or implied that you should approach this plan with black-and-white thinking or a lofty goal for perfection. If you temporarily fall back into old, unhealthy food patterns, you can gently bring yourself back to center the next day, or even with the next bite. *Never beat yourself up or think you have to start over.*

I encourage you to strive for progress, not perfection. Imagine leaving your house to go out for a walk. You get three blocks away from home, and you trip on a crack in the sidewalk and fall to the ground. What do you do? Do you stay down for years and blame the crack in the sidewalk for your slip? Do you get up and go all the way back home and start your walk over, negating the three blocks of progress you had already made? Or do you adopt a positive attitude, pick yourself up, dust yourself off, and continue on your committed path with the understanding that slips happen, and it is your healthy response to those slips that empower you to continue on from where you are? The latter attitude has allowed me to keep my weight off for twenty years. I have had my share of "slips," but I have never allowed them to completely derail me from my committed path, and neither should you.

"Starting over" thinking is one of the most damaging thought forms in any attempt to improve one's health. No one is perfect. Without changes in attitude, most people are unable to maintain a healthy lifestyle.

## Meaningful Fitness

The most important aspect of gaining health is choosing healthy foods. However, for true healing to occur, we have to balance our healthy food choices with moderate physical activity. Calorie burning aside, the value of exercise is more extensive than you ever imagined. Our body was designed to move— not sit around for hours and hours on "end" (rear end, that is)—and there is a very good reason for that. The quality of our health is entirely dependent upon how we move. Our circulatory system sends blood throughout our body, relying on our heart as the "pump" to make this action happen. Also within our body is a lesser-known secondary circulatory system underneath the skin, called the lymphatic system, which rids the body of toxins, bacteria, heavy metals, dead cells, cholesterol, trapped protein, and fat globules. The lymphatic system is basically the garbage disposal of the body.

## The River of Life

Like the cardiovascular system, the lymphatic system is made up of channels, or vessels, plus valves and filters (lymph nodes). Unlike the circulatory system, however, the lymphatic system has no "pump." Instead, the fluid (called lymph) that moves through the lymphatic system relies on us to move our body to stimulate the healthy flow of lymph. Muscle action, deep breathing, and gravitational pressure from exercise are what keep the lymph flowing freely. In other words, exercise is the only pump for the lymphatic system.

In 2001, a well-respected cardiologist from Philadelphia, Gerald M. Lemole, MD, wrote a book called *The Healing Diet*, which describes the link between the health of the lymphatic system and the overall health of the body. Once a skeptic about the power of lifestyle changes, he is now a strong believer in the philosophy of the venerated Greek healer Hippocrates, who said that "walking [exercise] is man's best medicine." In his book, Dr. Lemole calls the lymphatic system "our river of life."

According to Dr. Lemole, when the lymphatic system is flowing freely, our body works fine. When it becomes sluggish or backs up, we gain weight, get sick, or both. The lymphatic system slows down and becomes sluggish when we are inactive, and especially when we sit for long periods of time. The consequences of a sluggish lymphatic system can be serious, even life threatening. In addition to being part of the body's plumbing and repair system, the lymphatics are an essential part of our immune system. Besides filtering out toxic materials, the lymph nodes also produce substances that

## Swing Your Arms

The oldest physical activity of the human race can be expressed in one word—*walking*. A brisk two-mile walk every day (with long strides and vigorous arm movements) increases enzyme and metabolic activity and may increase calorie burning for up to twelve hours afterward![1]

fight off invading viruses and bacteria and destroy abnormal cells that develop within the body, such as cancer cells.

Conditioning and purifying the lymphatic system is essential for ridding the body of fat, especially the unsightly cellulite that builds up on our thighs and buttocks. Therefore, the Processed-Free Plan for Balanced Living emphasizes the types of fitness exercises that will condition and cleanse the lymphatic system—bouncing and swinging your arms while walking briskly.

Dr. Lemole may be the first doctor to truly explain the reason exercise has proved to be such a powerful remedy for lowering cholesterol and causing major reductions in heart disease. According to Dr. Lemole, clearing the lymphatic system can substantially reduce the risk of atherosclerosis, or blockage of the arteries. A study he performed on primates demonstrated that this allows the body to more efficiently clear excess cholesterol out of the arteries: the excess cholesterol is carried through the lymphatics to the veins and then to the liver, where it can be broken down and discarded. Furthermore, according to the results of two separate U.S. studies, brisk walking does the same job of lowering LDL (bad cholesterol) as do cholesterol-lowering drugs, and more besides. Exercise not only significantly reduces LDL, but also increases levels of HDL (good cholesterol). Researchers found that brisk walking more than twelve miles per week will lower LDL, but only sustained moderate exercise, such as jogging twenty miles per week, will raise HDL.[2]

Dr. Lemole says walking should be your first option for the purposes of keeping the lymphatic system healthy. As you remember, I *walked* my way to a 100-pound weight loss. Walking was my main form of fitness, for thirty to sixty minutes each day at least five days each week. I encourage you to do the same. Walk briskly, dramatically swinging your arms along with

## Your Daily Walk

Begin your walk with some light stretching and a warm-up period of normal-pace walking for about five minutes. Then begin to walk briskly. If you are just beginning a walking program, start out with twenty-minute brisk walks, and work your way up to thirty to sixty minutes as your body responds to your daily activity. You may walk outside in the sunshine (the preferred method), or indoors on a treadmill. The distance you walk is not as important as the length of time. As long as you are walking, you will benefit from the exercise in many ways.

The pace of brisk walking is different for each person. I like the recommendation of obesity specialist Gus Prosch Jr., MD, for determining how fast one should walk: "Imagine that you are wearing thin clothing and that the temperature outside is below freezing, the wind is blowing hard, and it is raining and you have to go to the bathroom very badly and you are a mile from home. How fast would you walk to get there? Now, that's brisk walking!" You should be walking at a pace that is so intense that it is difficult to carry on a conversation. Always give yourself a cooldown period as you decrease the pace of your walking.

your pace. Allowing your arms to hang limply at your sides does not keep the lymphatic system moving.

## Bounce Your Way to Health

A few years ago I attended a weight-loss convention where one of the featured speakers shared he had lost 200 pounds in eighteen months. He claimed that the only exercise he engaged in during his weight loss was jumping on a trampoline. He humorously revealed that he wore out five mini-trampolines by the time he reached his weight goal.

His story made sense to me, because the action of bouncing, or more recently known as rebounding, gives the lymphatic system a complete cellular cleansing. Dr. Gus J. Prosch was a big proponent of rebounding, or using a mini-trampoline, claiming that it may be one of the best forms of exercise for cleansing the lymphatic system. In an article "Twelve Vital Nutritional and Health Topics," he writes, "This form of exercise is different from other physical activities because it puts gravity to work in your favor. By subjecting each of the sixty trillion cells in your body to greater gravitation pull, waste products are squeezed out and nutritional elements and oxygen are drawn into the cells. The cells function more efficiently and the metabolism increases to its maximum. As the lymphatic vessels have one-way valves in them, and the lymph flows only one way (towards the heart) when one jumps up on the rebounder, the lymph is thrown up also and cannot go back down the vessels because of the one-way valves. This acts as a suction pump to pull out and suck out the lymph and return it back to the circulation where it is supposed to be."[3]

The exercise of rebounding has many other health benefits. In her book *The Fat Flush Plan*, author Ann Louise Gittleman espouses the benefits of rebounding:

> Use of a mini-trampoline (or rebounder) has proven to be an efficient form of exercise with virtually no harmful side effects. Your cardiovascular fitness will excel, and you will be toning your body at the same time. It fires up cellular metabolism, energizing every cell with fresh oxygen and nutrients. The low impact (such as the light pressure on the thighs) stimulates waste drainage, easing waste material out of the lymphatic system. In approximately two weeks, you should notice that your legs, buttocks, and ankles are becoming toned and those orange peel-like cellulite deposits are smoothing out.[4]

You can purchase a mini-trampoline at any sports store, some department stores, or online. They typically stand about eight inches off the ground and are anywhere from thirty-six to forty inches in diameter. They cost anywhere from $50 to $400, depending on the size and type.

Gittleman recommends bouncing every day for five minutes. Dr. Prosch suggests a more detailed rebounding routine (see sidebar).

One great thing about rebounding is that anyone can do it, regardless of age or physical challenges. Even those who can't walk can still benefit from the effects of rebounding by sitting on the rebounder while someone else bounces on it. Just the motion of bouncing stimulates the lymphatic system.

## Dr. Prosch's Recommended Use of a Rebounder

Jog on the rebounder for two minutes, then jump with both feet on the rebounder for two minutes. Repeat this process over and over for twenty minutes in all. If you get dizzy at first, this is because the toxins are being pulled out of the spaces between your cells too rapidly. You should slow down or stop for a few minutes before continuing, if this should happen.[5]

If you feel unsteady on the rebounder, place a high-backed chair next to the rebounder and hold on to it while you are bouncing.

### Getting Started

Traditional physiological science has proven that exercising in the morning is the best way to improve overall metabolism. After having slept all night, the lymphatic system is at its lowest rate; therefore, moving the body first thing in the morning stimulates the flow of lymph and keeps your metabolism burning all day. However, if you can't exercise in the morning, do not use that as an excuse not to exercise! Exercise at any time of the day is better than no exercise at all.

At the very least, you should do some running in place to the count of 100 every morning. This takes less than two or three minutes and gets your lymphatic system moving. If you can do ten to twenty-five jumping jacks, either on the rebounder on just on the ground, that is another excellent way to get things moving. The point is to just *move*.

During the Skinny Beginning phase, your exercise should be moderate—thirty-minute brisk walks five to six days per week. You should also rebound for at least five minutes each day. For the following two weeks, you should increase your walking time to forty or forty-five minutes each, and continue to rebound for five minutes each day. During these two weeks, you should begin to start thinking about what other form of exercise you want to add to your routine after the fourth week. I recommend a yoga class, an exercise boot camp, a gym membership, or exercise videos that will incorporate resistance training into your routine. Resistance training tones your muscles,

## Kristine's Story

I have been a fitness coach for over fourteen years and always strived to eat healthy foods. But after learning the things Dee taught me, I realized I was not eating as healthy as I thought. After making the switch to processed-free eating, I immediately noticed an increase in my energy level. I also noticed that after adding coconut oil to my meals, my muscles did not hurt as much after my workouts.

In the two years since adopting this plan, I feel better than ever. I teach all of my clients how to eat processed free, and have seen faster weight-loss results and amazing strength-endurance capabilities in those who follow the processed-free eating plan. This natural plan has been life changing—for me, my family, and everyone else I know who has earnestly jumped on board.

—*Kristine Heidrich, age 45, health and fitness coach*

increases your bone density, and burns fat more efficiently throughout the day. You should also engage in any other forms of physical activity you enjoy—roller skating, bicycling, hiking, swimming, dancing, and sports— as a part of your healthy lifestyle. Buddying with a friend in an exercise activity or gym membership might help both of you keep with it, if you tend to taper off taking an interest in such activities.

## Rejuvenating Rest

In addition to moving your body, allowing it to relax and regenerate is equally important. Relaxation and adequate sleep are as vital to good health as exercise. Quiet time, breathing exercises, or meditation, even for a minute, will bring strength, whether you are walking, standing still, or resting. Taking a long, hot bath or sitting in a hot tub is another way to relax your body and your mind. Put on some light music, light a candle, and soak for twenty to thirty minutes. Make time every day to do something restful and enjoyable.

Lack of sleep creates an acidic condition in the body, in addition to placing huge stress on your endocrine (hormonal) system. Make it a practice to get at least eight hours of sleep each night.

# Journaling

Writing became an invaluable tool that allowed me to overcome my emotional attachments to unhealthy foods. Writing in a journal can be a new form of comfort food without the calories, or as enlightening as a session with a psychologist without the hourly fee. It is more than an outlet for creativity. It's a meditative, stress-relieving experience as potent as any pill. Writing things down is a way of coping with life. It's a way of communing with yourself. A journal is a place of emotional freedom, where you can be completely honest.

Writing allows you to access feelings that you may not always be aware of until you start writing about them. The practice of writing in a journal on a regular basis will help you see patterns in our behaviors and thinking. Writing also strengthens and trains your mind to look for your motivations for wanting to eat when you're not hungry.

A journal can be used in any of the following ways:

- Write at least one page in a journal every day, preferably in the morning. Writing in the morning helps to ground you in your intentions for the coming day.
- Write out feelings rather than acting on them or avoiding them. Describe your feelings when you feel a lot of anything, even if you can't put names to your feelings.
- Use your journal to write down what you eat every day. This encourages honesty and accountability. I have included a daily checklist on page 310 to help you keep track of your food intake.
- Write about decisions you have to make. List pros and cons of your choices. This will help clear your thinking process.

Ask yourself questions that will help you change your thinking and behaviors. In her book *The Right Questions*, author Debbie Ford presented a set of ten essential questions to guide us to an extraordinary life. I found many of the questions can apply directly to situations where food and life choices are involved. For example, in any situation, you can ask yourself the following questions and then write your answers and feelings into a journal:

- Will this choice bring me closer to my goals or take me away from them?
- Will this choice bring me long-term fulfillment or short-term gratification?
- Will this choice add to my life force or rob me of my energy?
- Will I use this situation as a growth opportunity or to beat myself up?
- Does this choice empower or disempower me?
- Is this an act of self-love or self-sabotage?
- Am I acting out of commitment or emotion?[6]

Keeping a journal is easy. You can use a softbound composition notebook, loose-leaf paper, or a hardbound book with blank pages. It doesn't matter what you write on, it just matters that you write!

Living a balanced life is not always easy; I will be the first to admit that it is sometimes challenging to keep all the plates spinning. There will inevitably be times when it is impossible to do it all. That is why it's important to stay committed, rather than give up. Do what you can, when you can, as best you can. The more committed you are, you'll find yourself being able to do more than you thought you could. My bottom line is that I always eat processed free, no matter what else is going on in my life, and whether or not I have time for a workout or for journaling. Find your bottom line, and you will find your centering place. A Buddhist monk once told his students, "There is no good meditation; there is no bad meditation; there is just meditation." So if you find yourself falling away from your healthy routines one day, gently bring yourself back to center the next day, or even in the next minute. When you do this, you cannot fail.

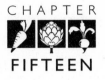

CHAPTER

FIFTEEN

# Cooking Tips and Recipes

*You don't have to cook fancy or complicated masterpieces—
just good food from fresh ingredients.*

—JULIA CHILD

In addition to planning and cooking processed-free meals for myself and my family, I have worked as a personal chef cooking processed-free meals for individuals and families with young children, and for a time Michael and I had our own organic processed-free meal delivery business called Dee's Healthy Gourmet, where I was the head chef de cuisine in charge of recipe creation and menu planning. I certainly know my way around a kitchen, and I hope to inspire you to try a few of these easy and tasty recipes. With a few exceptions, and with some preplanning, most of them can be prepared in thirty minutes or less.

I have tried to bring a variety of different types of recipes to the table, from easy breakfast ideas to salads and stews, grains, vegetables, meats, and meatless dishes. I have not forgotten about the kids, so there are some kid-friendly recipes here, too, such as Creamy Beef-Topped Baked Potatoes and Home-made Chocolate Syrup. I've included dressings and sauces that are versatile and can go with different items, such as Authentic Peanut Dressing/Dipping Sauce that can be used for dipping chicken nuggets or as the dressing for the

331

Asian Cold Noodle Salad. Also, the Basic Baked Sweet Potato recipe will provide you with baked sweet potatoes that can be enjoyed as is, or used as ingredients for some of the other recipes, such as the delectable Coconut–Sweet Potato Brownies. Speaking of brownies, yes, there are also some yummy baked goods and "occasional sweet treat" recipes here that will please most palates (homemade chocolate truffles, anyone?).

Most of the recipes are gluten free, or they can easily be made so by switching out breads, tortillas, and so on, for gluten-free versions. I've included many vegetarian-friendly items as well, and most diabetics will be safe eating these recipes. If you are diabetic, you will always want to use stevia or the lowest-glycemic sweeteners such as coconut sugar or xylitol, in place of raw unfiltered honey, pure maple syrup, and Sucanat. Although the latter are healthy and contain valuable enzymes and nutrients, the natural sugars contained in them can exacerbate a diabetic condition.

Some of the recipes call for white whole wheat flour—a lighter colored, sweeter-tasting variety of whole wheat. Hard white wheat berries are a naturally occurring albino variety of wheat that have less tannins and phenolic acid in their bran. The flour is not actually white; rather, a cream color. White whole wheat flour retains the entire grain and is just as nutritious as the more traditional whole wheat flour that is ground from hard red wheat berries. White whole wheat flour tastes and behaves more like refined white flour in baking, and is a preferred whole-grain flour for cookies, brownies, muffins, quick breads, and pancakes. You can find white whole wheat flour in natural food markets and some mainstream supermarkets.

In my cooking I use the best practice of not heating oils so high as to damage their health-promoting qualities. While I mentioned this earlier, it bears repeating that the *only* oils that can withstand temperatures above 350°F are butter and the tropical fats (coconut oil and palm oil), as they are very stable saturated fats. Therefore, most of the recipes call for coconut oil as the cooking oil. If you do not have coconut oil on hand, there are some instances where a monounsaturated oil such as extra-virgin olive oil, unrefined sesame oil, or unrefined peanut oil can be used, but only if you cover the bottom of the pan with water or broth to help cool your oil and protect it (see tips on page 248). If you're going to be baking anything above 300°F, you cannot safely use any oils other than the saturates. Extra-virgin olive oil oxidizes to free radicals at 302°F, so it is not a safe oil for roasting vegetables at high temperatures. And while we are on the topic of cooking oils, you should banish the nonstick spray oils from your kitchen, even the olive oil ones, for the reasons just mentioned. You may want to keep your own spray bottle of coconut oil in a warm place near your stove for easy spraying to keep foods from sticking to your pans. As for keeping foods from sticking to your bakeware, the good old-fashioned way of greasing pans is the best. Use butter, coconut oil, or palm oil shortening. Instead of greasing muffin pans or baking sheets, I recommend using Beyond Gourmet unbleached parchment paper and muffin liners. You can find them in most natural food markets and online.

If you do not have some of the ingredients listed, you can always switch them out with ingredients that you have on hand. I have learned that a cook's best skill is the ability to improvise. For instance, if you don't have any tamari sauce, you can use Bragg Liquid Aminos or soy sauce instead. And please remember, recipes are only guidelines; you can switch fruits, vegetables, seasonings, and so on, to suit your own tastes.

Here are some additional basic kitchen/cooking tips:

Just say no to Teflon. Avoid all Teflon-coated cookware and aluminum-containing pots, pans and foil, and opt for noncoated stainless-steel cookware instead. Teflon is a synthetic polymer called polytetrafluoroetheylene (PTFE), which releases toxic substances into the environment, and quite likely into food. Aluminum easily leaches into the food you are cooking, which is bad news as aluminum is known to inhibit the body's use of calcium and magnesium—the very minerals that are needed to build bones and neutralize acidity in the body. Although there is no definite link, researchers conducting autopsies on many Alzheimer's patients discovered higher levels of aluminum in their brains. The most common source of aluminum is from cookware. Although there are a growing number of new cookware options on the market, they haven't been in use long enough for us to know whether they're safe—even if they're advertised as "green" or "nonstick." I continue to recommend noncoated stainless-steel and cast-iron cookware for stovetop cooking and glass, CorningWare, or Pyrex for the oven. As mentioned, I cover cookie sheets with parchment paper to keep the food from sticking and also to place a barrier between the food and the metal. These cookware options might be a little harder to clean, but your health is worth it.

No steamer? No problem. Steaming is a great way to reheat food quickly, but you don't need a steamer to do it. When I have things like leftover chicken, rice, and vegetables, I put a small amount of water in a large skillet over medium heat, then place all my foods in the skillet, keeping them separated, and put the cover on the skillet to let the steam from the water heat the food. This takes less than five minutes to reheat in a safe manner.

Time-saving appliances. As you transition into preparing more of your own foods, you may want to invest in some time-saving kitchen appliances such as a rice cooker, a food processor, and a slow cooker.

Rice cookers. There are many rice cookers on the market, but not all are created equal. Most have aluminum and nonstick inner cooking pots. There are a few companies, such as Lotus Foods, that manufacture rice cookers and vegetable steamers with inner cooking pots made of stainless steel.

Food processors. These handy machines with S-shaped blades and grating attachments make chopping vegetables a snap, and can also blend and puree foods easily. Any food processor on the market will do the trick. The ultimate kitchen appliance is a Vitamix, a high-powered blender/food processor that can do everything from grind flaxseeds, coffee beans, and grains, to make ice cream and soups in a matter of minutes. It is the best blender for making smoothies, as it can blend whole fruits and vegetables, including stems and peels, into creamy drinks, retaining all of the valuable nutrients. The Vitamix is definitely a major purchase, it can cost about $400 and up, depending on the model and accessories, but is well worth the investment. I've had mine for many years and I don't know how I would live without it.

Slow cooker. These timesaving appliances are fairly inexpensive and quite versatile. They're great in winter months for cooking soups, beans, stews, casseroles, and even oatmeal, but are just as helpful during the hot summer months when you don't want to turn on the oven. It takes no time at all to fill up the slow cooker with chicken, a turkey breast, meat loaf, and even potatoes. Turn it on before leaving the house in the morning, and you'll have a meal ready to eat when you get home in the evening. Slow cookers are also great for cooking in bulk, then freezing the extra for future meals.

## A Word About Calorie Counts

As you know, I am not a fan of calorie counting, as it is a very inexact method and does not reflect what is truly going on in the body. However, some people find it helpful to know how many calories they are consuming, so I have included them for each recipe. You will find that most serving sizes have low to moderate numbers of calories, but some have a high fat count due to the healthy oils from nuts, seeds, avocados, coconut oil, or full-fat yogurt. Please let me remind you that these types of fats are the ones that you need to lose fat and get skinny, so don't be overly concerned by this. As long as your meals are balanced and full of alkaline-forming foods, the fats will be metabolized correctly. The goal is to enjoy great tasting healthy food, and let nature take care of the calories.

# Skinny Smoothies 🍇

## BERRY BLAST SMOOTHIE

Smoothies are highly nutritious and simple to prepare. They are also one of the easiest ways to incorporate the good, healthy oils into your meals.

### MAKES 1 SERVING

1 cup unsweetened almond milk
3 drops liquid stevia extract
1 tablespoon ground flaxseeds
1 tablespoon extra-virgin coconut oil
1 scoop vanilla whey protein powder or hemp protein powder
1 scoop alkalizing green superfood (optional)
1 cup fresh or frozen berries of your choosing

▶ Place all ingredients into a blender and blend until smooth and creamy. Drink immediately.

*Nutrition per serving: 350 calories; 19 g total fat; 11 g saturated fat; 10 g protein; 34 g carbohydrates; 7 g dietary fiber; 10 mg cholesterol; 259 mg sodium*

VARIATIONS: You can change the ingredients for different taste profiles:
- Use different fruits.
- Add half of an avocado.
- Use ground nuts, or ground seeds such as almonds, chia seeds, or sunflower seeds.
- Use coconut milk instead of almond milk (⅓ cup coconut milk plus ⅔ cup water)
- Replace the coconut oil with flaxseed oil.
- Add unsweetened carob powder or cacao powder.

The possibilities are endless!

## PUMPKIN SMOOTHIE

This smoothie is a great way to eat a serving of starchy vegetables for breakfast. Pumpkin is high in fiber, low in calories, and high in cancer fighting antioxidants.

### MAKES I SERVING

1 cup almond milk
3 drops liquid stevia extract
1 tablespoon ground flaxseeds
1 scoop vanilla whey protein powder or hemp protein powder
1 tablespoon pumpkin pie spice (see note)
½ cup cooked pumpkin, canned or fresh
1 tablespoon extra-virgin coconut oil

▶ Place all the ingredients into a blender and blend until smooth and creamy. Drink immediately.

**NOTE:** You can make your own pumpkin pie spice by combining the following:

1 ½ teaspoons ground cinnamon          ¼ teaspoon ground nutmeg
¾ teaspoon ground ginger               ¼ teaspoon ground cloves

*Nutrition per serving: 251 calories; 19 g total fat; 11.5 g saturated fat; 10 g protein; 17 g carbohydrates; 6 g dietary fiber; 10 mg cholesterol; 236 mg sodium*

## CHOCOLATE PB&B SMOOTHIE

The blending of chocolate, peanut butter, and bananas never gets old! This will appeal to kids and grown-ups alike.

### MAKES I SERVING

1 cup unsweetened almond milk
3 drops liquid stevia extract
1 scoop vanilla whey protein powder or hemp protein powder
1 medium-size banana
1 tablespoon natural peanut butter
1 tablespoon unsweetened cocoa powder

▶ Place all the ingredients in a blender and blend until smooth and creamy. Drink immediately.

*Nutrition per serving: 345 calories; 12 g total fat; 2 g saturated fat; 16 g protein; 42 g carbohydrates; 5 g dietary fiber; 10 mg cholesterol; 270 mg sodium*

# Skinny Breakfasts

## SKINNY YOGURT SUPREME

This meal packs a lot of nutrition into one small bowl!

### MAKES I SERVING

I cup plain whole-milk yogurt (preferably organic)
I teaspoon pure vanilla extract
3 drops liquid stevia extract
I tablespoon ground flaxseeds
¼ cup oat bran
I scoop alkalizing green superfood powder (optional)
I cup fresh fruit, such as blueberries, raspberries, kiwifruit,
    or sliced strawberries (or a medley of several different fruits)
6 raw almonds (about ¼ ounce), chopped

▶ Combine the yogurt, vanilla, and stevia in a small bowl. Stir until you no longer see
   the color of the vanilla. Add the flaxseeds, bran, and alkalizing green superfood (if
   using). Stir to combine thoroughly. Top with the fruit and chopped almonds. Enjoy!

NOTE: All of the fat grams in this recipe come from the type of oils that makes
your body burn more fat, so don't be alarmed by its high fat content. The heart-
healthy omega-3 from flaxseeds, the healthy saturated fat from yogurt, and the
cholesterol-lowering monounsaturated fat from almonds are all highly beneficial.
People who regularly include these types of oils in their meals safely lose weight
and are skinnier than those who don't!

*Nutrition per serving (without green superfood): 335 calories; 16 g total fat; 5 g satu-
rated fat; 15 g protein; 41 g carbohydrates; 7 g dietary fiber; 32 mg cholesterol; 113 mg
sodium.*

*Nutrition per serving (with green superfood): 370 calories; 16 g total fat; 5 g saturated
fat; 15 g protein; 49 g carbohydrates; 10 g dietary fiber; 32 mg cholesterol; 128 mg
sodium*

## OVER-EASY EGGS FLORENTINE

Leftover brown rice comes in handy for this quick skillet breakfast.

### MAKES I SERVING

1 tablespoon extra-virgin coconut oil
1 clove garlic, minced
½ cup cooked brown rice
2 cups baby spinach leaves or other greens, chopped
2 eggs, preferably organic
3 sprigs fresh parsley

▶ Heat a skillet over medium heat and place ½ tablespoon of the coconut oil, the garlic, and the brown rice in the pan. Sauté for 1 minute, then add the spinach and stir until it wilts lightly. Transfer everything to a plate, turn down the heat to medium-low, and return the skillet to the heat.

▶ Add the remaining coconut oil, and then crack the two eggs into the skillet. Cook until the whites are mostly set, then flip the eggs over gently, being careful not to break the yolks. Turn off the heat, let the eggs sit for a few more seconds, then transfer the eggs to the plate on top of the rice and spinach. Garnish with the parsley (which you will eat!). Serve immediately.

*Nutrition per serving: 411 calories; 24 g total fat; 14 g saturated fat; 18 g protein; 30 g carbohydrates; 1.5 g dietary fiber; 425 mg cholesterol; 219 mg sodium*

## BELL PEPPER, BASIL, AND SPINACH CRUSTLESS QUICHE

This quiche, packed with powerful liver-cleansing foods, makes a great meal for any time of day, and can be eaten warm or cold. A good timesaving strategy is to double the recipe and make two quiches—one to eat now and one to freeze for easy meals at another time.

### MAKES 4 SERVINGS (SERVING = ¼ QUICHE)

1 tablespoon coconut oil, plus more for coating the pie pan
½ red bell pepper, seeded and diced
½ cup chopped onion
2 cloves garlic, minced
½ cup fresh basil
1 cup spinach, well rinsed
8 organic eggs

¼ cup coconut milk
Sea salt and pepper (optional)
Fresh parsley sprigs, for garnish

► Preheat the oven to 350°F.
► Place the tablespoon of coconut oil in a skillet over medium heat. Sauté peppers, onion, and garlic until the peppers are soft, about 10 minutes. Add the spinach and basil and cook just until slightly wilted, 1 to 2 minutes. Remove from the heat.
► Whisk the eggs, coconut milk, and salt and pepper (if using) together in a large bowl, or place in a blender and blend until well mixed.
► Coat a 9-inch pie pan (deep dish works best) or an oven-safe skillet with coconut oil. Spread the cooked vegetables over the bottom of the pan. Pour the egg mixture over the vegetables. Place the pan on the center rack of the oven and bake for 20 to 30 minutes, or until the center of the quiche is set. Remove from the oven, let cool slightly, then cut into four equal pieces. Serve with fresh parsley sprigs.

NOTE: You can add more or different veggies to this recipe; just remember to cook them before adding to the quiche. If the veggies are not cooked first, your quiche may become too watery. Also, if you have some prebaked sweet potatoes on hand, you can layer them on the bottom of the pie pan before topping with the veggies and eggs. This will give you a nice sweet potato "crust."

*Nutrition per serving: 211 calories; 15 g total fat; 7 g saturated fat; 14 g protein; 6 g carbohydrates; 1 g dietary fiber; 425 mg cholesterol; 155 mg sodium*

## BREAKFAST WALDORF SALAD

This refreshing breakfast will keep you satisfied all morning. Try it with different fruits, nuts, or seeds.

### MAKES 2 SERVINGS

1 medium-size organic apple, cored and cut into ½-inch pieces
1 tablespoon freshly squeezed lemon juice
2 cups plain whole-milk organic yogurt
2 teaspoons raw honey
1 cup organic red seedless grapes, halved
14 walnut halves (about 1 ounce)

► Place the apple pieces in a bowl, add the lemon juice, and toss. This will keep the apples from turning brown if you want to save some of this salad to eat later or the next day.

▶ Add the yogurt, honey, grapes, and walnuts. Stir to combine. Eat immediately or store in the refrigerator.

---

*Nutrition per serving: 350 calories; 17 g total fat; 6 g saturated fat; 10 g protein; 42 g carbohydrates; 3 g dietary fiber; 32 mg cholesterol; 112 mg sodium*

## BREAKFAST BAKED APPLES

These warm apples pair well with yogurt for a very satisfying breakfast.

### MAKES 4 SERVINGS (SERVING = 1 APPLE)

4 organic apples, preferably red-skinned
4 dates, pitted
12 walnut or pecan halves
2 tablespoons freshly squeezed lemon juice
1 teaspoon ground cinnamon
4 tablespoons water

▶ Preheat the oven to 350°F.
▶ Slice the tops off the apples. Using a corer or paring knife, remove the core from each apple without cutting through the bottom. Place the apples in an 8-inch baking dish. Stuff each apple with one date and three walnut halves. Combine the lemon juice, cinnamon, and water in a small bowl, then pour the lemon juice mixture evenly into each apple. Fill the apples with more water if needed, and put the tops back on.
▶ Bake until soft, 15 to 20 minutes. Serve warm.

---

*Nutrition per serving: 187 calories; 5 g total fat; 0 g saturated fat; 1.5 g protein; 34 g carbohydrates; 5 g dietary fiber; 0 mg cholesterol; 0 mg sodium*

## SPROUTED FRENCH TOAST À LA MODE

High in fiber and protein—sans the powdered sugar—this French toast is a yummy way to start the day.

### MAKES 2 SERVINGS

2 eggs, preferably organic
1 tablespoon coconut milk
2 teaspoons ground cinnamon
2 slices flourless sprouted-grain bread (or gluten-free bread)
1 teaspoon extra-virgin coconut oil, for oiling the griddle

I cup plain whole-milk organic yogurt
2 tablespoons pure maple syrup, brown rice syrup, or coconut nectar

▶ Crack eggs into a medium-size bowl and beat with a wire whisk. Add the coconut milk and cinnamon. Whisk again to mix.
▶ Cut the slices of bread in half, making four halves. Place the bread in the egg mixture and let it soak until it is saturated, about 2 minutes.
▶ Heat the coconut oil in a skillet or griddle over medium heat. When the oil is hot, place the pieces of egg-soaked bread in the skillet. Pour the remaining egg mixture over the bread. Cook until golden, then flip and cook until the other side is golden and the egg is cooked through. Transfer to a plate.
▶ While the French toast is cooking, whisk the yogurt and syrup together in a small bowl. Top French toast with dollops of maple-sweetened yogurt.
▶ Serve immediately.

*Nutrition per serving: 289 calories; 13 g total fat; 7 g saturated fat; 15 g protein; 29 g carbohydrates; 4 g dietary fiber; 229 mg cholesterol; 253 mg sodium*

## LEMON-RICOTTA PANCAKES

These fluffy, fritterlike pancakes are a hit for special occasion breakfasts. Serve them with yogurt or turkey sausages.

### MAKES 10 SERVINGS (SERVING = I [4-INCH] PANCAKE)

I cup white whole wheat flour
2 teaspoons nonaluminum baking powder
½ teaspoon baking soda
¼ teaspoon sea salt
I cup organic whole-milk ricotta cheese
I organic egg
2 organic egg whites
½ cup freshly squeezed lemon juice
2 teaspoons lemon zest
I tablespoon coconut nectar or raw honey
I tablespoon coconut oil, warm enough to be in liquid form,
    plus more for oiling the griddle

▶ In a large bowl, whisk together the flour, baking powder, baking soda, and salt.
▶ In a medium-size bowl, whisk together the ricotta, egg, egg whites, lemon juice, lemon zest, coconut nectar, and the tablespoon of coconut oil. Using a rubber

spatula or wooden spoon, fold this mixture into the dry ingredients to make a thick batter.

▶ Brush a griddle or skillet with coconut oil, then heat over medium-low heat. With a ¼-cup measuring cup, drop the batter onto the griddle, spreading it slightly. Multiple pancakes can be cooked at once.

▶ Cook the pancakes until browned and beginning to set, about 2 minutes. Flip and cook until browned on the second side and cooked at the center, about 2 minutes longer.

▶ Repeat with the remaining batter. Serve immediately.

*Nutrition per serving: 118 calories; 5 g total fat; 3 g saturated fat; 6 g protein; 11 g carbohydrates; 1 g dietary fiber; 42 mg cholesterol; 218 mg sodium*

# Skinny Salads, Dressings, Sauces, and Seasonings

## SWEET SKINNY APPLE CIDER VINAIGRETTE

This sweet and tangy vinaigrette is a very powerful alkalizing salad dressing. It can be used on any salad or as a marinade. I typically double or triple the recipe and keep a big bottle of it in the refrigerator.

### MAKES ABOUT 1½ CUPS (SERVING = 1 TABLESPOON)

1 cup extra-virgin olive oil
½ cup raw, unfiltered apple cider vinegar
1 tablespoon freshly squeezed lemon juice
¼ teaspoon liquid stevia extract
2 cloves garlic
1 teaspoon dried parsley
1 teaspoon dried oregano
1 teaspoon dried basil
1 teaspoon dried thyme
¼ teaspoon Herbamare or sea salt

▶ Place all the ingredients in a blender and blend on high speed to combine thoroughly. Let the blender run for about 2 minutes for a creamy-type Italian vinaigrette. Place any leftover dressing in a glass jar or cruet.

*Nutrition per serving: 82 calories; 9 g total fat; 1 grams saturated fat; 0 g protein; 0 g carbohydrates; 0 grams dietary fiber; 0 mg cholesterol; 27 mg sodium*

## BALSAMIC-GINGER VINAIGRETTE

Make sure you are using a high-quality balsamic vinegar from Modena, Italy. Inexpensive grocery store varieties are sugary, fake versions of the real thing.

### MAKES ABOUT 1 CUP (SERVING = 1 TABLESPOON)

½ cup raw, unfiltered apple cider vinegar
2 tablespoons balsamic vinegar
4 tablespoons extra-virgin olive oil
2 cloves garlic, pressed, or 1 teaspoon garlic powder
1 (½-inch) piece fresh ginger, peeled and diced, or ½ teaspoon powdered ginger
Pinch of sea salt

▶ Whisk all the ingredients together in a medium-size bowl, or place everything in the blender and blend on high speed for 1 minute. Transfer the dressing to a glass jar and store in the refrigerator.

*Nutrition per serving: 30 calories; 3 g total fat; 0 g saturated fat; 0 g protein; 3 g carbohydrates; 0 g dietary fiber; 0 mg cholesterol; 108 mg sodium*

## CREAMY HONEY-MUSTARD DRESSING AND DIPPING SAUCE

Kids love dipping chicken nuggets in this sauce; grown-ups like it on salads and as a spread for sandwiches.

### MAKES 2 CUPS (SERVING = 1 TABLESPOON)

1 cup safflower mayonnaise
¼ cup Dijon mustard
¼ cup extra-virgin olive oil
¼ cup raw honey
⅛ teaspoon onion powder
⅛ teaspoon sea salt
¾ teaspoon raw, unfiltered apple cider vinegar
1 clove garlic, minced

▶ Place all the ingredients in a blender or mix by hand with a wire whisk until well blended. The dressing may be kept up to 3 weeks refrigerated.

*Nutrition per serving: 45 calories; 4 g total fat; 0 g saturated fat; 0 g protein; 3 g carbohydrates; 0 g dietary fiber; 0 mg cholesterol; 108 mg sodium*

# AUTHENTIC PEANUT DRESSING AND DIPPING SAUCE

Whereas most versions of peanut sauce are made with peanut butter, this recipe starts with real peanuts—and you'll taste the difference! This sauce can be used for a variety of purposes, from a dip for veggies or chicken nuggets, to a dressing for salads and a marinade for chicken or tempeh.

### MAKES 3 CUPS (SERVING = ¼ CUP)

⅓ cup water
⅓ cup coconut milk
1 cup unsalted dry-roasted peanuts
2 cloves garlic, minced
2 teaspoons unrefined toasted sesame oil
2 tablespoons plus 2 teaspoons wheat-free reduced-sodium tamari sauce
2 tablespoons coconut nectar or raw honey
½ tablespoon freshly squeezed lime juice
½ teaspoon cayenne (optional)

▶ Place all the ingredients in a blender or food processor in the order listed. Blend or process until the sauce is smooth. If you prefer a runnier peanut sauce, add a little more water or coconut milk. Do a taste test, adding more tamari sauce if it's not salty enough, or more cayenne if it's not spicy enough. If it's too salty, add a fresh squeeze of lime juice. Add a bit more nectar or honey if more sweetness is desired. Serve warm or at room temperature.

*Nutrition per serving: 108 calories; 8 g total fat; 2 g saturated fat; 3.5 g protein; 6 g carbohydrates; <1 g dietary fiber; 0 mg cholesterol; 246 mg sodium*

# ASIAN COLD NOODLE SALAD

This recipe includes lots of veggies to balance out the noodles. Add chicken or tempeh if desired.

### MAKES 2 SERVINGS (SERVING = ½ CUP NOODLES PLUS VEGGIES AND DRESSING)

2 ounces uncooked brown rice spaghetti noodles
1 cup napa cabbage, sliced thinly
½ medium-size red bell pepper, julienned
½ cup thinly sliced red cabbage
2 medium-size carrots, shredded
2 tablespoons chopped green onions
¼ cup chopped fresh cilantro

¼ cup chopped fresh mint leaves
I cup Authentic Peanut Dressing (page 345)
2 teaspoons dry-roasted peanuts

▶ Cook the spaghetti noodles according to the package directions. Drain and place in a large bowl.

▶ Add remaining ingredients to the bowl and toss together. Serve immediately or refrigerate.

*Nutrition per serving: 359 calories; 17 g total fat; 3 g saturated fat; 11.5 g protein; 41 g carbohydrates; 4 g dietary fiber; 0 mg cholesterol; 559 mg sodium*

## DEE'S EVERYDAY RAINBOW SALAD

I eat a version of this salad literally every day. The vegetables can vary depending on season and availability, but the goal is to get as many colors into the salad as possible. Sometimes I have it with turkey and sometimes I make it a vegetarian salad by replacing the turkey with ½ cup of black beans.

### MAKES I SERVING

I ½ cups chopped romaine lettuce
½ cup chopped kale
I cup mixed chopped assorted veggies (celery, red bell pepper, carrot, beet, raw red cabbage, cauliflower)
2 tablespoons Sweet Skinny Apple Cider Vinaigrette (page 343)
3 ounces cooked turkey, or ½ cup cooked black beans
½ cup cooked brown rice or cooked quinoa
I teaspoon raw pine nuts (about ¼ ounce)
¼ avocado, peeled and cubed
3 to 4 sprigs fresh parsley

▶ Place the romaine and kale on the bottom of a large bowl. Top with the chopped veggies. Add the vinaigrette and toss. Next, top with the turkey, brown rice, avocado, pine nuts, and parsley. Enjoy!

*Nutrition per serving (with turkey): 509 calories; 29 g total fat; 4 g saturated fat; 33 g protein; 37 g carbohydrates; 4 g dietary fiber; 71 mg cholesterol; 152 mg sodium*

*Nutrition per serving (with beans): 537 calories; 29 g total fat; 4 g saturated fat; 13 g protein; 57 g carbohydrates; 10 g dietary fiber; 0 mg cholesterol; 108 mg sodium*

# WILD ALASKAN SALMON–STUFFED TOMATOES

High-quality canned wild salmon can be just as nutritious as cooking it yourself. Salmon is one of the best sources of omega-3 essential fatty acids. The salmon can be replaced with canned tuna.

### MAKES 2 SERVINGS

1 tablespoon extra-virgin olive oil
1 tablespoon freshly squeezed lemon juice
1 teaspoon Dijon mustard
Sea salt and pepper
2 large beefsteak tomatoes
6 ounces baked wild salmon fillet, or 1 (6-ounce) can wild Alaskan salmon, drained
½ teaspoon dried dill
2 tablespoons finely chopped or grated carrot
2 tablespoons finely chopped celery

▶ To make the dressing, whisk the olive oil, lemon juice, and Dijon mustard in a small bowl. Season with sea salt and pepper as desired.

▶ To make the salad, cut the tomatoes in half crosswise; scoop out and discard the flesh and seeds. In a separate bowl, combine the salmon, carrot, celery, and parsley. Drizzle with the dressing and toss lightly.

▶ Fill each tomato half with the salmon mixture. Serve immediately.

*Nutrition per serving: 194 calories; 9 g total fat; 2 g saturated fat; 17 g protein; 11 g carbohydrates; 1.5 g dietary fiber; 30 mg cholesterol; 144 mg sodium*

# CUCUMBER-TOMATO SALAD WITH HONEY MUSTARD VINAIGRETTE

Serve this simple, easy salad over fresh lettuce or spring mix, or just eat it without the greens. It also makes a great snack food. You can add other veggies, too, such as shredded carrots or crunchy cauliflower.

### MAKES 4 SERVINGS (SERVING = 1 CUP)

¼ cup raw, unfiltered apple cider vinegar
1 tablespoon plus 1 teaspoon raw honey
1 teaspoon Dijon mustard
2 medium-size cucumbers, sliced
4 firm Roma tomatoes, quartered, then sliced
½ small red onion, sliced thinly

**4 radishes, sliced thinly**
**½ cup thinly sliced fresh basil**

▶ Combine the vinegar, honey, and Dijon in a bowl and whisk together. Add the rest of the ingredients. Toss well. Enjoy immediately, or cover and refrigerate for several hours to blend the flavors.

*Nutrition per serving: 62 calories; 0 g total fat; 0 g saturated fat; 1.5 g protein; 13 g carbohydrates; 1.5 g dietary fiber; 0 mg cholesterol; 41 mg sodium*

## FRESH BASIL PESTO

Use this pesto as a dip for raw veggies or mix it with shredded raw zucchini, carrots, and cabbage for a yummy quick salad.

### MAKES 8 SERVINGS (SERVING = I TABLESPOON)

**2 cups fresh basil leaves**
**¼ cup extra-virgin olive oil**
**I clove garlic, minced**
**¼ cup raw pine nuts**

▶ Place the basil, oil, and garlic in the bowl of a food processor and blend until the basil is chopped. Add the pine nuts and blend until smooth. Stop occasionally to scrape down the sides of the bowl with a rubber spatula. This pesto will keep for 5 days in the refrigerator.

**VARIATION:** For an omega-3 version, replace half or all of the olive oil with flaxseed oil or hemp oil.

*Nutrition per serving: 93 calories; 9 g total fat; 1 g saturated fat; 1 g protein; 2 g carbohydrates; 1 g dietary fiber; 0 mg cholesterol; 3 mg sodium*

## GREEN ENCHILADA SAUCE

I created this sauce because I could not find a commercially prepared enchilada sauce that didn't have hydrogenated oils or preservatives in it. It's great for enchiladas, but can also be used as a taco sauce, in burritos, or on top of eggs.

### MAKES I QUART (SERVING = ½ CUP)

**¼ cup extra-virgin olive oil**
**2 onions, chopped**

8 cloves garlic
3 cups reduced-sodium chicken broth or vegetable broth
I pound tomatillos
I ½ teaspoons ground cumin
I tablespoon chili powder
I (4-ounce) can mild diced green chiles

▶ Heat the oil in a skillet over medium heat. Add the onions and garlic and cook until soft and translucent. Add the broth, tomatillos, cumin, chili powder, and green chiles and bring to a boil.

▶ Lower the heat to a simmer and cover. Continue cooking until the tomatillos are soft. Remove from the heat and allow to cool. When cool enough to handle, transfer the sauce to a food processor or blender and blend until smooth.

▶ Use immediately or store the leftover sauce in the refrigerator or freezer to use another time.

*Nutrition per serving: 120 calories; 7 g total fat; 1 g saturated fat; 2 g protein; 11 g carbohydrates; 1 g dietary fiber; 0 mg cholesterol; 398 mg sodium*

## TACO SEASONING MIX

*Taco seasoning mixes that come in packets usually contain monosodium glutamate (MSG) and other undesirable additives. This one tastes identical to the commercial variety, without the chemical ingredients. Try it on ground beef, ground turkey, chicken, and beans.*

### MAKES ½ CUP (SERVING = I TEASPOON)

4 tablespoons chili powder
I teaspoon garlic powder
I teaspoon onion powder
¼ teaspoon cayenne
I teaspoon Mexican oregano
2 teaspoons paprika
2 tablespoons ground cumin
4 teaspoons ground coriander
2 teaspoons sea salt

▶ Mix all of the ingredients together in a small bowl. Store in an airtight container or spice jar.

*Nutrition per serving: 9 calories; 0 g total fat; 0 g saturated fat; 0 g protein; 1 g carbohydrates; 0 g dietary fiber; 0 mg cholesterol; 199 mg sodium*

## TOASTED SESAME SEEDS

Many of my recipes call for toasted sesame seeds, as they are one of the few alkaline-forming seeds. You may buy them already toasted, but they taste better and are more fragrant when you toast them yourself. Sprinkle them on salads, cooked vegetables, rice, or quinoa to boost the alkaline-forming quality of your meals.

### MAKES 8 SERVINGS (SERVING = I TEASPOON)

½ cup (or more) raw sesame seeds

▶ For stove-top toasting, place the raw sesame seeds in a dry skillet and heat over medium heat, shaking the pan occasionally or stirring with a flat spatula. Remove the seeds when they darken and become fragrant. Be careful not to burn them. It takes between 3 and 5 minutes to toast sesame seeds on the stove top.
▶ To toast in the oven, preheat the oven to 275°F. Spread out the seeds on a dry baking sheet. Bake until the seeds are brown and become fragrant. It takes 15 to 20 minutes to toast sesame seeds in the oven.
▶ For both methods, allow the toasted seeds to cool, then store at room temperature in a tightly covered jar with little air space. These will keep for several weeks.

*Nutrition per serving: 3 calories; 0 g total fat; 0 grams saturated fat; 0 g protein; 0 g carbohydrates; 0 grams dietary fiber; 0 mg cholesterol; 0 mg sodium*

# Skinny Veggies and Sides

## BASIC BAKED SWEET POTATOES

You'll want to make extras of these to add to meals later in the week.

### MAKES 4 SERVINGS (SERVING = ABOUT ½ CUP)

I pound sweet potatoes

▶ Preheat the oven to 375°F.
▶ Wash the sweet potatoes well under cool running water. Use a brush or scrubber to remove any dirt. Rinse, drain, and pat dry. Lift any small bruises or eyes from the sweet potatoes with the pointed end of a vegetable peeler. Remove any dark or black areas.

▶ Pierce the skin a few times with a fork to allow steam to escape and prevent possible bursting while baking.

▶ Place the potatoes on a baking sheet and bake for 45 to 55 minutes, depending on thickness and size of the potatoes. *Do not* wrap potatoes in foil, as the steam will not escape and you will end up with soggy potatoes.

▶ Test the potatoes for doneness by squeezing them gently. The potatoes are done when they are slightly soft.

▶ The potatoes can be served immediately. Cut open and eat them the same as you would a white baked potato.

▶ Extra baked potatoes can be stored in the refrigerator to be eaten later. They're great cold or reheated. Wrap a large lettuce leaf around a piece of cold sweet potato for a great nutritious snack.

**VARIATIONS:** The great news about sweet potatoes is that they are very sweet and delicious eaten just as they are, but you may add some of the following toppings:

I teaspoon organic butter or coconut oil
Ground cinnamon, paprika, nutmeg, or cloves
Chopped pecans or walnuts
Steamed broccoli or other veggies

*Nutrition per serving: 102 calories; 0 g total fat; 0 g saturated fat; 2 g protein; 24 g carbohydrates; 4 g dietary fiber; 0 mg cholesterol; 41 mg sodium*

## SWEET POTATO HUMMUS

Great as a veggie dip, or just eaten with a spoon!

### MAKES 4 SERVINGS (SERVING = ½ CUP)

I pound sweet potatoes, baked in skin (about I large or 2 small), cooled, or 2 cups canned sweet potato puree (make sure there are no chemical additives)
I teaspoon ground cumin
I tablespoon freshly squeezed lemon juice
¼ teaspoon sea salt
¼ teaspoon cayenne
⅛ teaspoon black pepper
I tablespoon tahini (sesame seed paste, available in gourmet food stores)
I tablespoon extra-virgin olive oil
Zest of I orange

▶ Scoop the flesh of the sweet potatoes into the bowl of a food processor. Discard the skins.

▶ Add the rest of the ingredients to the food processor and blend, stopping to scrape the sides of the bowl, until smooth and creamy. Serve immediately or refrigerate and enjoy later.

*Nutrition per serving: 159 calories; 5 g total fat; 0 g saturated fat; 3 g protein; 25 g carbohydrates; 4 g dietary fiber; 0 mg cholesterol; 206 mg sodium*

## PANFRIED SWEET POTATOES

These are great as a breakfast side dish with eggs, or they can be added to salads or wraps.

### MAKES 4 SERVINGS (SERVING = ½ CUP)

I pound sweet potatoes
2 tablespoons extra-virgin coconut oil

▶ Wash the sweet potatoes well under cool running water. Use a brush or scrubber to remove any dirt. Rinse, drain, and pat dry. Lift any small bruises or eyes from the sweet potatoes with the pointed end of a vegetable peeler. Remove any dark or black areas.

▶ Slice the sweet potatoes in half lengthwise. Holding the two halves together, slice them horizontally into thin slices, about ⅛ inch thick.

▶ Heat the oil in a large skillet over medium heat. Add the potato slices and toss them around with a spatula to coat them in the oil. Cover the skillet and lower the heat. After about 5 minutes, uncover and turn the potatoes with a spatula. Cover and continue to cook until tender, another 5 minutes. Check frequently (you want them to be browned on each side, but not burned). Uncover and cook for a few more minutes, to glaze the potatoes. The potatoes are done when they are tender enough to cut with a fork. Serve hot. Store leftovers in the refrigerator.

Note: Panfried sweet potatoes are also good cold. If you have any leftovers, they made great additions to salads.

*Nutrition per serving: 148 calories; 7 g total fat; 6 g saturated fat; 2 g protein; 24 g carbohydrates; 4 g dietary fiber; 0 mg cholesterol; 41 mg sodium*

## TAMARI SWEET POTATO WEDGES WITH ROSEMARY

These make great appetizers for parties, but they're great as a side dish also.

### MAKES 12 SERVINGS (SERVING = ¼ POUND)

3 pounds sweet potatoes
2 tablespoons coconut oil
1 teaspoon chili powder
1 teaspoon wheat-free reduced-sodium tamari sauce
1 heaping tablespoon chopped fresh rosemary

▶ Preheat the oven to 400°F.
▶ Wash the sweet potatoes well under cool running water. Use a brush or scrubber to remove any dirt. Rinse, drain, and pat dry. Lift any small bruises or eyes from the sweet potatoes with the pointed end of a vegetable peeler. Remove any dark or black areas.
▶ Halve the potatoes crosswise, then lengthwise, and cut each piece into four wedges. Place the potato wedges in a large bowl.
▶ In a smaller bowl, mix the coconut oil, chili powder, tamari sauce, and rosemary. Drizzle over the potatoes, and toss to coat.
▶ Arrange the potatoes skin side down in one layer on baking sheets.
▶ Bake for 20 minutes. Turn the slices, and bake until tender, 12 to 15 minutes more. Serve immediately.

*Nutrition per serving: 123 calories; 2 g total fat; 2 g saturated fat; 2 g protein; 24 g carbohydrates; 4 g dietary fiber; 0 mg cholesterol; 61 mg sodium*

## 15-MINUTE STEAMED BEETS AND SAUTÉED BEET GREENS WITH GOAT CHEESE

This is a great way to use every part of the fresh beets you buy. Both the beets and the greens are powerful cancer fighters and detoxifiers. Consuming both on a regular basis will make you super skinny! Serve this wonderful vegetable dish with quinoa, poultry, or fish.

### MAKES 2 SERVINGS

1 bunch beets with greens (about 3 beets, about 3 inches in diameter)
1 tablespoon extra-virgin olive oil
2 cloves garlic, minced
1 shallot, sliced thinly

**Salt and pepper (optional)**
**1 ounce soft goat cheese, plain or herbed**

▶ Wash the beets and greens gently under cool running water, taking care not to tear the skin of the beet—this tough outer layer helps keep most of the beets' pigment inside the vegetable.

▶ Cut off the greens, leaving 1 inch of stem attached to the beets, and also leave the root ends attached to the beets. Set the greens aside to drain and dry.

▶ Fill the bottom of a steamer with 2 inches of water. Cut the beets into quarters, but do not peel them. When the water is steaming, place the beets in the steamer basket, cover, and steam for 15 minutes. The beets are done cooking when you can easily insert a fork or the tip of a knife into a beet. Although some of their colorful phytonutrients are lost to the steaming water, there is plenty of color and nutrients still left in the beets. You can save this beet juice for adding to smoothies or just drinking as is.

▶ Set the beets in a bowl until they are cool enough to touch. Remove the skins using a paper towel, or just leave the skins on, as they are quite edible.

▶ Prepare the greens for sautéing by tearing them into 2- to 3-inch pieces. Heat a large skillet over medium heat and pour in a small amount of water to cover the bottom of the pan. Add the olive oil, garlic, and shallot. Cook for about 1 minute and then add the greens. Cook and stir until greens are wilted and tender. Season with salt and pepper, if desired. Serve the greens with the steamed beets and top them with crumbles of goat cheese.

Note: You may also use golden beets for this recipe. With either type of beet, don't peel beets until after they've been cooked, because the beet juice can stain your skin. If you do get some of the beet juice on your skin, you can rub some lemon juice on your hands to remove the stain.

---

*Nutrition per serving: 167 calories; 10 g total fat; 3 g saturated fat; 6 g protein; 15 g carbohydrates; 6 g dietary fiber; 6 mg cholesterol; 277 mg sodium*

## QUICK-BRAISED RED CABBAGE

The cabbage family of vegetables contains more phytochemicals with anticancer properties than any other vegetable family. Here's a tasty way to include cabbage in your meals. This goes nicely with quinoa, rice, and fish.

---

**MAKES 4 SERVINGS (SERVING = 1 CUP)**

3 tablespoons butter, preferably organic

1 medium-size clove garlic, smashed

2 pounds red cabbage heads, cored and cut into 1½-inch pieces

½ cup apple cider

½ teaspoon caraway seeds

½ teaspoon ground allspice

1½ tablespoons raw, unfiltered apple cider vinegar

▶ Heat a large skillet over medium heat. Place the butter and garlic in the pan and cook for 1 minute, stirring frequently. Add the cabbage, apple cider, caraway seeds, and allspice, and cook covered, stirring occasionally, until the cabbage is tender, 15 to 18 minutes.

▶ Add the vinegar and cook uncovered, stirring occasionally, until the liquid has evaporated, 2 to 3 minutes.

*Nutrition per serving: 167 calories; 9 g total fat; 5 g saturated fat; 3 g protein; 18 g carbohydrates; 2 g dietary fiber; 22 mg cholesterol; 110 mg sodium*

## EASY SAUTÉED GREENS

A flavorful twist on a Southern tradition, these greens can accompany any grain, legume, meat, fish, or poultry.

### MAKES 2 SERVINGS (SERVING = 1 CUP)

½ tablespoon extra-virgin coconut oil

2 cloves garlic, minced

1 (1-inch) piece fresh ginger, peeled and minced

1 tablespoon toasted sesame oil

2 (10-ounce) packages baby spinach or collard greens

1 tablespoon wheat-free reduced-sodium tamari sauce

1 tablespoon Toasted Sesame Seeds (page 350)

▶ Heat a large skillet over medium heat and place the coconut oil, garlic, and ginger in the pan. Sauté, stirring, until the garlic softens, about 1 minute. Add the sesame oil and greens, then cook until the leaves soften and heat through, about 1 minute. Add the tamari sauce and sesame seeds; toss to combine. Serve immediately.

*Nutrition per serving: 178 calories; 11 g total fat; 4 g saturated fat; 9 g protein; 12 g carbohydrates; 3 g dietary fiber; 0 mg cholesterol; 561 mg sodium*

## SKILLET-STEAMED LEMON AND BUTTER ASPARAGUS

Asparagus is one of the most alkaline-forming vegetables. This easy recipe ensures that you will eat it often. Asparagus pairs nicely with fish, rice, legumes, and squash.

### MAKES 2 SERVINGS

I to I ½ cups water
I tablespoon butter, preferably organic, plus more for serving (optional)
I pound asparagus
Lemon wedges

▶ Place the water in a large, lidded skillet and bring to a boil. Add the tablespoon of butter to the water and then add the asparagus. Stir to mix the butter evenly with the asparagus, then cover the skillet to allow the asparagus to steam. Cook for 3 to 4 minutes, checking frequently for doneness. The asparagus is done when you can easily pierce it with a fork but it is still firm.

▶ When the asparagus is done, immediately drain it in a colander, then place it on serving plates. Squeeze the lemon juice over the asparagus and add more butter as desired.

Note: Asparagus will continue to cook after it has been removed from the steam, therefore it is better to remove it before it is completely soft.

*Nutrition per serving: 83 calories; 2 g total fat; 1 g saturated fat; 7 g protein; 8.5 g carbohydrates; 2 g dietary fiber; 5 mg cholesterol; 23 mg sodium*

## SESAME SAUTÉED BRUSSELS SPROUTS

You've never had Brussels sprouts like these! The combination of garlic and sesame oil makes a delicious flavor profile.

### MAKES 2 SERVINGS

I pound Brussels sprouts, ends removed, cut in half
4 medium-size shallots, chopped finely
2 cloves garlic, minced
I tablespoon unrefined toasted sesame oil
I tablespoon Toasted Sesame Seeds (page 350)

▶ In a large, flat-bottomed skillet, pour in enough water to cover the bottom of the pan and heat over medium-high heat. Place the Brussels sprouts in the pan, cut side down, in a single layer. Scatter the chopped shallots and garlic over the sprouts.

▶ Allow the sprouts to cook for 3 to 4 minutes, then stir to turn them over, and cook for another 5 minutes or so. You may need to add more water if the pan goes dry.

▶ Continue stirring and then allow to steam-fry until all the liquid has cooked off and the sprouts are tender. Drizzle with the toasted sesame oil and toss. Sprinkle Toasted Sesame Seeds on top. Serve hot.

*Nutrition per serving: 83 calories; 2 g total fat; 1 g saturated fat; 7 g protein; 8.5 g carbohydrates; 2 g dietary fiber; 5 mg cholesterol; 23 mg sodium*

## SAUTÉED GREENS WITH GARLIC AND CANNELLINI BEANS

This is a great way to get your greens! It can be eaten as a main dish or as a side for fish or poultry.

### MAKES 4 SERVINGS

1 tablespoon extra-virgin coconut oil
2 tablespoons extra-virgin olive oil
4 cloves garlic, thinly sliced
¼ teaspoon red pepper flakes (add more for more spice)
1 pound fresh dark greens (kale, collards, etc.), thick stems removed
1 cup fat-free low-sodium chicken broth or vegetable broth
1 (15-ounce) can cannellini beans (white kidney beans), drained and rinsed
1 teaspoon raw, unfiltered apple cider vinegar, or to taste
Sea salt and pepper (optional)

▶ Place a lidded pan over medium heat and add the coconut oil, olive oil, garlic, and red pepper flakes to the pan. Stir until the garlic is just starting to lightly brown. Add the greens by large handfuls and stir just until they begin to wilt.

▶ Add the broth, cover the pan, and simmer on low heat until the greens are just tender, about 10 minutes.

▶ Add the cannellini beans to the pan and simmer uncovered, until the beans are heated through and the liquid is almost gone. Stir in the vinegar.

▶ Season with salt and pepper to taste, and add more vinegar, if desired.

*Nutrition per serving: 242 calories; 11 g total fat; 4 g saturated fat; 10 g protein; 28 g carbohydrates; 6 g dietary fiber; 0 mg cholesterol; 66 mg sodium*

## CREAMY SPAGHETTI SQUASH WITH ASPARAGUS AND ROSEMARY

Another great way to eat asparagus. Try this instead of eating pasta.

### MAKES 4 SERVINGS (SERVING = I CUP)

I small spaghetti squash
I tablespoon extra-virgin olive oil
Pinch of Herbamare
I tablespoon extra-virgin coconut oil
I pound thin asparagus, steamed until tender
4 cloves fresh garlic, minced
I tablespoon chopped fresh rosemary
I cup organic ricotta cheese
I tablespoon raw pine nuts

▶ Preheat the oven to 350°F.
▶ Fill a baking dish with about ½ inch of water. Cut the squash in half and scoop out the seeds. Place it face down in the baking dish. Bake about 30 minutes, or until tender when tested with a fork.
▶ Scrape out the squash with a fork and place the stringy squash in a mixing bowl. Drizzle with the olive oil, and season with Herbamare.
▶ Heat the coconut oil in a large skillet over medium heat. Slice the steamed asparagus into 1-inch pieces and sauté with the garlic and rosemary for I minute. Stir in the ricotta and squash. Sauté until hot and creamy. Top with the pine nuts.

*Nutrition per serving: 355 calories; 15 g total fat; 7 g saturated fat; 14 g protein; 40 g carbohydrates; 8 g dietary fiber; 19 mg cholesterol; 485 mg sodium*

## FARMERS' MARKET COCONUT CURRY

This dish can be made with any seasonal vegetables, and you can even use frozen vegetables to save time on chopping.

### MAKES 4 SERVINGS (SERVING = I CUP)

I tablespoon coconut oil
2 cups chopped onion
2 tablespoons brown rice flour
I cup light coconut milk
2 cups low-sodium vegetable broth
I cup thickly sliced carrot
I cup seeded and thinly sliced red bell pepper (or cut into chunks)

1 cup cubed sweet potato
2 tablespoons fresh mint leaves
½ tablespoon curry powder
1 teaspoon turmeric
1 cup cauliflower florets
1 cup broccoli florets

▶ In a large saucepan, heat the oil over medium heat. Add the onion and cook, stirring often, until soft and translucent, 4 to 5 minutes. Stir in the brown rice flour and cook, stirring, for 1 minute.

▶ Slowly stir in coconut milk, broth, carrots, sweet potato, mint leaves, turmeric, and curry. Cook the mixture until thick and bubbly, 2 to 3 minutes.

▶ Add the cauliflower and broccoli. Lower the heat to medium-low, cover and cook for 5 minutes more. Serve hot over brown rice or quinoa.

*Nutrition per serving: 210 calories; 8 g total fat; 6 g saturated fat; 5 g protein; 30 g carbohydrates; 3 g dietary fiber; 0 mg cholesterol; 125 mg sodium*

## SIMPLY SKINNY BROWN RICE

If you have the time, it's best to soak the rice in the cooking water with a small amount of vinegar overnight. The soaking and the vinegar make the nutrients in grains more digestible and alkaline forming. Use this simple brown rice for adding to salads, as a side dish, or as an ingredient for other recipes. To ensure always having cooked brown rice on hand, you can make a big batch and then freeze individual portions to reheat later.

### MAKES 4 SERVINGS (SERVING = ½ CUP)

2 cups plus two tablespoons water
1 cup brown rice
½ teaspoon raw, unfiltered apple cider vinegar, if soaking overnight before cooking

▶ Combine the water, rice, and vinegar in a saucepan. Bring to a boil over high heat. Boil for 5 minutes, stirring occasionally. Cover and lower the heat to a simmer. Cook slowly until all the water has been absorbed, about 50 minutes. Do not stir the rice after you have lowered the heat and covered the pan.

**NOTE:** A rice cooker or a steamer with a rice-cooking feature is a handy kitchen tool. Follow the manufacturer's instructions for rice cooking times.

*Nutrition per serving: 108 calories; <1 g total fat; 0 g saturated fat; 2 g protein; 23 g carbohydrates; <1 g dietary fiber; 0 mg cholesterol; 1 mg sodium*

## SESAME BROWN RICE

This is a flavorful variation for cooking brown rice.

### MAKES 4 SERVINGS (SERVING = ½ CUP)

I cup brown rice
2 cups water or low-sodium broth
I tablespoon wheat-free reduced-sodium tamari sauce
I tablespoon unrefined toasted sesame oil
2 teaspoons Toasted Sesame Seeds (page 350)
I tablespoon chopped green onions

▶ Combine the rice, water, tamari sauce, and sesame oil in a saucepan. Bring to a boil and boil for 5 minutes. Cover and lower the heat to a simmer. Cook slowly until all the water has been absorbed, about 50 minutes. Do not stir the rice after you have lowered the heat and covered the pan. Fluff with a fork and garnish with the green onions and sesame seeds.

*Nutrition per serving: 146 calories; 4 g total fat; <1 g saturated fat; 3 g protein; 24 g carbohydrates; <1 g dietary fiber; 0 mg cholesterol; 178 mg sodium*

## LEMON-DILL RICE

Jasmine brown rice is an aromatic, light, and fluffy variety of long grain rice. It lends nice flavor to this recipe, although any variety of brown rice can be used.

### MAKES 4 SERVINGS (SERVING = ½ CUP)

I cup jasmine brown rice
1¾ cup water
Zest of I large lemon
Juice of I large lemon
½ teaspoon dried dill
I teaspoon dried parsley, or I tablespoon chopped fresh
2 tablespoons organic butter
½ teaspoon sea salt

▶ Combine all the ingredients in a saucepan. Bring to a boil and boil for 5 minutes. Stir to mix evenly. Cover and lower the heat to a simmer. Cook slowly until all the water has been absorbed, about 50 minutes. Do not stir the rice after you have lowered the heat and covered the pan. Fluff with a fork and serve.

*Nutrition per serving: 146 calories; 4 g total fat; <1 g saturated fat; 3 g protein; 24 g carbohydrates; <1 g dietary fiber; 0 mg cholesterol; 178 mg sodium*

## BASIC QUINOA

From this basic recipe of cooked quinoa, you can use it to make salads, add to other dishes, stuff bell peppers, or toss with vegetables. A light and fluffy grain, quinoa resembles couscous and can be eaten in the same way.

### MAKES 5 SERVINGS (SERVING = ½ CUP)

I cup quinoa, soaked and rinsed (see notes)
2 cups water

▶ For perfectly cooked quinoa, simply add one part quinoa to two parts water or clear broth in a saucepan. After the mixture is brought to a boil, lower the heat to a simmer and cover the pan.

▶ One cup of quinoa cooked using this method usually takes 15 to 20 minutes to prepare, which is less time than brown rice. The grains become translucent at the end of the cooking process, and the white germ partially detaches from the main body of the grain, appearing like a white spiral tail.

NOTES: One cup of dry quinoa cooked in 2 cups of liquid will typically yield 2½ cups of cooked quinoa.

Soaking quinoa prior to cooking helps to loosen up the outer coating of saponin, which can give a bitter taste if not removed. A typical soaking time is 30 minutes or more, but if you don't have that long, you can soak it for 5 minutes in hot water prior to cooking. After soaking, strain off the soaking water by pouring the quinoa into a fine-mesh sieve and rinsing it under running water.

To obtain a nuttier flavor, you can dry toast the quinoa for 5 minutes in a skillet before adding the water for cooking.

*Nutrition per serving: 65 calories; 1 g total fat; 0 g saturated fat; 2 g protein; 12 g carbohydrates; 1 g dietary fiber; 0 mg cholesterol; 4 mg sodium*

## MINTY QUINOA

Here's a great way to use your cooked quinoa!

### MAKES 4 SERVINGS (SERVING = ½ CUP)

2 cups cooked quinoa, warm or cold
2 teaspoons wheat-free reduced-sodium tamari sauce
⅓ cup pine nuts
2½ tablespoons chopped fresh mint leaves
½ cup frozen peas, thawed

▶ Place the quinoa in a bowl. Sprinkle with tamari sauce, pine nuts, mint, and peas. Mix and serve.

*Nutrition per serving: 200 calories; 8 g total fat; 1 g saturated fat; 6 g protein; 25 g carbohydrates; 3 g dietary fiber; 0 mg cholesterol; 128 mg sodium*

## QUINOA TABBOULEH

This is a gluten-free version of the favorite bulgur-based salad. Makes a great snack or lunchbox item.

### MAKES 6 SERVINGS (SERVING = ½ CUP)

1 cup cooked quinoa, cold or room temperature
⅓ cup chopped fresh parsley
2 tablespoons chopped fresh mint leaves
2 plum tomatoes, seeded and chopped very finely
½ red bell pepper, seeded and chopped very finely
½ teaspoon Herbamare or sea salt
2 tablespoons extra-virgin olive oil
2 tablespoons freshly squeezed lemon juice

▶ Place all the ingredients in a bowl and toss to mix well. Enjoy immediately or place in the refrigerator for 1 hour or more before eating, to let the flavors meld.

*Nutrition per serving: 159 calories; 6 g total fat; 0 g saturated fat; 4 g protein; 22 g carbohydrates; 2 g dietary fiber; 0 mg cholesterol; 228 mg sodium*

# Skinny Soups, Wraps, Breads, and Meatless Main Dishes

## SKINNY NO-HAM SPLIT PEA SOUP

My vegetarian clients rave about this soup because it's loaded with flavor without the ham.

### MAKES 8 SERVINGS (SERVING = 1 CUP)

8 cups water
1 pound dried green split peas, sorted and rinsed
3 medium-size carrots, sliced thickly (1½ cups)
2 medium-size stalks celery, chopped (1 cup)
1 medium-size onion, chopped (½ cup)

2 cloves fresh garlic, minced
2 bay leaves
1 teaspoon sea salt
1 teaspoon dried thyme
1 teaspoon dried basil
1 teaspoon dried oregano
1 teaspoon dried rosemary
¼ teaspoon black pepper

▶ Mix all the ingredients in a large stockpot and bring to a boil. Lower the heat to medium and simmer until done, about 1½ hours. Stir and add more water as needed.

*Nutrition per serving: 232 calories; <1 g total fat; 0 g saturated fat; 15 g protein; 41 g carbohydrates; 3 g dietary fiber; 0 mg cholesterol; 309 mg sodium*

## CARROT-GINGER SOUP

Carrots and ginger are highly alkaline forming as well as liver cleansing. This soup can be eaten hot or cold.

### MAKES 8 SERVINGS (SERVING = ½ CUP)

2 tablespoons coconut oil
2 small yellow onions, peeled and diced
2 to 3 cloves garlic, crushed
2 pounds carrots, peeled and diced (16 medium-size)
3 tablespoons chopped green onions
1 tablespoon minced fresh ginger
3 cups fat-free chicken or vegetable broth
½ cup coconut milk
Sea salt and toasted crushed peppercorns

▶ Heat the oil over medium heat in a stockpot. Sauté the onions, garlic, carrots, green onions, and ginger over medium heat for about 10 minutes. Add the broth, bring to boil, and simmer for 5 minutes. Transfer the soup in batches to a food processor and puree until smooth. Pour it back into the stockpot and stir in the coconut milk. Bring to a slow simmer but do not boil. Season to taste with salt and crushed peppercorns.
▶ Remove from the heat and serve.

*Nutrition per serving: 174 calories; 9 g total fat; 6 g saturated fat; 3 g protein; 20 g carbohydrates; 2 g dietary fiber; 0 mg cholesterol; 222 mg sodium*

# CREAMY PUMPKIN SOUP

This warming soup is creamy, sweet, and filling. Pumpkin soup is traditionally made from fresh pie pumpkin. You can use canned pumpkin puree if fresh pumpkin is not available. Using fresh pumpkin is preferred for the antioxidant value. You can use the flavorful pumpkin seeds as a garnish or snack, and a pumpkin shell makes a great tureen for serving the soup.

### MAKES 6 SERVINGS (SERVING = 1 CUP)

1 cup chopped yellow onion
2 tablespoons organic butter
4 cups fat-free low-sodium chicken broth or vegetable broth
1 pound fresh pie pumpkin, peeled and cubed, or 1 (15-ounce)
    can pure pumpkin puree
1 cup light coconut milk
½ teaspoon sea salt
⅛ teaspoon ground black pepper
¼ teaspoon ground cinnamon
½ teaspoon pumpkin pie spice (see note, page 337)
1 tablespoon raw organic whole cane sugar or Sucanat
½ teaspoon ground ginger
2 tablespoons arrowroot powder
¼ cup water
¼ cup chopped fresh parsley, for garnish

▶ Sauté the onion in the butter until tender. If using fresh cubed pumpkin, add the broth and pumpkin, stir and bring to a boil. Lower the heat to a simmer and cook for about 25 minutes, or until the pumpkin is tender. Remove from the heat.

▶ If using canned pumpkin, add the broth and pumpkin puree to the sautéed onion and bring to a simmer. Remove from the heat.

▶ Add the coconut milk, sea salt, pepper, cinnamon, pumpkin pie spice, sugar, and ginger to the soup. Transfer the soup to a food processor or a blender and blend until it is smooth. Transfer the blended soup back to the pan and bring it to a boil. Lower the heat, cover the pan, and let the pumpkin soup simmer for no longer than 10 minutes.

▶ While the soup is simmering, place the arrowroot into a small bowl and add the water. Stir to dissolve the arrowroot. Add the arrowroot mixture to the soup and stir until the soup thickens. Remove from the heat.

▶ Pour the soup into your pumpkin tureen or just ladle into soup bowls. Garnish with the chopped parsley.

*Nutrition per serving: 126 calories; 6 g total fat; 4 g saturated fat; 2 g protein; 14 g carbohydrates; 1.5 g dietary fiber; 10 mg cholesterol; 346 mg sodium*

## TOO-EASY CHICKEN AND RICE SOUP

As long as you have some cooked brown rice and chicken on hand, this is the perfect soup for those days when you don't have time to cook. Kids love this simple classic.

### MAKES 4 SERVINGS (SERVING = 1 CUP)

4 cups low-sodium chicken broth
1 large carrot, diced
1 large celery stalk, diced
4 ounces cooked chicken, shredded or cut into chunks
1 cup cooked brown rice

▶ Heat the broth to a boil in a saucepan. Add the carrot and celery. Lower the heat and simmer until the vegetables are soft. Add the chicken and rice and simmer a few more minutes. Serve.

*Nutrition per serving: 120 calories; 2 g total fat; 0 g saturated fat; 12 g protein; 14 g carbohydrates; <1 g dietary fiber; 24 mg cholesterol; 138 mg sodium*

## AVOCADO–BLACK BEAN VEGGIE WRAP

The black beans and the tortilla in this recipe form a complete vegetarian protein. The avocado and veggies bump the fiber of this little wrap up to a whopping 13 grams (nearly half your daily requirement)!

### MAKES 4 SERVINGS (SERVING = 1 WRAP)

1 ripe large avocado, pitted and peeled
1½ cups cooked black beans (about 1 [15-ounce] can), drained, rinsed, and patted dry
½ cup fresh salsa or diced tomatoes
4 (8-inch) Dee's Naturals whole wheat flour tortillas (or use sprouted-grain or gluten-free tortillas)
2 cups spring mix or shredded dark green lettuce
1 cup shredded red cabbage
2 carrots, shredded
½ cup diced cucumber
2 tablespoons minced red onion
½ cup chopped fresh cilantro

▶ Place the avocado flesh in a large bowl. Add the black beans and mash with a potato masher or your hands, until it sticks together (you will still have some whole beans in the mixture). Add the salsa and stir to mix.

▸ Warm the tortillas by placing them one at a time on a griddle or skillet over medium-high heat. Heat one side for 30 to 60 seconds, or until the tortilla starts to puff up. Flip the tortilla and heat the other side for about 30 seconds. Transfer to a plate. Repeat with remaining tortillas.

▸ To assemble the wraps, divide the avocado mixture among the four tortillas and top with equal amounts of the veggies. Roll up and then cut the wraps in half to serve.

*Nutrition per serving: 310 calories; 7.5 g total fat; 1.6 g saturated fat; 13 g protein; 52 g carbohydrates; 13 g dietary fiber; 0 mg cholesterol; 168 mg sodium*

## CHEDDAR SWEET POTATO WRAPS

These wraps are a staple in our house. Half of a wrap is very filling and usually enough for one meal. The wraps can be cut in half, wrapped individually, and frozen for re-heating later.

### MAKES 12 SERVINGS (SERVING = ½ WRAP)

1½ cups baked sweet potatoes (about 1 pound)
1 tablespoon extra-virgin coconut oil
½ yellow onion, chopped
½ cup seeded and diced red bell pepper
2 cloves garlic, minced
2 (15-ounce) cans red kidney beans (preferably organic), drained and rinsed
1 cup water
1½ tablespoons chili powder
1 teaspoon ground cumin
2 teaspoons prepared yellow mustard
Pinch of cayenne, or to taste
1½ tablespoons wheat-free reduced-sodium tamari sauce
6 (8-inch) Dee's Naturals whole wheat flour tortillas (or sprouted-grain tortillas)
4 ounces raw organic Cheddar cheese (or other cheese), shredded
    (about 1 cup)

▸ Cut open the baked sweet potatoes and scrape out the inner flesh into a bowl. Discard the peels. Mash the potatoes with a potato masher. They can still be slightly lumpy. Set aside.

▸ Heat the coconut oil in a large skillet over medium heat. Add the onion and bell pepper and sauté until soft. Add the garlic and sauté for 1 minute more. Stir in the kidney beans, and mash them with a masher. Gradually stir in the water, and heat until warm. Stir in the chili powder, cumin, mustard, cayenne, and tamari sauce.

Add the mashed sweet potatoes and stir. Bring to a low simmer, just enough to heat the sweet potatoes, then remove from the heat.

▶ Warm the tortillas by placing them one at a time in a dry skillet or griddle over medium heat. Heat for 15 to 20 seconds on each side, or until warm to the touch. Transfer the tortilla to a flat surface, such as a cutting board or a plate. Add one-sixth of the sweet potato mixture down the center of the tortilla. Top each with one-sixth of the cheese. Roll up the tortilla burrito style, cut in half, and serve. Repeat with remaining tortillas. These are best accompanied with a large salad of leafy greens.

*Nutrition per serving: 206 calories; 6 g total fat; 3 g saturated fat; 10 g protein; 28 g carbohydrates; 6 g dietary fiber; 10 mg cholesterol; 232 mg sodium*

## SEASONED CREAMY CHEESE AND CHICKEN PINWHEELS

Neufchâtel is softer than regular cream cheese and has 33 percent less fat. Use the organic version if possible, which is the healthiest option. The seasoning in this recipe is reminiscent of dry ranch dressing mixes that come in packets, sans the MSG. You can replace the poultry with hummus for a vegetarian version. This is a great lunchbox item for kids and adults alike.

### MAKES 6 SERVINGS (SERVING = 1 WRAP, CUT INTO PINWHEELS)

1 (8-ounce) package Neufchâtel, preferably organic
1 teaspoon dried parsley, or 1 tablespoon chopped fresh
1 teaspoon dried chives, or 1 tablespoon chopped fresh
¼ teaspoon dried dill
½ teaspoon garlic powder
¼ teaspoon onion powder
⅛ teaspoon dried thyme
¼ teaspoon ground black pepper
6 (8-inch) Dee's Naturals whole wheat flour tortillas (or sprouted-grain or gluten-free tortillas)
12 ounces thinly sliced or shredded cooked chicken or turkey (or nitrate-free sliced deli turkey), or 1½ cups hummus
½ sweet red bell pepper, sliced lengthwise very thinly
1 cup baby spinach leaves, washed and dried

▶ Using a rubber spatula, combine the cheese, parsley, chives, dill, garlic powder, onion powder, thyme, and pepper in a bowl. Stir until creamy and well mixed.

▶ Warm the tortillas if desired in a dry skillet over medium heat, or just use them cold. Spread each tortilla with a thin layer (about 2 tablespoons) of the cream cheese mixture. Place 2 ounces of the chicken over two-thirds of a tortilla. If using hummus, place ¼ cup of hummus down the center of each tortilla. Place three or four red bell pepper strips along one edge. Top with the spinach. Roll the tortillas as tightly as possible. Place seam side down on a cutting board and slice into 1-inch pieces.

**NOTE:** To pack for kids' lunches, place the pinwheels in a container as if they are sushi. Add some baby carrots or other fun veggies for munching.

---

*Nutrition per serving (with poultry): 286 calories; 11 g total fat; 5g saturated fat; 22 g protein; 26 g carbohydrates; 5 g dietary fiber; 53 mg cholesterol; 268 mg sodium*

---

*Nutrition per serving (with hummus): 252 calories; 11 g total fat; 5g saturated fat; 10 g protein; 28 g carbohydrates; 6 g dietary fiber; 23 mg cholesterol; 281 mg sodium*

---

# FOUR-BEAN CHILI FOR THE STOVE TOP OR SLOW COOKER

Beans are one of the most nutritious foods we can eat. They're high in fiber and a rich source of vegetarian protein.

### MAKES 12 SERVINGS (SERVING = 1 CUP)

1 tablespoon extra-virgin coconut oil
1 onion, chopped
1 red bell pepper, seeded and chopped
1 green bell pepper, seeded and chopped
5 cloves garlic, minced
1 cup chopped carrot
1 (28-ounce) can diced tomatoes, including liquid
1 (14-ounce) can reduced-sodium tomato sauce
1 (6-ounce) can tomato paste
2 cups water
3 tablespoons chili powder
1 teaspoon dried oregano
2 teaspoons ground cumin
1 (15-ounce) can pinto beans, drained and rinsed
1 (15-ounce) can red kidney beans, drained and rinsed
1 (15-ounce) can black beans, drained and rinsed
1 (15-ounce) can white beans, drained and rinsed

▶ Place the oil, onion, bell peppers, and garlic in a large stockpot and cook over medium heat until the onion is translucent. Add the carrot, tomatoes with liquid, tomato sauce, tomato paste, and water. Increase the heat to medium-high and cook until the mixture starts to boil. Add the chili powder, oregano, cumin, and beans. Lower the heat to medium and simmer for 45 minutes, stirring occasionally.

▶ Alternatively, after sautéing the onion, garlic, and peppers, put all of the ingredients into a slow cooker and cook on LOW for 8 hours.

▶ Refrigerate the leftover chili to eat the next day. It tastes even better when the spices have released their flavor overnight!

▶ Serve with a fresh green salad.

*Nutrition per serving: 180 calories; 2 g total fat; 1 g saturated fat; 9 g protein; 34 g carbohydrates; 7 g dietary fiber; 0 mg cholesterol; 249 mg sodium*

## SMOKY BLACK BEAN AND AVOCADO PITAS

Putting veggies into pitas is the best way to eat a salad!

### MAKES 4 SERVINGS (SERVING = 1 WHOLE PITA)

1 tablespoon extra-virgin olive oil
1 small yellow onion, diced (about 1 cup)
2 cloves garlic, minced
2 (15-ounce) cans black beans, drained and rinsed
2 teaspoons smoked paprika
½ teaspoon dried oregano
4 sprouted-grain or whole wheat pita breads
1 cup shredded carrot
1 avocado, pitted, peeled, and sliced
2 cups spring mix or other fresh raw greens

▶ Heat the oil in a skillet over medium heat. Add the onion and garlic and cook for 5 minutes, or until soft. Add the beans, paprika, and oregano. Lower the heat to medium-low and cook for 10 minutes. Remove from the heat and mash the beans with a masher or the back of a spoon. There can still be some whole beans.

▶ Cut the pitas in half and split open. Divide the bean mixture among the pita halves. Add the carrot, avocado slices, and spring mix. Enjoy immediately or pack for the lunchbox.

*Nutrition per serving: 349 calories; 10 g total fat; 1g saturated fat; 16 g protein; 53 g carbohydrates; 13 g dietary fiber; 0 mg cholesterol; 133 mg sodium*

## HOMEMADE SUNSHINE BURGERS

Not exactly the same as the wonderful commercially available Sunshine Burgers, but they're pretty darn good in their own right. Eat these on salads, with cooked veggies, or on a sprouted grain bun with all the fixings.

### MAKES 5 SERVINGS

1 cup raw sunflower seeds, ground in a coffee grinder, spice mill, or Vitamix
2 tablespoons ground flaxseeds
1 cup cooked brown rice
½ teaspoon garlic powder
½ teaspoon onion powder
1 teaspoon Herbamare
¼ cup water
⅔ cup finely chopped or grated carrot
⅔ cup finely chopped celery
¼ cup chopped fresh parsley
Coconut oil, for brushing pan

▶ Preheat the oven to 375°F.
▶ Place the ground sunflower seeds, ground flaxseeds, cooked rice, garlic powder, onion powder, Herbamare, and water in the bowl of a food processor fitted with an S blade. Process until the mixture is smooth (it can still have chunks of brown rice in it).
▶ Add the carrots, celery, and parsley, and pulse until the mixture is well blended, but chunks of carrot and celery should still be visible. If the texture is too dry and thick, add a bit more water to moisten it. It should be moist enough to form into patties.
▶ Divide the mixture into five balls of equal size, then shape them into patties. Place them on a parchment-lined baking sheet brushed with coconut oil. Bake for about 35 minutes, flipping halfway through, until both sides are golden brown and the patties are firm. These patties can be frozen for up to 1 month.

*Nutrition per serving: 250 calories; 17 g total fat; 2 g saturated fat; 7 g protein; 17 g carbohydrates; 2 g dietary fiber; 0 mg cholesterol; 544 mg sodium*

# CREAMY BUTTERNUT MAC AND CHEESE

Everyone's favorite comfort food gets a bit of a healthy makeover . . . well almost! This is definitely not an everyday food, but adding a low-calorie vegetable to take the place of some of the cheese makes this a healthier indulgence. Kids and grown-ups love this recipe, but I suggest pairing it with lots of raw veggies to help balance the meal.

### MAKES 8 SERVINGS (SERVING = 1 CUP)

8 ounces brown rice elbow macaroni
1½ tablespoons organic butter
1 small onion, chopped
1½ tablespoons brown rice flour
1 cup light coconut milk
2 cups butternut puree (canned or frozen; see note)
12 ounces raw Cheddar cheese, shredded
⅛ teaspoon grated nutmeg
⅛ teaspoon white pepper
1 teaspoon prepared yellow mustard

► Cook the macaroni according to the package directions. Drain in a colander.
► To make the cheese sauce, heat the butter on medium heat in a large stockpot. Add the onion and sauté until the onion is translucent. Add the flour, and cook, stirring constantly, until the mixture resembles a thick paste but has not browned, 1 to 2 minutes.
► Add the coconut milk and cook, stirring until the mixture begins to thicken, 3 to 4 minutes. Add the butternut puree, cheese, seasonings, and mustard, and stir until the cheese is melted and the sauce is smooth. Stir in the macaroni and cook just long enough for the whole mixture to warm. Remove from the heat and serve.

NOTE: Some grocery stores carry small bags of raw, cubed butternut squash ready for steaming, which would be best for this recipe. You may also bake butternut squash and use some of it for this recipe.

*Nutrition per serving: 350 calories; 18 g total fat; 12 g saturated fat; 14 g protein; 32 g carbohydrates; 2 g dietary fiber; 51 mg cholesterol; 316 mg sodium*

## SWEET POTATO AND SPINACH ENCHILADAS

These enchiladas are an absolute favorite. Another way to eat your dark green leafies!

---
### MAKES 10 SERVINGS (SERVING = 1 ENCHILADA)
---

1 ½ pounds baked sweet potato
1 tablespoon coconut oil
1 small onion, chopped
4 cloves garlic, minced
1 (10 ounce) package frozen spinach, thawed and drained
2 tablespoons Taco Seasoning Mix (page 349)
10 stone-ground corn tortillas
2½ cups Green Enchilada Sauce (page 348)
1 cup shredded raw Jack cheese

► Preheat the oven to 350°F.
► Place the baked sweet potato flesh in a large bowl and mash with a spoon (discard the skins). Set aside.
► Heat the oil in a skillet over medium heat. Add the onion and garlic; cook for a few minutes until fragrant but not brown. Stir in the spinach and taco seasoning, and cook for about 5 more minutes. Remove from the heat and add to the sweet potatoes in the bowl. Mix well.
► Warm the enchilada sauce in a saucepan over medium heat until it bubbles, then lower the heat to low.
► Cover the bottom of a 9-inch by 13-inch baking dish with a thin layer of the enchilada sauce. Set aside.
► Using tongs or your fingers, dip one tortilla into the remaining hot enchilada sauce, making sure it gets fully coated and flexible, about 15 seconds, then place the sauce-covered tortilla on a plate.
► Spoon about ⅓ cup of the spinach mixture onto the center of the tortilla. Roll up and place seam side down in the baking dish. Repeat with remaining tortillas.
► When all enchiladas are in the baking dish, pour the remaining enchilada sauce over the top, and sprinkle with the cheese.
► Bake for 15 to 20 minutes, until the sauce is bubbling and the cheese is melted.

---

*Nutrition per serving: 216 calories; 7 g total fat; 3 g saturated fat; 6 g protein; 32 g carbohydrates; 3 g dietary fiber; 10 mg cholesterol; 209 mg sodium*

# Meats, Poultry, Fish, and Main Dishes 🧅

## EXTREMELY EASY OVEN-BAKED SALMON

This is the most amazing and easy way to cook salmon. The low temperature for cooking this fish keeps the olive oil safe, and also produces a wonderfully moist and tender fish. You can use leftover salmon for adding to salads, or for making some of the other salmon recipes in this book.

### MAKES 4 SERVINGS (SERVING = 4 OUNCES COOKED SALMON)

1 wild Alaskan salmon fillet (about 1 pound)
2 to 4 tablespoons fresh dill, thyme, or parsley
    (or any herbs you like; see note)
½ teaspoon sea salt
1 teaspoon extra-virgin olive oil

► Preheat the oven to 200°F (not a typo).
► Rub the olive oil onto an ovenproof serving platter or large plate. If the fillet is skinned, sprinkle a small amount of sea salt on both sides. If the skin is still on the fillet, no salt is needed. Place the fillet skin side down on the platter. Run your oily hand over the top of the salmon to help the herbs stick. Sprinkle the herbs on top of the salmon and pat down.
► Bake for 40 to 45 minutes, until the salmon flakes easily with a fork. It will be very moist and tender. Serve with Skillet-Steamed Lemon and Butter Asparagus (page 356) and Lemon-Dill Rice (page 360).

**NOTE:** You may also used dried herbs if you don't have any fresh; just use less of them.

*Nutrition per serving: 177 calories; 9 g total fat; 2 g saturated fat; 23 g protein; 0 g carbohydrates; 0 g dietary fiber; 74 mg cholesterol; 56 mg sodium*

## BASIC BAKED CHICKEN OR TURKEY BREASTS

Baking up a batch of chicken or turkey parts ensures that you'll have lean healthy protein for meals during the week. Add to salads, sandwiches, or soups, or wrap in lettuce leaves for a healthy snack.

### MAKES 5 SERVINGS (SERVING = 3 OUNCES COOKED CHICKEN)

1 pound boneless and skinless chicken or turkey breast
1 teaspoon Herbamare or sea salt
2 teaspoons garlic powder
½ teaspoon pepper
1 tablespoon dried or fresh chopped parsley

▶ Preheat the oven to 350°F.
▶ Rinse the poultry breasts and place them in a glass baking dish. Sprinkle evenly on both sides with the seasonings.
▶ To prevent the poultry from drying out while baking, fill the baking dish a quarter of the way full with water. Bake the poultry for 20 minutes, then turn each piece over and bake for 10 to 20 more minutes, or until no longer pink in the center (test with a fork). When done, remove from the oven and remove from the baking dish so that the poultry won't continue to cook in the hot water. Serve immediately or refrigerate to use for other meals during the week.

NOTE: You can bake other poultry parts, such as legs or thighs, in the same way, and you can also cook these in a slow cooker for 6 to 8 hours.

*Nutrition per serving: 118 calories; 3 g total fat; <1 g saturated fat; 23 g protein; 0 g carbohydrates; 0 g dietary fiber; 62 mg cholesterol; 577 mg sodium*

## DIJON-GARLIC CHICKEN

The tangy sauce on this chicken excites the taste buds in a natural way. You can also use the sauce as a marinade for tofu or tempeh. Serve with brown rice and steamed vegetables.

### MAKES 4 SERVINGS (SERVING = 3 OUNCES COOKED CHICKEN)

3 to 4 boneless, skinless chicken breasts (12 to 16 ounces)
4 cloves garlic, minced
¼ cup Dijon mustard
¼ cup fat-free low-sodium chicken broth
2 tablespoons extra-virgin olive oil
2 tablespoons wheat-free reduced-sodium tamari sauce
Pinch of cayenne
Pinch of Italian seasoning
Sea salt and pepper

▶ Place the chicken in a single layer in a baking dish. Whisk together all of the other ingredients in a bowl, then pour the mixture over the chicken. Use your hands or a spoon to thoroughly coat all sides of the chicken with the sauce. Cover the dish with plastic wrap and marinate the chicken in the refrigerator for 2 hours or overnight.

▶ When ready to bake the chicken, preheat the oven to 350°F. Remove the baking dish from the refrigerator and let it sit out while the oven comes to temperature.

▶ When the oven is ready, place the chicken in the oven and bake for 30 to 40 minutes, or until the juices run clear. Serve hot.

---

*Nutrition per serving: 197 calories; 10 g total fat; 2 g saturated fat; 23 g protein; 3 g carbohydrates; 0 g dietary fiber; 58 mg cholesterol; 771 mg sodium*

## GRASS-FED BEEF AND VEGETABLE STEW FOR THE SLOW COOKER

The slow cooker is an excellent time-saving kitchen tool for preparing meals with little effort. This delicious stew is wonderful for lunch or dinner.

---
**MAKES 10 SERVINGS (SERVING = 3 OUNCES BEEF PLUS VEGETABLES)**

2 pounds organic grass-fed beef stew meat
2 medium-size russet potatoes, cut into chunks
5 medium-size carrots, cut into thick slices
1 large onion, chopped
2 cloves garlic, minced
3 medium-size celery stalks, chopped
1 (8-ounce) can tomato sauce
1 (28-ounce) can diced tomatoes
2 tablespoons pure maple syrup
1 bay leaf
1 teaspoon dried oregano
1 teaspoon dried basil
1 teaspoon dried parsley
Sea salt and ground black pepper
3 tablespoons arrowroot powder
3 tablespoons water

▶ Put all the ingredients except the arrowroot and water in a slow cooker; mix thoroughly. Cover and cook on the LOW setting for 12 hours or on the HIGH setting for 5 to 6 hours.

▶ After the stew has cooked, mix the arrowroot and water in a small bowl and stir to dissolve the arrowroot. Add the arrowroot mixture to the slow cooker and stir until the stew begins to thicken, 1 to 2 minutes. Once the stew has thickened, it is ready to serve. Leftovers can be frozen.

**NOTE:** If you'd like to cook this stew on the stove top, you should first brown the beef in the stockpot you will be using, with a small amount of water and coconut oil. Then add all the ingredients, except the arrowroot and water, to the stockpot and bring to a boil. Lower the heat to low, cover, and simmer gently, stirring occasionally, for 1½ hours. Uncover the pot and continue simmering for up to 30 minutes more, until the meat is nicely tender but still holds its shape. Add the arrowroot mixture to the stew and stir until the stew begins to thicken, then turn off the heat.

*Nutrition per serving: 271 calories; 3.5 g total fat; 1 g saturated fat; 31 g protein; 30 g carbohydrates; 3 g dietary fiber; 69 mg cholesterol; 95 mg sodium*

## CREAMY BEEF AND CARROT–TOPPED BAKED POTATOES

Baked potatoes take about an hour or more to cook, so plan your time for this recipe accordingly. The potatoes may be baked ahead of time and then reheated just before the meat mixture is ready. Serve this dish with some steamed broccoli, green beans, or a nice green salad.

### MAKES 5 SERVINGS (SERVING = 1 SMALL POTATO, 3 OUNCES BEEF)

5 small russet potatoes (about 6 ounces each)
Small amount of water, for the pan
1 tablespoon extra-virgin olive oil
2 large carrots, sliced
½ cup chopped onion
1 pound organic grass-fed ground beef
¼ cup brown rice flour
¼ teaspoon sea salt
¼ teaspoon ground pepper
2 cups organic low-sodium beef broth
1 teaspoon natural Worcestershire sauce (such as Annie's Organic)

► Preheat the oven to 350°F.
► Wash the potatoes well under cool running water. Use a brush or scrubber to remove any dirt. Rinse, drain, and pat dry. Lift any small bruises or eyes from the potatoes with the pointed end of a vegetable peeler. Remove any dark or black areas.
► Pierce the skin a few times with a fork to allow steam to escape while baking. Place the potatoes directly on the center rack of the oven, and place a large baking sheet on the rack just underneath the potatoes to catch any drippings. The cooking time will vary from 1 hour and up, depending on the size and quantity of the potatoes

you bake. To test for doneness, the skin should be puffed up and golden brown, and the potatoes should squish easily and be very soft on the inside.

▶ While potatoes are baking, heat a skillet over medium heat. Pour in enough water to cover the bottom of the skillet, and then add the olive oil. Add the carrots and onion. Cook, stirring, until tender. Add the beef, salt, and pepper. Cook until the meat is browned, stirring occasionally. Drain the meat mixture in a colander and return it to the skillet. Sprinkle the brown rice flour over the meat mixture and stir until well blended. It will start to thicken.

▶ Add the broth and Worcestershire sauce to the meat mixture and stir until thickened. Bring to a simmer, then turn off heat.

▶ Place the baked potatoes on serving plate. Split. Push the ends toward the center to open. Spoon about ½ cup of the meat mixture into each potato.

*Nutrition per serving: 371 calories; 9 g total fat; 3 g saturated fat; 30 g protein; 41 g carbohydrates; 4 g dietary fiber; 69 mg cholesterol; 293 mg sodium*

## WILD ALASKAN SALMON CROQUETTES

My young clients, kids between the ages of three and twelve, *love* these croquettes. Make small slider-size croquettes for the kids, and larger patties for the grown-ups. They last for several days in the refrigerator and can be eaten cold or reheated. Serve with baked sweet potatoes and vegetables, or place them on whole-grain buns and eat like a sandwich. They can also be added to salads.

### MAKES 4 SERVINGS (SERVING = I [3-INCH-DIAMETER] PATTY

1 ½ pounds baked wild salmon fillet (or three 6-ounce cans wild Alaskan salmon, drained)
2 teaspoons dried dill
½ teaspoon Herbamare or sea salt
2 green onions, chopped
2 tablespoons freshly squeezed lemon juice
¼ cup raw oat bran
I egg, preferably organic
3 tablespoons safflower mayonnaise
I teaspoon Dijon mustard
Coconut oil, for the pan (optional)

▶ Preheat the oven to 350°F.

▶ Place the salmon in a large bowl and flake it with a fork. Add the dill, Herbamare, green onions, lemon juice, and oat bran. Stir with the fork to combine. Add the egg, mayonnaise, and mustard. Mix well with a large spoon or rubber scraper.

▶ Shape the mixture into patties. Line a baking sheet with parchment paper or coat with coconut oil to prevent the patties from sticking. Place the salmon croquettes on the baking sheet. Bake for 10 minutes, flip over, then bake for another 10 minutes. Remove from the oven and serve.

---

*Nutrition per serving: 219 calories; 11 g total fat; 2 g saturated fat; 23 g protein; 9 g carbohydrates; 1 g dietary fiber; 127 mg cholesterol; 360 mg sodium*

## TURKEY MEATLOAF OR MEATBALLS

This is Michael's favorite comfort food; we make it several times a month. This recipe works for grass-fed ground beef as well, and can also be used to make meatballs.

---

### MAKES 6 SERVINGS (SERVING = 5 OUNCES MEAT LOAF)

1½ pounds hormone-free ground turkey
1 cup chopped onion
3 cloves garlic, minced
½ cup seeded and chopped red bell pepper
1 large egg
½ cup raw oat bran
1 teaspoon dried basil, or 1 tablespoon chopped fresh
1 teaspoon dried parsley, or 1 tablespoon chopped fresh
1 teaspoon dried oregano, or 1 tablespoon chopped fresh
1 teaspoon sea salt
½ teaspoon black pepper
1 (8-ounce) can tomato sauce
Coconut oil, for coating the pan

▶ Heat oven to 350°F.
▶ In a large bowl, combine all the ingredients, except the coconut oil, and mix well with a wooden spoon. Form into a loaf and place in a glass baking dish or loaf pan coated with coconut oil. Bake for 45 to 50 minutes, or until no longer pink in center. Let stand at room temperature for 5 minutes before slicing.

---

*Nutrition per serving: 224 calories; 12 g total fat; 2.5 g saturated fat; 21 g protein; 13 g carbohydrates; 2 g dietary fiber; 146 mg cholesterol; 324 mg sodium*

# SKINNY SWEET-AND-SOUR MEATBALLS

The secret ingredient in these meatballs, which are always a hit with kids and grown-ups, is the apricot jam. They make great party appetizers, but are also a great meal. Try the sauce on chicken, tempeh, and tofu as well.

---

**MAKES 8 SERVINGS (SERVING = ¼ CUP SAUCE PLUS 3 OUNCES COOKED MEATBALLS)**

*Meatballs:*

1 ½ pounds hormone-free ground turkey
1 teaspoon garlic powder
1 teaspoon dried basil
1 teaspoon dried parsley
1 teaspoon dried oregano
1 teaspoon sea salt
¼ teaspoon pepper
2 green onions, white and green parts, chopped
1 egg
½ cup oat bran

*Sauce:*

¼ cup brown rice vinegar
¾ cup 100% fruit apricot jam
1 cup bottled unsweetened ketchup plus ¼ teaspoon liquid stevia
1 teaspoon dried oregano
¼ cup unrefined expeller-pressed peanut oil
¼ cup diced onion
Small amount of water, for sautéing the onion

▶ Preheat the oven to 350°F.

▶ Combine all the meatball ingredients in a large bowl and mix together. Form the mixture into balls no greater than 1 level tablespoon in size. Place the meatballs on a parchment-lined baking sheet. Bake for 20 minutes. Remove from the oven.

▶ While the meatballs are baking, make the sauce. In a large bowl, whisk together the vinegar, apricot jam, ketchup, oregano, and all but 1 tablespoon of the peanut oil. Set aside.

▶ Heat a stockpot over medium heat, and pour in a small amount of water and the remaining tablespoon of peanut oil. Add the onion and sauté until it is translucent. Add the remaining sauce ingredients. Cook until bubbling, then lower the heat and simmer until thick, stirring occasionally, about 5 minutes. Add the meatballs to the sauce and stir to coat.

▶ Serve hot. They go well with brown rice and steamed broccoli.

---

*Nutrition per serving: 267 calories; 13 g total fat; 2 g saturated fat; 19 g protein; 19 g carbohydrates; 1 g dietary fiber; 87 mg cholesterol; 399 mg sodium*

## PERFECT CORN BREAD

This golden corn bread is moist and lightly sweet. It's a delightful accompaniment to any meal.

---
**MAKES 10 SERVINGS (SERVING = 1 PIECE)**
---

Coconut oil, butter, or palm shortening, for pan
1 cup whole wheat pastry flour
4 teaspoons baking powder
¾ teaspoon salt
1 cup whole-grain yellow cornmeal
2 eggs
1 cup light coconut milk
4 tablespoons butter, melted
½ cup raw unfiltered honey

▶ Preheat the oven to 425°F and oil a 9-inch square by 2-inch-high baking pan.
▶ Sift together the flour, baking powder, and salt into a bowl. Add the cornmeal, eggs, and coconut milk. Blend thoroughly. Stir in the melted butter and honey. Beat together until the batter is smooth.
▶ Pour the batter into the prepared pan, and bake for 20 to 25 minutes, or until golden brown.

---
*Nutrition per serving: 207 calories; 8 g total fat; 4 g saturated fat; 4 g protein; 32 g carbohydrates; 2 g dietary fiber; 55 mg cholesterol; 364 mg sodium*

# Skinny Snacks and Sweets

## ALLOWABLE SIN

Looking to get your daily dose of cacao? These alkaline-forming allowable truffles are the ticket—they're loaded with protein, beneficial fat, fiber, and of course all the antioxidant power of chocolate. *And* they're sugar free. To make them super skinny, use raw cacao powder. Oh, and beware—these morsels can be addicting!

---
**MAKES 28 TO 32 PIECES (SERVING = 1 PIECE; 2 PIECES CONTAIN ABOUT 6.7 GRAMS OF DARK CHOCOLATE)**
---

¼ cup extra-virgin coconut oil
2 ounces 100% cacao unsweetened baking chocolate
¼ cup vanilla-flavored whey protein powder

2 tablespoons unsweetened cocoa powder or
   unsweetened raw cacao powder
½ cup finely chopped raw almonds
¼ cup dried unsweetened shredded coconut
¼ cup finely chopped dates or raisins
½ cup natural peanut or almond butter
1 teaspoon liquid stevia
   (vanilla or chocolate flavors work well here)
1 teaspoon pure vanilla extract
   (can be omitted if using flavored stevia)

▶ Place the coconut oil in a small saucepan over the lowest setting on the stove top. Use a chef's knife to chop the chocolate into very small pieces for easy melting. Add the chopped chocolate to the coconut oil and stir with a heatproof rubber spatula. Allow the chocolate to slowly melt, stirring frequently. This will take only a few minutes. Turn off the heat and set the pan aside.

▶ In a large mixing bowl, combine the protein powder, cocoa powder, almonds, coconut, and dates. Stir well. Add the peanut butter and mix thoroughly. At this point, the mixture should be somewhat crumbly.

▶ Add the stevia and the vanilla extract (if using) to the melted chocolate mixture in the saucepan and stir to mix thoroughly. Transfer the melted chocolate mixture to the bowl, using the rubber spatula to scrape out the saucepan.

▶ Stir the mixture thoroughly, scraping the sides of the bowl to make sure you have a good blend of all the ingredients.

▶ Use a small measuring spoon, such as a teaspoon, to scoop and fill thirty-two truffle cups or mini muffin liners with the chocolate mixture. Place in a single layer in a baking dish or other large, flat container and place in the freezer until the truffles harden, 20 to 30 minutes. Keep these in the freezer or refrigerator until ready to eat.

NOTE: When frozen, the truffle cups will peel off easily and you will have a chocolate delight that resembles a mini Reese's Peanut Butter Cup (without the sugar and trans fats)! You can use any size cupcake liner for these, but you should be careful not to overindulge.

---

*Nutrition per serving: 72 calories; 6 g total fat; 3 g saturated fat; 2 g protein; 4 g carbohydrates; 1.5 g dietary fiber; 0 mg cholesterol; 10 mg sodium*

## SPELT CHOCOLATE CHIP COOKIES

These cookies are wheat free and dairy free. You will not believe how good they are!

### MAKES 12 SERVINGS (SERVING = 1 COOKIE)

1 1/4 cups whole spelt flour
1/4 teaspoon sea salt
1 teaspoon nonaluminum baking powder
1/2 teaspoon baking soda
1/4 cup organic whole cane sugar
1/3 cup pure maple syrup
1/3 cup coconut oil, warm enough to be in a liquid state
1 1/2 teaspoons pure vanilla extract
1/2 cup grain-sweetened chocolate chips (SunSpire brand)

▶ Preheat oven to 350°F and line a baking sheet with parchment paper.
▶ Use a wire whisk to thoroughly mix together the spelt flour, salt, baking powder, baking soda, and sugar in a large bowl.
▶ In a second large bowl, whisk together the maple syrup, coconut oil, and vanilla. Whisk until the entire mixture is thick and syrupy.
▶ Add half of the flour mixture to the syrup mixture. Use a rubber spatula to mix until blended. The mixture will be very wet. Add the chocolate chips and stir.
▶ Add the rest of the flour mixture and stir, making sure to scrape the sides of the bowl with the rubber spatula to get all of the flour mixed in. At this point, the dough should be soft but not overly oily or wet.
▶ Break off tablespoon-size pieces of dough and place them 1 inch apart on the prepared baking sheet. You do not need to roll the dough into balls; however, the dough pieces should be somewhat round.
▶ Bake for 11 to 15 minutes. The cookies should be slightly puffy when removed from the oven, but will flatten out a little during cooling. Let cool on the cookie sheet for 5 minutes and then transfer to a wire rack to cool completely. The cookies will be chewy when completely cooled.

*Nutrition per serving: 155 calories; 8 g total fat; 6 g saturated fat; 2 g protein; 21 g carbohydrates; 2 grams dietary fiber; 0 mg cholesterol; 108 mg sodium*

# COCONUT–SWEET POTATO BROWNIES

Pureed baked sweet potato, unsweetened cocoa powder, coconut flour, and eggs yield rich, dense, and fudgy brownies that will knock your socks off! The original recipe called for white sugar, bittersweet chocolate, and soy milk. I made a few changes to make it a truly processed-free recipe!

---

### MAKES 16 SERVINGS (SERVING = 1 BROWNIE)

---

Coconut oil, butter, or palm shortening, for pan
1 cup cooked and mashed orange-fleshed sweet potato or
    canned sweet potato puree
1½ cup organic whole cane raw sugar or Sucanat
1 cup coconut flour (or almond meal, if desired)
½ cup unsweetened cocoa powder
⅛ teaspoon sea salt
4 large eggs

▶ Preheat the oven to 375°F. Coat an 8-inch square glass baking dish with coconut oil, butter, or palm shortening.

▶ Blend the sweet potato, 1 cup of the sugar, and the coconut flour, cocoa powder, and salt in a food processor for 30 seconds, or until smooth, scraping the bowl as necessary. Leave in the food processor bowl.

▶ Separate three of the eggs, placing the whites in a large bowl, preferably of a stand mixer. Add the three yolks and remaining whole egg to the sweet potato mixture; pulse to combine. Transfer the sweet potato mixture to a large bowl.

▶ Beat the egg whites at high speed with an electric mixer until soft peaks form. Add the remaining ½ cup of sugar; beat for 2 minutes more, or until stiff, glossy peaks form.

▶ Fold one-third of the egg white mixture into the sweet potato mixture, using a spatula. Gently fold in the remaining whites. Pour the batter into the prepared pan. Bake for 45 minutes, or until a toothpick inserted into the center comes out clean.

▶ Remove from the oven and let cool completely before serving.

---

*Nutrition per serving: 142 calories; 3 g total fat; 1 g saturated fat; 4 g protein; 26 g carbohydrates; 3 g dietary fiber; 74 mg cholesterol; 63 mg sodium*

## OAT BRAN–PUMPKIN MUFFINS

These muffins have been a staple in my diet for twenty years. The oat bran and pumpkin are the secret to their healthy fiber and amazingly low number of calories. Delicious and filling, these muffins make a great breakfast food or snack.

### MAKES 12 MUFFINS (SERVING = 1 MUFFIN)

Coconut oil or butter, for pan (optional)
2¼ cups oat bran
2⅛ teaspoons nonaluminum baking powder
1 tablespoon pumpkin pie spice (see variations)
½ teaspoon sea salt
½ cup cooked or canned pure pumpkin puree (see variations)
2 tablespoons extra-virgin coconut oil
3 egg whites
1 cup unsweetened almond milk
½ teaspoon liquid stevia
1 teaspoon pure vanilla extract
½ cup raw honey or coconut nectar

▶ Preheat the oven to 400°F. Line twelve muffin cups with paper liners or coat with coconut oil or butter.

▶ Combine the dry ingredients in a large mixing bowl and mix together thoroughly with a wire whisk. In a separate mixing bowl, combine the pumpkin, coconut oil, egg whites, almond milk, stevia, and vanilla with the wire whisk until the mixture becomes somewhat frothy.

▶ Slowly add the wet ingredients to the dry ingredients and mix thoroughly with a spoon.

▶ Add the honey very slowly to the mixture while stirring. The batter should become lighter in texture.

▶ Fill the muffin cups and bake for 15 minutes, or until the muffins are golden brown and a knife inserted into the center comes out clean.

▶ Remove from the oven and let cool for 10 minutes in the pan, then transfer to a wire rack to cool completely.

**VARIATIONS:** You may replace the pumpkin with ½ cup of mashed banana or unsweetened applesauce, and replace the pumpkin pie spice with 1 tablespoon of ground cinnamon and ½ teaspoon of grated nutmeg. Add nuts or raisins to this recipe, if desired.

*Nutrition per serving: 107 calories; 4 g total fat; 2 g saturated fat; 4 g protein; 21 g carbohydrates; 3 g dietary fiber; 0 mg cholesterol; 167 mg sodium*

# WHOLE WHEAT BANANA BREAD

Whole wheat flour is not typically used in quick breads, but it really adds to the flavor and nutrition in this classic favorite.

---
**MAKES 16 SERVINGS (SERVING = 1 SLICE OR 1 MUFFIN)**
---

Coconut oil, for pan
8 tablespoons organic butter, softened
¼ cup coconut oil, warm enough to be in a liquid state
½ cup organic whole cane sugar
2 eggs
3 large ripe bananas, mashed
¼ cup honey or coconut nectar
1 teaspoon vanilla extract
2 cups stone-ground whole wheat flour
1 teaspoon baking soda
¼ cup ground flaxseeds
1 teaspoon sea salt

▶ Preheat the oven to 350°F. Coat a 9-inch by 5-inch loaf pan with coconut oil, or if making muffins, line muffin cups with paper muffin cups or coat with coconut oil.
▶ In a large bowl, cream the butter, coconut oil, and cane sugar with an electric mixer. Add the eggs, bananas, honey, and vanilla. Beat well.
▶ In a separate bowl, mix together the flour, baking soda, flaxseeds, and salt.
▶ Stir the banana mixture into the flour mixture and mix well. At this point, the batter will be fairly thick. Pour the batter into the prepared loaf pan. If making muffins, fill each muffin cup about three-quarters full.
▶ Bake for 1 hour for a loaf, or 20 to 30 minutes for muffins, or until a knife inserted in the center comes out clean. Let cool in the pan for 10 minutes, then transfer to a wire rack to cool completely.

---
*Nutrition per serving: 185 calories; 9 g total fat; 5 g saturated fat; 4 g protein; 21 g carbohydrates; 2 g dietary fiber; 53 mg cholesterol; 260 mg sodium*

## SUGAR-FREE STRAWBERRY FROZEN YOGURT

Even if you don't have an ice-cream maker, you can still enjoy homemade frozen yogurt that is healthier than store-bought. The trick is to start with unsweetened frozen fruit and whirl it in a food processor with yogurt. You can try this recipe with other frozen fruits as desired.

### MAKES 4 SERVINGS (SERVING = ¾ CUP)

1 (16-ounce) package frozen unsweetened organic strawberries
  (about 3½ cups)
½ cup plain whole-milk organic yogurt
½ teaspoon liquid stevia (vanilla crème flavor works great here)
1 tablespoon freshly squeezed lemon juice

▶ Place the frozen strawberries in a food processor. Pulse until coarsely chopped. Combine the yogurt, stevia, and lemon juice in a bowl; with the machine running, gradually pour the mixture through the feed tube of the processor.

▶ Process until smooth and creamy, scraping down the sides of the bowl once or twice. (The frozen yogurt should be firm enough to be served directly from the food processor, but if it is a little soft, let it harden in the freezer for about 30 minutes.)

*Nutrition per serving: 69 calories; 1 g total fat; <1 g saturated fat; 1.5 g protein; 14 g carbohydrates; 1 g dietary fiber; 4 mg cholesterol; 16 mg sodium*

## HOMEMADE ALMOND MILK
## (CHOCOLATE MILK, TOO!)

Making your own almond milk is easy, cost effective, and far superior to the commercially available almond milk (which has a lot of things added to it so it can sit on a shelf). Almond milk is versatile and can be used to replace regular milk in nearly all recipes. Try this with vanilla or chocolate added to it.

### MAKES 3 TO 4 SERVINGS (SERVING = 1 CUP)

1 cup raw almonds, soaked in water for 8 hours or overnight
3 cups water, plus water to soak (see notes)

▶ Place the almonds in a large bowl and add enough water to cover them well. Cover the bowl with a towel and leave it in a cool place or in the refrigerator to let the almonds soak for at least 6 hours or overnight. Soaking will plump the almonds and soften them, in addition to increasing the nutritional value of the milk.

▶ When ready to make the almond milk, drain the almonds in a colander and rinse them well with water. Shake as much water off the almonds as possible.

▶ Place 3 cups of fresh water in a blender and add the soaked almonds. Blend on high speed for a few minutes, until the mixture is well blended and smooth. You will see the almond pulp suspended in the milk, and when you remove the cover of your blender, the top of the milk will be frothy.

▶ Strain the almond milk through a fine-mesh sieve, cheesecloth, or a nut-milk bag strainer (see notes) into your original bowl or another large container, such as a pitcher. Press or squeeze as much of the milk from the almond pulp as possible. You can discard the almond pulp or save it for a variety of uses, such as adding to smoothies, yogurt, or muffin batter, or dehydrate it and turn it into almond flour.

▶ At this point, the almond milk is done and can be drunk or used as is. Store it in a tightly sealed container in the refrigerator and try to use it within a week. You will need to stir or shake the almond milk every time you bring it out of the refrigerator, since it does settle. Use it with cereal or in recipes calling for milk.

▶ If you want flavored or sweetened almond milk for drinking, you can put the almond milk back into your blender along with two pitted Medjool dates (or other natural sweetener), vanilla extract, or unsweetened cacao powder and blend.

**NOTES:** Make sure to use good-quality water, such as reverse-osmosis, bottled water, or pitcher-filtered water.

You may want to invest in a nut-milk strainer bag (about $7 to $12 online; see appendix)—a fine-mesh nylon bag that makes straining the almond pulp easy and is highly recommended. Once you have blended your almond milk and removed the cover from your blender, the nut-milk strainer bag slips over the top of your blender so you can just invert the contents into the bag and collect the almond milk in another large container. The nut bag has a drawstring to keep it closed and makes squeezing all of the almond milk out of the bag clean and efficient. Nut-milk strainer bags are easy to clean and can be reused many times.

---

*Nutrition per serving: 40 calories; 3 g total fat; 0 g saturated fat; 2 g protein; 1 g carbohydrates; 1 g dietary fiber; 0 mg cholesterol; 2 mg sodium*

## HOMEMADE CHOCOLATE SYRUP

Ditch the premade sugary chocolate syrups with all those additives for this extremely low-glycemic, high-antioxidant version that your kids will *love*! Mix in with your favorite milk, use as a dip for fruits, or drizzle on top of ice cream.

### MAKES ABOUT ½ CUP (SERVING = 1 TABLESPOON)

½ cup coconut nectar or honey
2 tablespoons unsweetened cocoa powder

▶ Place the coconut nectar in a glass jar or plastic container. Add the cocoa powder. Stir, breaking up any lumps, until all of the cocoa powder is dissolved. Allow it to sit. The longer it sits, the thicker it gets. Store covered in the refrigerator. The recipe may be doubled.

*Nutrition per serving: 69 calories; 0 g total fat; 0 g saturated fat; <1 g protein; 15 g carbohydrates; 1 g dietary fiber; 0 mg cholesterol; 22 mg sodium*

## THE WORLD'S BEST POPCORN

I learned to make popcorn from scratch from a pro—my mom! Here's my healthy version of Mom's classic technique for making sure every kernel pops without burning.

### MAKES ABOUT 10 CUPS (SERVING = 3 CUPS POPPED CORN)

2 tablespoons extra-virgin coconut oil
½ cup organic popcorn kernels
Pinch of sea salt (optional)

▶ Cover the bottom of a medium-size stockpot with the coconut oil. Place the pot (without the cover) on the stove top over medium-high heat.
▶ Add three popcorn kernels to the pot, cover, and allow them to pop. Once the three kernels have popped, remove the cover and quickly add the rest of the popcorn kernels in an even layer. Put the cover back on and remove the pot from the heat for 30 seconds. (This allows the oil to heat evenly, and brings all of the kernels to a near-popping temperature so that when you return the pot to the heat, they will all pop at about the same time.)
▶ Return the pot to the heat. If you don't have a cover with a steam-release hole in it, leave the lid slightly ajar to let the steam release (this will produce drier and crunchier popcorn). Very soon, the popcorn will begin to pop rapidly and all at

once. Shake the pot by moving it back and forth over the burner to prevent the popcorn from burning. When the popping starts to taper off (several seconds between pops), take the pot off the heat, remove the cover, and quickly transfer the popcorn to a large bowl. Season with a pinch of sea salt, if desired.

**NOTE:** To distribute the salt more evenly, you can add it to the oil in the pot before popping.

**VARIATION:** You may want to try some other fun toppings, such as Taco Seasoning (page 349), Parmesan cheese, nutritional yeast, curry powder, or smoked paprika.

*Nutrition per serving: 50 calories; 3 g total fat; 2 g saturated fat; 1 g protein; 6 g carbohydrates; 1 g dietary fiber; 0 mg cholesterol; 0 mg sodium*

## SIMPLY SKINNY ALMOND CRUNCH GRANOLA

Most commercial granolas contain canola oil, soybean oil, high amounts of sugar, or all three! This simple version is one of the best granolas you can eat.

### MAKES 5 CUPS (SERVING = ¼ CUP)

⅓ cup extra-virgin coconut oil
½ cup raw honey or coconut nectar
I teaspoon vanilla extract
I teaspoon almond extract
I tablespoon ground cinnamon
4 cups rolled oats
I cup raw almonds

▶ Preheat the oven to 300°F.
▶ In a large bowl, mix together the coconut oil, honey, vanilla and almond extracts, and cinnamon. Add the oats and almonds; mix well. Spread the mixture on two ungreased baking sheets.
▶ Bake for 10 minutes and then stir the granola around on the baking sheet to make sure it gets baked evenly. Continue to bake for another 10 minutes or longer, until the granola is golden.
▶ Remove it from the oven and let it cool on the baking sheets. If it looks moist when you first remove it from the oven, don't worry; it will become crunchier as it cools. Let cool to room temperature, then store in a tightly sealed container.

**VARIATIONS:** You can add other ingredients to this granola, such as raisins, dried fruit, dried coconut, seeds, other nuts, and so on. You'll have to adjust the oil and the baking time. An easier way would be to just stir in the additional ingredients after you've baked the basic recipe.

---

*Nutrition per serving: 154 calories; 8 g total fat; 4 g saturated fat; 4 g protein; 18 g carbohydrates; 3 g dietary fiber; 0 mg cholesterol; 9 mg sodium*

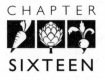
# Skinny on the Go

When eating out or traveling, you've got to have a strategy ahead of time. If you fail to plan, you plan to fail. Don't leave your healthy-eating commitment in the hands of others. You must take charge!

We live in a world that doesn't support processed-free eating, so you've got to support yourself! My motto is: *Always bring your own.* Follow this rule as often as possible and your chances of sticking with healthy choices are vastly improved.

## Social Events: Potlucks, Celebrations, Dinner Parties

Always bring something to a potluck that is healthy for you and that others will enjoy eating. This way, you know your needs will be taken care of. If there are other dishes at the potluck that are healthy and that you enjoy, that's a great bonus!

When people invite you for a meal at their home, ask what they'll be serving. If it doesn't suit your needs, ask for what you need or whether you can bring something.

Despite what you may feel, it is not rude to exempt yourself from any food. There are many people who do not eat certain foods for various reasons, and you can be one of them!

## Restaurants and Fast Food

Your best bets for breakfast will be oatmeal or other whole-grain cereal, eggs, fruit or veggies, cheese or cottage cheese, and milk or plain yogurt. Eggs can be poached or boiled (hard or soft), or have them as an omelet with veggies.

One of the biggest challenges with eating out is avoiding the trans fats. Basically, most anything that is cooked in oil in a restaurant is cooked in unhealthy oil. Ask how the food is cooked, so you can avoid the bad oils.

When it comes to oils, some cuisines are better than others—olive oil and sesame oil are usually readily available in Italian, Greek, Spanish, Chinese, and Thai restaurants. Some Japanese and Chinese dishes use peanut oil for stir-frying. This is acceptable.

Hold back on mayonnaise because most commercially prepared mayonnaise products are made with partially hydrogenated soybean oil. That leaves out tuna, egg, shrimp, and chicken salads, as well as coleslaw and potato salad.

When it comes to bread, muffins, crackers, and rolls, any made with refined white flour should be avoided. You will find that you just have to skip the bread basket in most restaurants because they just don't serve high-quality bread. This would also be the case for pastas, which are almost always made from white flour.

Choose whole-grain foods such as brown rice and whole-grain pastas.

Ask for no croutons on salads (much better than picking them out).

Seafood is always a great choice, and you can get salmon pretty much anywhere these days. Salmon and other fish should be grilled, broiled, poached, or baked in wine and seasoned with lots of garlic (specify fresh garlic, otherwise garlic salt will be used) and onions.

A smart choice in Mexican restaurants is fajitas (grilled meats and vegetables) with corn tortillas. Guacamole, as long as there is no mayonnaise added to it, is also a good choice. Avocados are a great source of healthy fat. Always ask for lemon wedges so you can squeeze the juice over veggies or salads. The lemon juice helps to cut the fats in the meal and assists in metabolism. Always ask for soft corn tortillas instead of white flour tortillas. Get whole beans instead of refried, and don't eat the rice; it's usually white rice that's been fried in vegetable oil.

Vegetables should be steamed without any seasonings or sauces.

Always order a green salad without dressing and ask for olive oil, lemon wedges, and balsamic vinegar on the side. This way you avoid the sugar that is usually in prepared vinaigrettes. You can add your own oil and vinegar and squeeze the lemon juice over the salad as well.

Herbal teas are also good choices when eating out.

Here are some more tips for eating out:

- Plan ahead as much as possible.
- If possible, check the menu online ahead of time.
- Go with a plan in mind (either choose your meal beforehand, or if no online menu is available, tell yourself, "Wherever I go tonight, I'm going to have grilled fish, vegetables, and a baked potato").
- Ask a lot of questions: How is the food prepared (e.g., grilled, fried, battered, or breaded)? Can you get extra vegetables? Can you substitute salad, vegetables, or a baked potato (butter or sour cream on the side) for French fries?
- If others in your party don't mind, ask the server not to bring bread or chips to the table. If others in your party want the bread and chips, place the basket away from you so that it's not within your easy reach.
- Always ask for whole wheat bread when menu items come on or are made with bread (e.g., sandwiches, burgers, toast, etc.)
- Always ask for real butter. Most restaurants use margarines in sauces and on toast.
- Avoid greasy fast-food joints such as burger places, taco stands, "express" or buffet-style Chinese restaurants, and fried chicken restaurants.

## Traveling

Whether traveling by car or plane, it is always advisable to scout out the supermarkets and natural foods stores at your destination, which often have healthy take-out options for meals and snacks. If you are traveling out of the country, it is useful to (a) look up the foreign terms for the kinds of foods you are seeking (e.g., the French for "whole-grain"), and also (b) to carry a card in the appropriate language explaining the criteria of your special requests. Letting the chef know that you don't want breading, sugar, oil, and so on, in your meal can take away anxiety or uncertainty about your dining experience.

## By Car (this is easy, you can bring most of your own food)

Pack a small cooler with fresh fruit, cut-up veggies, small cartons of milk, yogurts, cheese, or tuna or egg salad. Pack a bag with baked or dried foods such as oat bran muffins, dry cereal, ak-mak crackers, Ezekiel bread, peanut or almond butter, and raw nuts and seeds (or make your own trail mix). Bringing your own food reduces the need to eat fast food.

For long trips, bring enough food for most meals, and then stop at a sit-down restaurant for the main meal.

## By Plane (this is not as easy, due to the poor quality of airport food and the security restrictions for bringing some of your own food, but still doable)

My motto applies here: Bring your own as much as possible. I usually pack a small soft-sided cooler (lunchbox size) to carry on the plane, containing a lunch (or dinner) made ahead of time. Make sure you bring plastic cutlery and napkins. Beverages are usually available on the plane.

Early-morning flights are easy. I bring fruit and sometimes a muffin or cereal. These fit easily in my purse or carry-on.

The same types of food that you take in the car can apply here also (crackers, nuts, fruit, and veggies, etc.). When you have healthy snacks in your bag, you reduce the need to eat junk food.

Some airports have great eating establishments, others don't. If you don't know the airport, you'd better be prepared! Check ahead of time online.

## Staying in Other's Homes

Bring your own. I can't stress it enough! I always bring a few things that I know may be difficult to get, such as whole-grain cereals and crackers.

When you arrive, ask your host if you can make a trip to the grocery store to get a few things.

If meals will be shared, make sure you have input on what will be served. Offering to cook or help out in the kitchen is a good way to go, too.

Taking care of your healthy food needs when in social situations, in restaurants, and while traveling is vital to your success. This is the greatest act of self-care you can give to yourself. For most of us, relying on convenience and poor-quality food to take care of our needs has been our downfall. For long-term health and weight reduction, you have to be prepared!

## Karen's Story

I was always chubby and cannot recall ever weighing less than 100 pounds, even as a grade-schooler. Dieting over the years (off and on) left my metabolism in shreds; nothing I did seemed to affect my weight, and I tried every diet you've ever heard of. My library of diet books can rival any bookstore.

Exercise only made me hungrier. Attempting a new exercise plan would usually result in my injuring something, requiring surgery and bed rest. More pounds. Three back surgeries in 2003 and a hip replacement in 2005 (and I wasn't even 50!) clearly showed my future. Not pretty, and not healthy. Sedentary, obese, on ten prescription meds for diabetes, hypertension, depression, triglycerides, arthritis, you name it! What a sad state!

Discovering my biological half-siblings and learning about both my bio-parents' deaths (both from diabetes, compounded with renal failure and heart disease) was a wake-up call not to be ignored. Seeing some of my half-siblings, aunts, and great-aunts struggling with weight, diabetes, gastric bypasses, and all the ailments that go with obesity was frightening. Changes were imperative. I heard about this processed-free eating plan, and thought, "Oh, heck, it's worth a try." It was the most fortunate impulse of my life! At 200 pounds, I started going processed free. Between this plan (and a medically supervised supplement) I've dropped 60 pounds and plan to keep them off! I have energy, I feel and look great, and have a whole new outlook on life and my impending "golden years."

I've been on cruises and have traveled all over the world while eating processed free—it really is doable when you know how to plan and what to ask for in restaurants. This plan *works* for me.

*—Karen Brown, age 56, nurse educator*

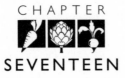
# What Now?
# Nutritional Responsibility
# and Staying Informed

When I gave up eating refined sugar and flour, I was not out to change the world. In the beginning, I applied the things I learned about food (both good and bad) solely to my own life. But the more I learned, it became clear that processed foods are not good for *any* human body. I wanted to be able to share the things that I learned with others, so that they could make their own decisions about what to eat and not eat. It's been said, "What you don't know won't hurt you," but in our world of tainted food, that statement doesn't hold true.

Now that *you* know much of the information I know about processed foods, what are you going to do? If you're like most people, you'll be shocked. Next may come anger, then perhaps outrage, and maybe a deep sense of sadness. The day I completed writing the chapter on sugar for this book, I broke down in tears at the thought of how so many people are obese and sick because of one food gone mad. I was also crying for the sugarcane, at how badly we've treated it and how we've lost our reverence for the life-giving plant that was so beautifully designed for us.

If you're overwhelmed, I know how you feel. I've had my share of meltdowns in the middle of a grocery store because every ingredient list of the items I wanted to purchase had high-fructose corn syrup, MSG, or some other undesirable additive in it. And when I think about how we got here, I realize that it's not any one person or company's fault, it just snowballed without anyone realizing how devastating it was going to get. Making changes to the food supply can do that in reverse. It won't be just one person who makes the change; it will be many people doing their small part.

It begins when something resonates with you, and you want to tell someone you care for about what you've learned. Everything you learned in this book, even a special recipe, is something to be shared with another person. And there are a few more things you can do, either for yourself, or for others.

## Stay Educated

**Processed-Free America**
**www.processedfreeamerica.org**
Processed-Free America is a great resource for you to continue to learn more. We have podcasts, videos, an e-newsletter, support groups, and a message board forum where you can interact with others who are living processed free.

Here are a few more websites you may find educational as well.

**The Weston A. Price Foundation**
**www.westonaprice.org**
The Weston A. Price Foundation supports the use of modern technology to promote the use of science and traditional farming methods as a force to help improve our environment and human health. Per this website, information is provided about "accurate nutrition instruction, organic and biodynamic farming, pasture-feeding of livestock, community-supported farms, honest and informative labeling, prepared parenting and nurturing therapies."

**Dr. Mercola's Optimal Wellness Newsletter**
**www.mercola.com**

Dr. Mercola provides cutting-edge information in the areas of health and fitness. His free biweekly e-newsletter is received by over 200,000 people. Dr. Mercola's website is one of the most popular alternative health websites in the world.

**Environmental Working Group (EWG)**
**www.ewg.org**

EWG is a nonprofit organization whose mission is to help protect our environment and public health by the distribution of public information. The EWG staff investigates data that relates to potential health and environmental threats and shares this information with the general public. As explained on its website, EWG provides practical information that will assist your efforts to protect the health and well-being of your family and community.

You can download the printable wallet guide of the EWG's "Dirty Dozen" and "Clean 15 Shopper's Guide to Pesticides in Produce" at www.foodnews .org. Carry the list in your purse or pocket when you go shopping.

# Other Ways to Become Involved

## Sign a Petition

Let the FDA know that you support a ban on the most egregious of food additives. There's a link on Processed-Free America's website (www.processed freeamerica.org). But don't stop there. There are many other meaningful petitions active with reputable organizations, such as the Center for Science in the Public Interest.

## Join or Start a Support Group

The Processed-Free Support Groups allow us to come together to support, affirm, and uphold our choice, and our right, to eat processed free. If you'd like support with eating processed free, a group may be just what you need.

Groups have formed in cities across the United States and Canada. If there is not a group in your area, you can start one. To find a group, log on to www.processedfreeamerica.org.

## Vote with Your Dollars

Processed foods only exist because people buy them! You can vote yes or no with your dollars. Every dollar you *don't* spend on processed foods is a no vote. Each one of us can contribute to big changes in small ways. Buy local and support organic farmers, so we all can have access to healthier foods.

## Be an Example

It's never a good idea to shout from the rooftops to people who don't care to hear what you have to say. Especially when it comes to the highly charged and emotional topic of food. It you are passionate about educating someone who doesn't want to hear, the best way for you to get their attention is to just be an example. Your glowing health will attract others who want what you have, and that is when you can help. Which leads me to my next suggestion . . .

## Become a Processed-Free Facilitator

Be part of the revolution! Be an agent for change! If you want to teach adults and children how to eat processed free, I have an online certification training program that will prepare you to teach others in your community, both adults and children, with age-appropriate curricula that are educational and engaging. Find out more at www.processedfreeamerica.org.

# METRIC CONVERSION CHART

- The recipes in this book have not been tested with metric measurements, so some variations might occur.
- Remember that the weight of dry ingredients varies according to the volume or density factor: 1 cup of flour weighs far less than 1 cup of sugar, and 1 tablespoon doesn't necessarily hold 3 teaspoons.

## General Formulas for Metric Conversion

| | |
|---|---|
| Ounces to grams | ➡ ounces $\times$ 28.35 = grams |
| Grams to ounces | ➡ grams $\times$ 0.035 = ounces |
| Pounds to grams | ➡ pounds $\times$ 453.5 = grams |
| Pounds to kilograms | ➡ pounds $\times$ 0.45 = kilograms |
| Cups to liters | ➡ cups $\times$ 0.24 = liters |
| Fahrenheit to Celsius | ➡ (°F − 32) $\times$ 5 ÷ 9 = °C |
| Celsius to Fahrenheit | ➡ (°C $\times$ 9) ÷ 5 + 32 = °F |

## Linear Measurements

| | | |
|---|---|---|
| $\frac{1}{2}$ inch | = | 1$\frac{1}{2}$ cm |
| 1 inch | = | 2$\frac{1}{2}$ cm |
| 6 inches | = | 15 cm |
| 8 inches | = | 20 cm |
| 10 inches | = | 25 cm |
| 12 inches | = | 30 cm |
| 20 inches | = | 50 cm |

## Volume (Dry) Measurements

$\frac{1}{4}$ teaspoon = 1 milliliter
$\frac{1}{2}$ teaspoon = 2 milliliters
$\frac{3}{4}$ teaspoon = 4 milliliters
1 teaspoon = 5 milliliters
1 tablespoon = 15 milliliters
$\frac{1}{4}$ cup = 59 milliliters
$\frac{1}{3}$ cup = 79 milliliters
$\frac{1}{2}$ cup = 118 milliliters
$\frac{2}{3}$ cup = 158 milliliters
$\frac{3}{4}$ cup = 177 milliliters
1 cup = 225 milliliters
4 cups or 1 quart = 1 liter
$\frac{1}{2}$ gallon = 2 liters
1 gallon = 4 liters

## Volume (Liquid) Measurements

1 teaspoon = $\frac{1}{6}$ fluid ounce = 5 milliliters
1 tablespoon = $\frac{1}{2}$ fluid ounce = 15 milliliters
2 tablespoons = 1 fluid ounce = 30 milliliters
$\frac{1}{4}$ cup = 2 fluid ounces = 60 milliliters
$\frac{1}{3}$ cup = 2$\frac{2}{3}$ fluid ounces = 79 milliliters
$\frac{1}{2}$ cup = 4 fluid ounces = 118 milliliters
1 cup or $\frac{1}{2}$ pint = 8 fluid ounces = 250 milliliters
2 cups or 1 pint = 16 fluid ounces = 500 milliliters
4 cups or 1 quart = 32 fluid ounces = 1,000 milliliters
1 gallon = 4 liters

## Oven Temperature Equivalents, Fahrenheit (F) and Celsius (C)

100°F = 38°C
200°F = 95°C
250°F = 120°C
300°F = 150°C
350°F = 180°C
400°F = 205°C
450°F = 230°C

## Weight (Mass) Measurements

1 ounce = 30 grams
2 ounces = 55 grams
3 ounces = 85 grams
4 ounces = $\frac{1}{4}$ pound = 125 grams
8 ounces = $\frac{1}{2}$ pound = 240 grams
12 ounces = $\frac{3}{4}$ pound = 375 grams
16 ounces = 1 pound = 454 grams

# Acknowledgments

Transforming this book into *The Science of Skinny* has been an amazing journey. Along the way I have been deeply touched and supported by many people in numerous ways. I would like to first give thanks to my mother, Carol, who always quietly supports me with love and strength. I felt you with me every day I was writing. I would also like to thank my sister, Rene; my brother, Derek; my father, John; and his wife, Sophia—your love is always with me.

I am also more grateful than I can express to:

Kristine Heidrich, whose support of my work over the past few years has been moving and deeply appreciated. You are an incredible gift to me on so many levels. Thank you for your beautiful patience and love.

Bob Cash, my first editor, for taking time to read my story for the millionth time and still find something beautiful to say about it. You are my literary hero.

My literary agent, Andrea Somberg, who heard the message and saw the promise of my book. I'm so glad you didn't miss the boat.

My editor at Da Capo Press, Renée Sedliar, whose patience and kind soul has been of great comfort throughout this process.

My truest friend, Rossi Mako, who supports me from afar, and inspires me to live my dreams.

All of the Processed-Free Support Group leaders around the country—your devotion and time to our mission is greatly appreciated.

My faithful supporters, followers, podcast listeners, message board members, clients, and students, whose e-mails, contributions, recipes, and testimonials have inspired me to continue on the processed-free path. Thank you for all the specialness you have brought to my life.

Most important, I give my deepest appreciation and gratitude to my husband and true love, Michael, who endured my absence from our home and business through the many days, weeks, and months of writing this work. This book truly would not be possible without your unwavering love and support. It was you who conceived of its title and it is you who deserves a million thank-yous for carrying me through to its completion. I am forever and deeply grateful for you.

# Appendix

## Recommended Processed-Free Food Products

The products listed in this section are known companies dedicated to providing high-quality products to health-conscious consumers. Not all of these products are available in stores; some must be purchased from online sources.

### Alkalizing and Liver-izing Supplements

Amazing Grass Green SuperFood drink
Dee's Naturals Alkalizing Green Superfood
Dee's Naturals Alkalizing Berry Fizzy Drink
Livatone
Nature's Answer alcohol-free dandelion root extract
Nature's Answer alcohol-free milk thistle extract
Phion Diagnosis pH Test Strips

### Beverages

Bragg Apple Cider Vinegar Drinks, in several flavors
Synergy Kombucha Tea, in several flavors
Teeccino Herbal Coffee, in several flavors
Virgil's Diet Sodas, in several flavors, sweetened with stevia
Zico Coconut Water

## *Breads/Cereals/Grains/Pastas*

Alvarado Street Bakery, sprouted-grain bread products
Ancient Harvest Quinoa and Quinoa Pasta
Bob's Red Mill Mighty Tasty GF Hot Cereal
Dee's Naturals Flourless Oat Bran Muffins, several varieties
Dee's Naturals Whole-Grain Tortillas
Erewhon Crispy Brown Rice Cereal
Food for Life, Ezekiel 4:9 Sprouted Whole-Grain Cereals
Food for Life, Ezekiel 4:9 Sprouted Whole-Grain Bread products
Galaxy Granola Not Sweet Vanilla Munch
Kashi 7 Whole-Grain Puffs (this is the only sugar-free Kashi cereal)
Tinkyada Pasta Joy Brown Rice Pastas
Uncle Sam Cereal
VitaSpelt Whole-Grain Spelt Pastas

## *Cacao/Chocolate*

Dagoba Unsweetened Cacao Powder
Navitas Naturals Organic Raw Cacao Powder and Raw Cacao Nibs
Righteously Raw dark chocolate bars
SunSpire 100% Cacao Baking Bar and Grain Sweetened Chocolate Chips
Theo Dark Chocolate Bars

## *Condiments/Salad Dressing*

Annie's Naturals Organic Yellow Mustard
Bragg Raw Unfiltered Apple Cider Vinegar
Bragg Salad Dressings, several varieties
Hain Pure Foods Safflower Mayonnaise
San-J Wheat-Free Tamari Soy Sauce
Santa Cruz 100% Organic Lemon Juice and Organic Lime Juice
Westbrae Unsweetened Ketchup
Wilderness Family Naturals Organic Mayonnaise

## *Cheese, Raw and Organic*

Organic Valley

## *Cookies/Crackers*

ak-mak crackers
Back to Nature Harvest Whole Wheats

Dee's Naturals Gluten-Free Oatmeal Raisin Cookies
Dee's Naturals Gluten-Free Peanut Butter Cookies
Lundberg Farms Brown Rice Cakes
Mary's Gone Crackers
RYVITA Crackers
San-J Tamari Brown Rice Crackers

### Deli Meat (nitrate-free)

Applegate Farms, lunch meats, hot dogs
Shelton's, sausages, hot dogs, jerky

### Miscellaneous

Amy's Organics, frozen meals
Eden Foods, canned beans
Organic Bistro, frozen dinners
Shelton's Broths
Sunshine Burger, frozen vegetarian patties, no soy

### Nondairy Milk

Almond Breeze Unsweetened Almond Milk
Living Harvest Unsweetened Hemp Milk
Nutiva Unsweetened Hemp Milk
Thai Kitchen Coconut Milk
Trader Joe's Lite Coconut Milk

### Oils

Barlean's Flax Oil and Extra-Virgin Coconut Oil
Garden of Life Extra-Virgin Coconut Oil and Fish Oils
Living Harvest Hemp Oil
Renew Life Norwegian Gold Ultimate Fish Oils
Spectrum Organic Shortening
Tropical Traditions Virgin Coconut Oil, all types
Udo's Choice Oil

### Probiotics

Garden of Life Raw Probiotics
Dr. Ohhira's Probiotics
Renew Life Ultimate Flora Probiotics

### Protein Powder/Whole Food Nutrition Bars

Action Whey Protein Concentrate Powder
Coconut Secret Coconut Bars, several varieties
Garden of Life Living Food Bars, several varieties
Larabars, several varieties (all except those containing chocolate chips)
Nutiva Hemp Protein Powder
NutriBiotic Brown Rice Protein Powder
Source Naturals The True Whey Protein Concentrate Powder
Vega Protein Powder

### Sweeteners

Coconut Secret Coconut Crystals
Coconut Secret Coconut Nectar
Rapunzel Organic Whole Cane Sugar, Unrefined and Unbleached
Smart Sweet Xylitol
Sweet Leaf Liquid Stevia Clear Extracts, several flavors
Sweet Leaf Powdered Stevia
Wholesome Sweeteners Organic Zero Erythritol
Wholesome Sweeteners Organic Sucanat

### Vitamins, Whole Food Supplements

Garden of Life Raw Vitamin Code
New Chapter Whole Food Vitamins

### Yogurt, Organic

Nancy's
Oikos
Stonyfield

## Companies and Organizations with Special Mention

**Action Whey / http://www.actionwhey.com**
This is one of the highest-quality whey protein powders available. It is cold-processed whey from the raw organic milk of grass-fed cows. Naturally sweetened with *luo han guo*, it comes in two flavors—vanilla and chocolate, made from real vanilla beans and untempered, alkali-free organic chocolate. It also contains coconut oil as an added source of medium-chain fats.

American Grass-Fed Beef / http://www.americangrassfedbeef.com

A great source of grass-fed beef roasts, steaks, and ground beef. Shipped frozen. They offer buyer club discounts and have a host of recipes on the website.

Dee's Naturals / http://www.deesnaturals.com

This is my line of healthy food products, including flourless oat bran muffins, whole wheat tortillas, and gluten-free cookies. All of my products are made from high-quality ingredients and do not contain preservatives or any artificial food additives. These products are sold in select natural food markets. If you would like your local natural food market to carry my products, please let the store manager know, and then send us an e-mail.

Vermont Fiddle Heads / http://vt-fiddle.com
The Raw Gourmet / http://rawgourmet.com

Nut-milk bags are available on Amazon, but these are my favorite online shops for them. The nut-milk bag has many different uses, which makes it a good investment. It can be a real hassle when you are using a strainer or cheesecloth to strain your nut milk. With a nut-milk bag, all you have to do is slip the bag over the top of your blender and pour your mixture through it. You can either hang it by the drawstring to drain out the nut milk, or you can squeeze it to get out every delicious drop. The fine nylon mesh bag leaves little residue, is easy to clean, and can be used time after time.

Righteously Raw Chocolate / http://www.righteouslyrawchocolate.com

Truly some of the best gourmet raw cacao bars available. The flavor varieties are unique, including açai, goji, and maca. They only use the best natural sweeteners: Their dark cacao is lightly sweetened with one or more of these low-glycemic ingredients: coconut sugar, coconut nectar, dates, figs, and raisins. Available at Whole Foods Markets.

SunSpire Chocolate / http://www.sunspire.com

One of the nation's leading producers of all-natural chocolate, with a reputation for crafting rich and indulgent confections that contain no refined sugars or artificial additives of any kind. SunSpire provides an assortment of innovative all-natural chocolate products, including baking morsels that are organic, Fair Trade Certified, dairy free and gluten free, vegan, and carob. They pioneered the use of healthful alternative sweeteners, including developing their own all-natural sweetening methods that eliminate the need for refined sugars, using malted grains instead. Their grain-sweetened chocolate chips contain half the amount of sugars per serving as do regular chocolate chips.

## To Your Health Sprouted Flour Company /
http://www.organicsproutedflour.net

You can order sprouted grains and sprouted grain flour from this family-owned business located in a small farm setting in rural Alabama. Their sprouted flour is freshly milled from organic grains—wheat, spelt, and rye. The grains are sprouted, dried, and milled at a very low temperature to maintain enzymes, vitamins, and minerals. The sprouted flour is milled to order. It never sits on the shelf or in a warehouse. This ensures the freshest, most nutritious whole-grain flour possible.

## Tropical Traditions / http://www.tropicaltraditions.com

This is the ideal source for the purchase of coconut oil and all things coconut at bulk discount prices. They offer many other products, such as sweeteners, rebounders, nontoxic cleaning products, personal care products, and more. The company e-mails weekly sales notices and always offers two-for-the-price-of-one deals.

## Vitacost / http://www.vitacost.com

This site offers top name-brand nutritional supplements, such as those I recommend, at significantly lower prices than retail. They also offer food products and personal care products.

## Vital Choice Wild Seafood and Organics / http://www.vitalchoice.com

Vital Choice offers home delivery of the world's finest wild seafood and organic fare, harvested from healthy, well-managed wild fisheries and farms. They offer premium frozen, canned, and pouched fish products, including many no-salt-added and kosher options.

## Wilderness Family Naturals / http://www.wildernessfamilynaturals.com

A great online store with many natural food products not found in natural food markets.

Of special note, they have the best and most pure organic mayonnaise available, made from a special oil blend based on the writings of Dr. Mary Enig. It contains organic extra-virgin olive oil, organic coconut oil, organic sesame tahini, organic eggs, organic spices, and organic vinegar. The only downside is that it also includes organic evaporated cane juice, but it's a very minimal amount.

# Notes

Introduction

1. Trust for America's Health, "F as in Fat: How Obesity Threatens America's Future 2011," July 2011, http://healthyamericans.org/report/88/ (July 13, 2011).
2. Ibid.


Chapter I

1. Leon Festinger, *A Theory of Cognitive Dissonance* (Palo Alto, California: Stanford University Press, 1957), 3.
2. Jordan S. Rubin, NMD, PhD, *The Maker's Diet* (Lake Mary, Florida: Siloam, 2004), 29.
3. Ronald F. Schmid, ND, *Traditional Foods Are Your Best Medicine* (Rochester, Vermont: Healing Arts Press, 1997), xiv.


Chapter 2

1. Kelly D. Brownell and Katherine Battle Horgen, *Food Fight: The Inside Story of the Food Industry, America's Obesity Crisis and What We Can Do About It,* (New York, New York: McGraw-Hill, September 2004), 6.
2. Elizabeth Lipski, PhD, CCN, "Traditional Non-Western Diets," *Nutrition in Clinical Practice*, 25, no. 6 (December 2010): 585–593.
3. Ronald F. Schmid, ND, *Traditional Foods Are Your Best Medicine* (Rochester, Vermont: Healing Arts Press, 1997), 8.

4. Ibid., 31.

5. Dr. Stephen Byrnes, "The Neglected Nutritional Research of Dr. Weston Price, DDS," Mercola.com, January 2001, http://www.mercola.com/2001/jan/21 /weston_price.htm (August 21, 2011).

6. Schmid, 9.

7. Ibid., 39.


Chapter 3

1. Massoud Arvanaghi, PhD, and Mike Yorkey, *The Vitamin Code* (West Palm Beach, Florida: Garden of Life, Inc., 2008), 25.

2. Michael Murray, ND, Joseph Pizzorno, ND, Lara Pizzorno, MA, LMT, *The Encyclopedia of Healing Foods* (New York: Atria Books, 2005), 17.

3. Hope Egan, *Holy Cow!* (Littleton, Colorado: First Fruits of Zion, 2005), 12.

4. Society of Chemical Industry, "Cocoa 'Vitamin' Health Benefits Could Outshine Penicillin," March 12, 1007, *ScienceDaily*. http://www.sciencedaily.com /releases/2007/03/070311202024.htm (August 12, 2011).

5. Jim Howenstien, MD, "Does Aspirin Prevent Heart Attacks and Strokes?" NewsWithViews.com, April 21, 2004, http://www.newswithviews.com/Howenstine /james10.htm (January 17, 2012).

6. Harvard School of Public Health, "Vegetables and Fruits: Get Plenty Every Day," *The Nutrition Source*, http://www.hsph.harvard.edu/nutritionsource/what -should-you-eat/vegetables-full-story/ (January 19, 2012).

7. The World's Healthiest Foods, "Broccoli," http://www.whfoods.com/gen page.php?tname=foodspice&dbid=9 (January 17, 2012).

8. Phyllis Balch, CNC, *Prescription for Nutritional Healing*, 4th ed. (New York: Avery Publishing Group, 2006), 12.

9. Ibid.

10. Frank J. Hurd, DC, MD, and Rosalie Hurd, BS, *A Good Cook . . . Ten Talents* (Chisholm, Minnesota: Dr. and Mrs. Frank J. Hurd, 1968), 7.


Chapter 4

1. Associated Press, "Cut Back, Way Back, on Sugar, Says Heart Group: American Adults Eat 24 Teaspoons of Sugar a Day; Teens 34 Teaspoons," msnbc.com, August 24, 2009, http://www.msnbc.msn.com/id/32543288/ns/health-diet_and _nutrition/t/cut-back-way-back-sugar-says-heart-group/ (August 25, 2011).

2. Nancy Appleton, PhD, *Lick the Sugar Habit* (New York: Avery Penguin Putnam, 1996), 10–11.

3. Dr. Michael Saska and Dr. Chung Chi Chou, "Antioxidant Properties of Sugarcane Extracts" (paper presented at Proceedings of First Biannual World Confer-

ence on Recent Developments in Sugar Technologies, Delray Beach, Florida, May 16–17, 2002), http://www.esugartech.com/documents/Properties%20Sugarcane %20Extracts.pdf (August 26, 2011).

4. Ibid.

5. R. S. Weisinger, et al., "Sugarcane-Derived Polyphenols Decrease Diet-Induced Obesity" (paper presented at International Symposium on Traditional Medicine, Toyoma, Japan, October 26, 2007), http://www.inm.u-toyoma.ac.jp/en //TM_sympo/abstract/16.pdf (August 26, 2011).

6. Appleton, 10–11.

7. Ibid., 17–18.

8. Nicole M. Avena, Pedro Rada, and Bartley G. Hoebe, "Sugar and Fat Binge-ing Have Notable Differences in Addictive-like Behavior," *Journal of Nutrition* 139, no. 3 (March 2009): 623–28, http://www.ncbi.nlm.nih.gov/pmc/articles/PMC 2714381/ (August 28, 2011).

9. Leah Ariniello, "Sugar Addiction," *Brain Briefings* (newsletter of the Society for Neuroscience, October 2003), http://faculty.haas.berkeley.edu/tetlock/Vita /Philip%20Tetlock/Phil%20Tetlock/BrainBriefings_Oct2003.pdf (August 28, 2011).

10. A. Sanchez, J. Reeser, H. Lau, et al., "Role of Sugars in Human Neutrophilic Phagocytosis.," *American Journal of Clinical Nutrition* 26, no.11 (November 1973): 1180–84.

11. UCTV, *Sugar: The Bitter Truth*, University of California Television, July 27, 2009.

12. Gary Taubes, "Is Sugar Toxic?" *The New York Times*, April 13, 2011, http:// www.nytimes.com/2011/04/17/magazine/mag-17Sugar-t.html?pagewanted=all (August 29, 2011).

13. P. B. Jeppesen, et al., "Stevioside Acts Directly on Pancreatic Beta Cells to Secrete Insulin: Actions Independent of Cyclic Adenosine Monophosphate and Adenosine Triphosphate-Sensitive K+-Channel Activity," *Metabolism*, 49, no. 2 (February 2000): 208–214.

14. Ray Sahelian, MD, and Donna Gates, *The Stevia Cookbook* (New York: Avery, 1999), 41–47.

15. The World's Healthiest Foods, "Honey," http://www.whfoods.com/genpage .php?tname=foodspice&dbid=96 (September 21, 2011).

16. M. Ukiya, T. Akihisa, H. Tokuda, et al., "Inhibitory Effects of Cucurbitane Glycosides and Other Triterpenoids from the Fruit of Momordica Grosvenori on Epstein-Barr Virus Early Antigen Induced by Tumor Promoter 12-O-Tetra-decanoylphorbol-13-Acetate," *Journal of Agricultural Food Chemistry*, 50 no. 23 (November 6, 2002): 6710–6715.

17. E. Takeo, H. Yoshida, N. Tada, et al., "Sweet Elements of Siraitia Grosvenori Inhibit Oxidative Modification of Low-Density Lipoprotein," *Journal of Athero-sclerosis and Thrombosis*, 9 no. 2 (2002): 114–120.

18. Y. A. Suzuki, et al., "Triterpene Glycosides of Siraitia Grosvenori Inhibit Rat Intestinal Maltase and Suppress the Rise in Blood Glucose Level After a Single Oral Administration of Maltose in Rats," *Journal of Agricultural Food Chemistry*, 53, no. 8 (April 20, 2005): 2941–2946.

19. Takeo et al.

20. Melanie Warner, "Does This Goo Make You Groan?" *The New York Times*, July 2, 2006, section 3, 8.

21. Ibid.

22. Ibid.

23. Duke University Medical Center, "High-Fructose Corn Syrup Linked to Liver Scarring, Research Suggests," *ScienceDaily*, March 22, 2010, http://www.sciencedaily.com/releases/2010/03/100322204628.htm (October 29, 2011).

24. Sally Fallon Morell and Rami Nagel, "Agave Nectar: Worse Than We Thought," Weston A. Price Foundation, April 30, 2009, http://www.westonaprice.org/modern-foods/agave-nectar-worse-than-we-thought (October 5, 2011).

25. Sugar.org, "What Is Crystalline Fructose?" http://www.sugar.org/other-sweeteners/other-caloric-sweeteners.html#crystalline-fructose (August 30, 2011).

26. Dr. Joseph Mercola and Dr. Kendra Degan Pearsall, *Sweet Deception: Why Splenda, Nutrasweet and the FDA May Be Hazardous to Your Health* (Nashville, Tennessee: Thomas Nelson, Inc., 2006), 19.

27. Ibid., 21.

28. Center for Science in the Public Interest, "Chemical Cuisine, Saccharin," http://www.cspinet.org/reports/chemcuisine.htm#saccharin (September 29, 2011).

29. Mercola and Pearsall, *Sweet Deception*, 38.

30. Ibid., 41.

31. Ibid., 239.

32. Ademir Barianni Rodero, Lucas de Souza Rodero, and Reinaldo Azoubel, "Toxicity of Sucralose in Humans: A Review," *International Journal Morphol* 27, no. 1 (2009): 239–244, http://www.scielo.cl/pdf/ijmorphol/v27n1/art40.pdf (September 29, 2011).

33. Dr. Janet Starr Hull, *Splenda: Is It Safe or Not?* (Dallas, Texas: The Pickle Press, 2004), 21.

## Chapter 5

1. Fran McCullough, *The Good Fat Cookbook* (New York: Scribner, 2003), 13.

2. Dr. Joseph Mercola, interview with Gary Taubes, mercola.com, August 20, 2011, http://articles.mercola.com/sites/articles/archive/2011/08/20/what-if-its-all-been-a-big-fat-lie-part-1.aspx (August 30, 2011).

3. Sally W. Fallon, MA, and Mary Enig, PhD, "Butter Is Better," *Health Freedom News* (December 1995), 58.

4. Sally Fallon, MA, and Mary Enig, PhD, "The Truth About Saturated Fats," mercola.com, August 17, 2002, http://articles.mercola.com/sites/articles/archive /2002/08/17/saturated-fat1.aspx (August 30, 2011).

5. Ibid.

6. Ibid.

7. Ibid.

8. Ibid.

9. Sally Fallon, MA, and Mary Enig, PhD, "The Great Con-ola," mercola.com, August 14, 2002, http://articles.mercola.com/sites/articles/archive/2002/08/14 /con-ola1.aspx (August 30, 2011).

10. Ibid.

11. Ibid.

12. Ibid.

13. Ibid.

14. Ibid.

15. McCullough, 25.

16. Ibid.

17. Udo Erasmus, *Fats That Heal, Fats That Kill* (Burnaby, BC, Canada: Alive Books, 1994), 127–129.

18. Fallon and Enig, "The Truth About Saturated Fats."

19. Ibid.

20. Ibid.

21. Erasmus, 43–44.

22. BBC News World Edition, "Fish Oil Keeps Arteries Clear," February 7, 2003, http://news.bbc.co.uk/2/hi/health/2732647.stm (August 30, 2011).

23. Fallon and Enig, "The Truth About Saturated Fats."

24. Erasmus, 52–53.

25. The World's Healthiest Foods, "Omega-3 Fatty Acids," http://www.whfoods .com/genpage.php?tname=nutrient&dbid=84 (January 17, 2012).

26. H. K. Kim, M. Della-Fera, J. Lin, and C. A. Baile, "Docosahexaenoic Acid Inhibits Adipocyte Differentiation and Induces Apoptosis in 3T3-L1 Preadipocytes," *The Journal of Nutrition*, 136, no. 12 (December 2006): 2965–2969.

## Chapter 6

1. David Lawrence Dewey, "Hydrogenated Oils—Silent Killers," http://www .dldewey.com/hydroil.htm, 1996, (January 19, 2012).

2. Sally Fallon, MA, and Mary Enig, PhD, "The Truth About Saturated Fats," mercola.com, August 17, 2002, http://articles.mercola.com/sites/articles/archive /2002/08/17/saturated-fat1.aspx (August 30, 2011).

3. Fran McCullough, *The Good Fat Cookbook* (New York: Scribner, 2003), 35.

4. Ibid., 36.

5. Ibid., 34–35.

6. Ibid., 37.


Chapter 7

1. Susan Carpenter, "Want to Reduce BPA Exposure? Cut Canned Foods from Your Diet, Report Says," *Los Angeles Times,* March 30, 2011, http://latimesblogs .latimes.com/greenspace/2011/03/bpa-canned-food.html (August 31, 2011).

2. Kristin Wartman, "Our Daily, Deadly, Chemical Cocktail," *The Huffington Post,* April 29, 2011, http://www.huffingtonpost.com/kristin-wartman/food-additives _b_853751.html (August 31, 2011).

3. "FDA Should Strengthen Its Oversight of Food Ingredients Determined to Be Generally Recognized as Safe (GRAS)" (United States Government Accountability Office, February 2010). http://www.gao.gov/new.items/d10246.pdf (August 31, 2011).

4. Food Additives Booklet, published by the International Food Additives Council, 2007, http://www.foodadditives.org/pdf/Food_Additives_Booklet.pdf (September 29, 2011).

5. Food Additives, published by Learning Seed, 2008, http://www.learning seed.com/_guides/1206_Food_Additives_Guide.pdf (September 29, 2011).

6. Wartman.

7. Eric Schlosser, *Fast Food Nation: The Dark Side of the All-American Meal* (New York: Harper Perennial, 2002), 126.

8. Lawrence Wilson, "Food Additives," *Arizona Networking News,* December/ January 2005, 1–2.

9. John Olney, "Brain Lesions, Obesity, and Other Disturbances in Mice Treated with Monosodium Glutamate," *Science* 164, no. 3880 (May 9, 1969): 719–721.

10. Martin Hickman, "Caution: Some Soft Drinks May Seriously Harm Your Health, Expert Links Additive to Cell Damage," *The Independent,* May 27, 2007, http://www.independent.co.uk/life-style/health-and-families/health-news/caution -some-soft-drinks-may-seriously-harm-your-health-450593.html (September 1, 2011).

11. Chemical Cuisine, "Acesulfame-K," Center for Science in the Public Interest, http://www.cspinet.org/reports/chemcuisine.htm#acesulfamek (January 19, 2012).

12. Gardiner Harris, "F.D.A. Panel to Consider Warnings for Artificial Food Colorings," *The New York Times,* March 29, 2011, http://www.nytimes.com /2011/03/30/health/policy/30fda.html (January 19, 2012).

13. Chemical Cuisine, "Blue 1," Center for Science in the Public Interest, http://www.cspinet.org/reports/chemcuisine.htm#blue1 (January 19, 2012).

14. Chemical Cuisine, "Blue 2," Center for Science in the Public Interest, http://www.cspinet.org/reports/chemcuisine.htm#blue2 (January 19, 2012).

15. Chemical Cuisine, "Green 3," Center for Science in the Public Interest, http://www.cspinet.org/reports/chemcuisine.htm#green3 (January 19, 2012).

16. Chemical Cuisine, "Orange B," Center for Science in the Public Interest, http://www.cspinet.org/reports/chemcuisine.htm#orangeb (January 19, 2012).

17. Chemical Cuisine, "Red 3," Center for Science in the Public Interest, http://www.cspinet.org/reports/chemcuisine.htm#red3 (January 19, 2012).

18. Chemical Cuisine, "Red 40," Center for Science in the Public Interest, http://www.cspinet.org/reports/chemcuisine.htm#red40 (January 19, 2012).

19. Chemical Cuisine, "Yellow 5," Center for Science in the Public Interest, http://www.cspinet.org/reports/chemcuisine.htm#yellow5 (January 19, 2012).

20. Chemical Cuisine, "Yellow 6," Center for Science in the Public Interest, http://www.cspinet.org/reports/chemcuisine.htm#yellow6 (January 19, 2012).

21. Kate Murphy, "Do Food Additives Subtract from Health?" *Business Week*, May 6, 1996, http://www.businessweek.com/1996/19/b3474101.htm (January 19, 2012).

22. "Final Report on the Safety Assessment of Sodium Lauryl Sulfate," *Journal of the American College of Toxicology* 2, no. 7 (1983).

23. Ibid.

Chapter 8

1. Barbara L. Minton, "Fermented Soy Is Only Soy Fit for Human Consumption," Natural News.com, February, 3, 2009, http://www.naturalnews.com/025513 _soy_food_soybeans.html (October 13, 2011).

2. Ibid.

3. William J. Cromie, "Growth Factor Raises Cancer Risk," *The Harvard University Gazette*, April 22, 1999, http://news.harvard.edu/gazette/1999/04.22/igf1 .story.html (January 19, 2012).

4. T. R. Dhiman, "Role of Diet on Conjugated Linoleic Acid Content of Milk and Meat," *Journal of Animal Science* 79, Suppl. 1 (2001): 241, http://www.adsa .org=/jointabs/iaafs108.pdf (October 25, 2011).

5. Fran McCullough, *The Good Fat Cookbook* (New York: Scribner, 2003), 120.

6. RawMilkFacts.com, http://www.raw-milk-facts.com/Raw_Milk_FAQ.html (January 19, 2012).

7. The World's Healthiest Foods, "Homogenization," http://www.whfoods .com/genpage.php?tname=george&dbid=150 (January 19, 2012).

8. Jo Johnson, "Why Grass-Fed Is Best," AmericanGrassFedBeef.com, http:// www.americangrassfedbeef.com/grass-fed-natural-beef.asp (January 20, 2012).

9. Ann Louise Gittleman, MS, CNS, *The Fat Flush Plan* (New York: McGraw-Hill, 2002), 32.

10. Arizona Center For Advanced Medicine, "Salmon and Red Meat," http:// arizonaadvancedmedicine.com/articles/salmon_and_red_meat.html (January 20, 2012).

11. Lois Swirsky Gold, Thomas H. Slone, and Bruce N. Ames, "Pesticide Residues in Food and Cancer Risk: A Critical Analysis," *Handbook of Pesticide Toxicolology*, 2nd ed. (San Diego, CA: Academic Press, 2001), 799–843, http://potency.berkeley.edu/pdfs/handbook.pesticide.toxicology.pdf (January 20, 2012).

12. Jeffrey Smith, "Genetically Modified Foods: Just Say No," *HealthKeepers Magazine* 11, no. 1 (Spring 2009): 31.

13. Ibid.

14. Institute for Responsible Technology, "10 Reasons to Avoid GMOs," http://www.responsibletechnology.org/10-Reasons-to-Avoid-GMOs (January 20, 2012).

15. *The Popcorn Agri-Chemical Handbook,* published by the Popcorn Board, 2011 Edition, http://www.popcorn.org/handbook/handbook.cfm (September 1, 2011).

16. A. Schecter et al., "Congener-Specific Levels of Dioxins and Dibenzofurans in U.S. Food and Estimated Daily Dioxin Toxic Equivalent Intake," *Environmental Health Perspectives* 102 (1994): 962–966.

## Chapter 9

1. Michael Murray, ND, Joseph Pizzorno, ND, and Lara Pizzorno, MA, LMT, *The Encyclopedia of Healing Foods* (New York: Atria Books, 2005), 777.

2. Robert O. Young, PhD, and Shelley Redford Young, *The pH Miracle* (New York: Warner Books, 2002), 24–33.

3. Ibid.

4. Otto Warburg, "The Prime Cause and Prevention of Cancer" (revised lecture at the meeting of the Nobel-Laureates, Lindau, Lake Constance, Germany, June 30, 1966), http://curezone.com/upload/Members/droxygen/PrimeCause.pdf (January 20, 2012).

5. Murray et al., 777.

6. USDA Agricultural Research Service, "Phytochemical Profilers Investigate Potato Benefits," http://www.ars.usda.gov/is/AR/archive/sep07/potato0907.htm (August 9, 2011).

7. Ibid.

8. Ann Louise Gittleman, MS, CNS, *The Fat Flush Plan* (New York: McGraw-Hill, 2002), 14.

## Chapter 10

1. Food and Agriculture Organization of the United Nations, "Calculation of the Energy Content of Foods-Energy Conversion Factors," http://www.fao.org/DOCREP/006/Y5022E/y5022e04.htm (January 20, 2012).

2. Dorchester County Health Department, *The Health Benefits of Water*, http://www.dorchesterhealth.org/water.htm (October 21, 2011).

Chapter 11

1. Michael Murray, ND, Joseph Pizzorno, ND, and Lara Pizzorno, MA, LMT, *The Encyclopedia of Healing Foods* (New York: Atria Books, 2005), 18.

2. The World's Healthiest Foods, "Parsley," http://www.whfoods.com/genpage.php?tname=foodspice&dbid=100 (October 15, 2011).

3. The World's Healthiest Foods, "Sweet Potatoes," http://whfoods.org/genpage.php?tname=foodspice&dbid=64 (October 15, 2011).

4. Ibid.

5. Murray et al., 180.

6. Ibid., 202.

7. Ibid., 218.

8. All-About-Lowering-Cholesterol.com, "Lowering Cholesterol with Avocado Fat," http://www.all-about-lowering-cholesterol.com/avocado-cholesterol-and-avocado-fat.html (September 1, 2011).

9. Ibid.

10. Murray et al., 252.

11. Ibid., 272.

12. The World's Healthiest Foods, "Watermelon," http://www.whfoods.com/genpage.php?tname=foodspice&dbid=31 (October 28, 2011).

13. Frances Katz, "New Sources of Resistant Starch," *FoodProcessing.com*, August 29, 2006, http://www.foodprocessing.com/articles/2006/162.html (October 29, 2011).

14. Ibid.

15. Carol S. Johnston, PhD, RD, and Cindy A. Gaas, BS, "Vinegar: Medicinal Uses and Antiglycemic Effect," *Medscape General Medicine* 8, no. 2 (2006): 61, published online May 30, 2006, http://www.ncbi.nlm.nih.gov/pmc/articles/PMC1785201/ (October 15, 2011).

16. Ibid.

17. Fran McCullough, *The Good Fat Cookbook* (New York: Scribner, 2003), 58.

18. Murray et al., 422.

19. Sally W. Fallon, MA, and Mary Enig, PhD, "Butter Is Better," *Health Freedom News* (December 1995), 58.

20. Ibid., 59.

21. The World's Healthiest Foods, "Almonds," http://whfoods.org/genpage.php?tname=foodspice&dbid=20 (October 28, 2011).

22. The World's Healthiest Foods, "Eggs," http://www.whfoods.com/genpage.php?tname=foodspice&dbid=92 (October 28, 2011).

23. Murray et al., 589–590.

24. Ibid.

25. Murray et al., 328–329.

26. Whole Grains Council, "Sprouted Whole Grains," http://www.wholegrains council.org/whole-grains-101/sprouted-whole-grains (October 28, 2011).

27. Stephen J. Crozier et al., "Cacao Seeds Are a 'Super Fruit': A Comparative Analysis of Various Fruit Powders and Products," *Chemistry Central Journal* 5, no. 5 (February 2011): doi:10.1186/1752–153X-5–5, http://journal.chemistry central.com/content/5/1/5 (August 15, 2011).

28. Mary B. Engler, PhD, et al., "Flavonoid-Rich Dark Chocolate Improves Endothelial Function and Increases Plasma Epicatechin Concentrations in Healthy Adults," *Journal of the American College of Nutrition* 23 (June 2004): 197–204, http://www.jacn.org/content/23/3/197.abstract (August 16, 2011).

29. Aviva, "Yerba Maté Is Packed with Naturally Occurring Nutrients and Antioxidants!" http://www.yerbamate.com/health.htm (January 9, 2012).

## Chapter 12

1. Ann Louise Gittleman, *The Fat Flush Plan* (New York: McGraw Hill, 2002), 170.

## Chapter 14

1. Jordan Rubin, NMD, PhD, *The Maker's Diet* (Lake Mary, FL: Siloam, 2004), 174.

2. Health World Online, "Exercise Better Than Drugs to Lower Cholesterol," *What Doctors Don't Tell You* 13, no. 10 (2002), http://www.healthy.net/scr/article .asp?Id=2893 (September 1, 2011).

3. Gus J. Prosch, Jr., MD, "Twelve Vital Nutritional and Health Topics," hbci.com, http://www.hbci.com/~wenonah/riddick/prosch12.htm (September 1, 2011).

4. Ann Louise Gittleman, MS, CNS, *The Fat Flush Plan* (New York: McGraw-Hill, 2002), 93.

5. Prosch.

6. Debbie Ford, *The Right Questions* (San Francisco, CA: Harper San Francisco, 2003), 7–8.

# Index